Imaging-Guided Interventional Breast Techniques

Springer
New York
Berlin
Heidelberg
Hong Kong
London
Milan
Paris
Tokyo

D. David Dershaw, M.D.
Memorial Sloan-Kettering Cancer Center
New York, New York

Editor

Imaging-Guided Interventional Breast Techniques

Introduction by D. David Dershaw

With 304 Illustrations

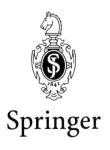

Springer

D. David Dershaw, M.D.
Memorial Sloan-Kettering Cancer Center
1275 York Avenue
New York, NY 10021
USA

Cover illustrations: Clockwise from upper left: Core biopsy histology specimen; stereotactic vacuum assisted biopsy of calcifications, ultrasound guided core biopsy of mass; specimen radiograph of preoperatively wire-localized calcifications.

Library of Congress Cataloging-in-Publication Data
Imaging-guided interventional breast techniques / editor, D. David Dershaw.
    p.; cm.
  Includes bibliographical references and index.
  ISBN 0-387-95454-6 (h/c : alk. paper)
  1. Breast—Cancer—Diagnosis. 2. Breast—Diseases—Diagnosis. 3. Diagnostic imaging.
4. Image analysis. I. Dershaw, D. David.
  [DNLM: 1. Breast Neoplasms—diagnosis. 2. Diagnostic Imaging—methods.
3. Diagnostic Techniques and Procedures. WP 870 I314 2002]
RG493.5.D52 I46 2002
616.99′449075—dc21   2002017663

ISBN 0-387-95454-6

Printed on acid-free paper.

Printed in the United States of America.

9 8 7 6 5 4 3 2 1   SPIN 10868109

www.springer-ny.com

Springer-Verlag   New York Berlin Heidelberg
A member of BertelsmannSpringer Science+Business Media GmbH

To Ryan Hunka
for giving special meaning to this project

Introduction

The techniques described in this book have been developed over several decades. The discovery that mammography could reveal nonpalpable disease within the breast led to the need to develop technology for the localization and documentation of the removal of worrisome tissue during the 1960s and 1970s. Refinement of the techniques used for preoperative localization occurred in the following decades. During the early 1990s the widespread use of imaging-guided large-gauge needle biopsy of the breast began, and in the decade that followed rapid improvement of these techniques occurred. The incorporation of new technologies, most importantly magnetic resonance imaging, into the algorithm for the diagnosis of breast disease has resulted in the development of further techniques for localization and biopsy.

Although these techniques continue to evolve, the rapid modification of this technology during the last decade of the twentieth century has slowed. This plateau in the development of new equipment and the understanding of the usefulness of these techniques in the diagnosis and treatment of breast disease has been taken as the opportunity to generate a new text for those performing and participating in the care of women undergoing these procedures. A large body of clinical experience and peer-reviewed literature is now available to support the use of these procedures and to assist in the selection of appropriate patients and incorporation of histopathologic results of these interventions in patient management. This text has been designed to make these data easily available and understandable to the reader.

This text also addresses some special concerns of those involved in these procedures. The incorporation of these techniques into a breast imaging practice necessitates the acquisition of equipment beyond that needed for imaging. Although some of this equipment can be obtained with minimal expense, some technology can be acquired only with considerable financial outlay. Issues of equipment selection and maintenance are of concern to those involved in its acquisition and are pivotal in the successful performance of some of these procedures. Therefore, these issues have been addressed throughout this book. Programs of quality control and quality assurance are also described.

Unlike the removal of large, obvious lesions, the retrieval of small lesions or small volumes of tissue from areas of concern results in unique problems for histopathologic diagnosis. The physician performing needle biopsies needs to understand which lesions are readily diagnosed with a single core of tissue and which lesions are better assessed with large volumes of tissue. The successful performance of fine needle aspiration can also present problems with adequacy of sampling and interpretation of results. An understanding of these issues is as important for the pathologist faced with interpreting the submitted tissue as it is for the physician performing these biopsies. Therefore, special attention has been paid to these issues. It is hoped that these discussions will be valuable to pathologists as well as radiologists and surgeons involved in these biopsies.

For radiologists performing these procedures, special skills beyond those generally required in radiology are needed. Anyone participating in a breast imaging practice appreciates that the patient interaction required for women undergoing imaging involves care, sensitivity, and patience in the communication of results to patients. Additionally, a general knowledge about cancer risks, limitations of imaging, and treatment of breast cancer is often required in discussions with women and their families. This is particularly important in the discussion of biopsy options to patients and the communication of biopsy results. The willingness and ability of the radiologist to have these discussions in a compassionate manner is as important to the patient and her family as the skillful performance of these procedures. It is impossible to overemphasize the importance of a warm, supportive, honest interaction with the patient as part of these procedures. They are best performed on patients who trust and are comforted by the physician doing these interventions. The physician must also be honest with the patient about their limitations and their failure to obtain a definitive result, thereby requiring repeat biopsy, when this occurs.

Physicians performing these procedures need to understand that they are often considerably more time consuming than just performing the procedure itself. When radiologists incorporate these procedures into their practice, there is a need to provide for the time and support required to communicate results and to maintain quality control. The success of these procedures is only assured when results of the pathologic analysis are correlated with the imaging studies. Specimen radiographs and biopsy results need to be reassessed with the pathology report in each case. Personal communication with the pathologist or surgeon is sometimes required to optimize quality of care. Radiologists need to appreciate that these procedures should not be considered completed until the pathology report addresses the lesion that has been biopsied, the specimen radiograph shows adequacy of excision of the area of concern, the results have been communicated to the patient and/or her clinician, and this has been documented in the report of the procedure.

Performance of these procedures also requires extra time, effort, and experience for the technologist who assists with them. Participation in these procedures involves dedication and skills that are beyond those needed for the performance of general radiography, sectional imaging, or noninterventional breast imaging. Patient anxiety is higher and requires special patience and compassion by the technologist. Training in infection control is also needed. The maintenance and quality control of new equipment must also be learned. Radiologists need to recognize these special skills and supply their technologists with the time necessary to learn and apply them.

When any intervention is performed, there is a possibility of complications. This is true with the procedures described in this text. Before performing any of these procedures, the physician should have in place a method for treating them. Whether they are treated by the radiologist or the patient is referred to a surgeon for treatment, the way in which treatment is delivered should be arranged before the physician is confronted, for example, with a large hematoma, pneumothorax or infection.

It is hoped that this text will encourage new physicians to perform these procedures and assist those who have incorporated them into their practices. Thousands of women require each of the interventions described in this text each year. The proliferation of skills needed to perform them will only result in the advantage inherent in each of these procedures being made available to larger numbers of women. It will make it possible to diagnose breast diseases more quickly, less expensively, and with less cosmetic deformity. The performance of these techniques will also enhance the sense of satisfaction derived from a breast imaging practice.

This text has only been possible because of the generosity of numerous, distinguished authors and their willingness to contribute. The demand on the time of each is profound, and I am extremely grateful and honored that they have been willing to participate in the production of this work. Inherent in the development of a multiauthored text is some diversity of opinion. It is hoped that the reader will appreciate that this diversity represents a spectrum of philosophies about these procedures and a variety of approaches for the performance and clinical application of these interventions. It is also hoped that the reader understands that this text has been designed to reflect the authors' knowledge of the state of the art in this field at the time this text was written. As experience with these techniques continues to accumulate, the appropriateness of some statements in this text may change.

I am deeply indebted to colleagues, family, and friends for their support while this book was being prepared. My colleagues and friends in the Breast Imaging Section of the Department of Radiology at Memorial Sloan-Kettering Cancer Center deserve particular mention. Drs. Andrea Abramson, Linda LaTrenta, Laura Liberman, and Elizabeth Morris have been a constant inspiration and have become a group where intellectual pursuit (and emotional support) has become part of our daily activity. I thank them for tolerating me. The faculty of the Department of Radiology and its chair, Dr. Hedwig Hricak, have been generous in their support of the time and effort required to undertake projects such as these and the clinical research upon which this work is based. Our fellows, past and present, have been a constant inspiration. None of this work would have been possible without the skills and compassion of our technologists. Thank you Cynthia Thornton, Dey Rizzo, Youngduk Paik, and Karen Larson. Finally, let me thank those who share in the pleasure and satisfaction in the completion of this work: Beckie, Bruce, Brewster, John, Renato, Alan, Wendy, Odette, and Ryan.

D. DAVID DERSHAW, M.D.
New York, New York
July, 2002

Preface

The practice of breast imaging has evolved from the interpretation of mammograms to the incorporation of a variety of imaging techniques into the armamentarium of the breast imager in discovering and staging the possible extent of tumor within the breast. This has become widely appreciated among our patients and colleagues. Informing a patient that she needs a biopsy often results in her questioning the radiologist if he or she "can do it today". Just as frequently, the scheduling of a patient for biopsy or possible breast conserving surgery depends on the availability of the radiologist to localize the lesion or mark the extent of tumor within the breast preoperatively.

Because of this, the success of breast imaging technology is increasingly interrelated with the ability of the radiologist to successfully retrieve or assist in the retrieval of tissue that has been deemed suspicious. Failure to achieve successful excision of this tissue will render an elegant imaging workup valueless. Therefore, the performance of the procedures described in this text has become as important in the care of women with breast disease as obtaining high quality images and interpreting them accurately.

Any radiologist, surgeon, pathologist or other physician involved in the care of women undergoing these interventions understands that knowledge about these procedures and an appreciation of the limitations inherent in them is a necessary part of adeptly caring for their patients. They also understand that the ability of each of us to successfully abort the natural history of breast cancer is truly a multidisciplinary effort. We need to accept the limitations of each discipline and to clearly communicate to each other and to our patients the advantages and limitations of our specialties.

The primary goal of this text is to assist those learning and performing the procedures described in this book to do them safely and successfully. Issues of equipment, quality control, accreditation of facilities, and legal concerns are addressed. The advantages, disadvantages, and limitations of each intervention are also discussed. These chapters will be of value to technologists and nurses assisting with these interventions, as well as to physicians performing them.

Additionally, it is hoped that this text will be of value to pathologists, surgeons, and others caring for women with breast disease to help them understand what patients will undergo when these procedures are performed and how these techniques can assist in the care of women. The limitations of each procedure in terms of patient selection, tissue retrieval, and diagnosis are also described and may be particularly valuable to these physicians.

The production of this text has been the work of multiple authors. I am most grateful to them for accepting the invitation to contribute to this book and making the time in their busy practices to generate these chapters. The contributors represent a distinguished group of physicians in the radiology and pathology community. Many have been pivotal in the development of the procedures they describe. It is hoped that their insights will be valuable to the reader.

D. DAVID DERSHAW, M.D.
New York, New York
July, 2002

Contents

Contributors

D. DAVID DERSHAW, M.D.
Department of Radiology
Memorial Sloan-Kettering Cancer Center
1275 York Avenue
New York, NY 10021
Telephone: (212) 639-7295
Fax: (212) 717-3056
Email: dershawd@mskcc.org

LAWRENCE W. BASSETT, M.D.
Department of Radiological Sciences
200 UCLA Medical Plaza
Los Angeles, CA 90095-1721
Telephone: (310) 206-9608
Fax: (310) 794-1428
Email: lbassett@mednet.ucla.edu

R. JAMES BRENNER, M.D., J.D.
Eisenberg Keffer Breast Center
John Wayne Cancer Center
St. John's Health Center
1328 22nd St.
Santa Monica, CA 90404
Telephone: (310) 582-7105
Fax: (310) 582-7110
Email: james.brenner@st.johns.org

ELLEN SHAW DEPAREDES, M.D.
Department of Radiology
Medical College of Virginia
Box 980615
Richmond, VA 23298
Telephone: (804) 828-0526
Fax: (804) 828-7989
Email: esshawde@hsc.vcu.edu

LINDA R. LATRENTA, M.D.
Department of Radiology
Memorial Sloan-Kettering Cancer Center
1275 York Avenue
New York, NY 10021
Telephone: (212) 639-8248
Fax: (212) 717-3056
Email: latrentl@mskcc.org

LAURA LIBERMAN, M.D.
Department of Radiology
Memorial Sloan-Kettering Cancer Center
1275 York Avenue
New York, NY 10021
Telephone: (212) 639-7289
Fax: (212) 717-3056
Email: libermal@mskcc.org

ELIZABETH A. MORRIS
Department of Radiology
Memorial Sloan-Kettering Cancer Center
1275 York Avenue
New York, NY 10021
Telephone: (212) 639-2236
Fax: (212) 717-3056
Email: morrise@mskcc.org

LIANE E. PHILPOTTS, M.D.
Department of Diagnostic Imaging
Yale University School of Medicine
333 Cedar St.
New Haven, CT 06501-3206
Telephone: (203) 785-2425
Fax: (203) 737-1688
Email: philpotts@biomed.med.yale.edu

HANDEL E. REYNOLDS, M.D.
Department of Radiology
Indiana University Hospital
550 N. University Blvd.
Indianapolis, IN 46202-5253
Telephone: (317) 274-4304
Fax: (317) 278-0214
Email: hreynold@xray.indyrad.IupuI.edu

P. PETER ROSEN, M.D.
Department of Pathology
New York Presbyterian Hospital
525 East 68th St.
New York, NY 10021
Telephone: (212) 746-6482
Fax: (212) 746-6484

EVA RUBIN, M.D.
Department of Radiology
University of Alabama Birmingham
1619 S. 19th St.
Birmingham, AL 35233
Telephone: (205) 823-0484
Email: evarubin@aol.com

CHAPTER 1

Ductography

Lawrence W. Bassett and Christine H. Kim

Ductography, also referred to as galactography or contrast mammography, is the radiographic examination of a mammary duct system following the injection of radiopaque contrast agent into a lactiferous duct orifice at the nipple. Ductography has long been utilized for the evaluation of nipple discharge. During the 1930s, Ries[1] and Hicken et al.[2] reported on "contrast ductograms." A few years after its introduction, ductography was discouraged due to reports of severe local tissue toxicity and infections.[3,4] These complications were related to the contrast agents used, including oil-based lipiodol and colloidal thorium dioxide. However, ductography performed with water soluble contrast agents, as originally described by Hicken et al.[2], later proved to be safe. In 1953, Leborgne[5] devoted a significant portion of his famous textbook *The Breast in Roentgen Diagnosis* to "Contrast Mammography." Leborgne defined abnormal ductography patterns and described the preoperative injection of methylene blue to guide the surgeon to intraductal lesions. Later, numerous other studies were published corroborating the diagnostic value of ductography.[6–10] Nonetheless, ductography is still not widely performed in the United States today. A recent survey of members of the American College of Radiology revealed that only 36% of radiologists utilized ductography in their practices.[11]

CAUSES OF NIPPLE DISCHARGE

The function of the breast is to produce fluid, specifically milk. Nipple discharge is not uncommon in nonlactating women. Bilateral discharge is particularly likely to be physiologic or due to other benign etiologies. The causes of benign nipple discharge are numerous.[12] They include the use of birth control pills, certain antihypertensive medications, major tranquilizers, antidepressants and other medications that increase prolactin levels. Endocrine abnormalities can also lead to bilateral nipple discharge secondary to elevated prolactin. Finally, benign fibrocystic changes and ductal ectasia can cause bilateral or unilateral nipple discharge. Benign discharges, whether bilateral or unilateral, are usually gray, green, brown, or white. Tabár et al. reported that greenish brown, gray, and milky discharges involving multiple ducts are always due to benign fibrocystic disease or ductal ectasia and therefore not an indication for ductography.[13]

Considering that the breast ducts normally contain fluid, it is not surprising that squeezing the nipple can produce a unilateral or bilateral discharge in many normal women.[14] Therefore, discharges that are elicited by squeezing the duct are generally not worrisome. However, spontaneous and persistent unilateral discharges require further evaluation. Those of greatest concern are bloody, serous, or serosanguineous unilateral discharges. Tabár et al.'s review of nine published articles reporting on 1628 cases that underwent both ductography and surgery identified the most common causes of nipple discharges as papillomas (34%) (Figure 1.1), fibrocystic changes (27%), ductal ectasia (13%) and carcinomas (10%) (Figure 1.2). A review by the same author of 11 articles reporting on 113 cancers detected by ductography found that 76% of the cancers were associated with a bloody discharge and 24% with a serous discharge.[13]

INDICATIONS FOR DUCTOGRAPHY

Based on the above information, the most important indication for ductography is a unilateral spontaneous, persistent nipple discharge that is bloody, serous (clear or watery), or serosanguineous (Figure 1.3).[13,15–17] Typically the patient reports periodic staining of the bra, blouse, or night-

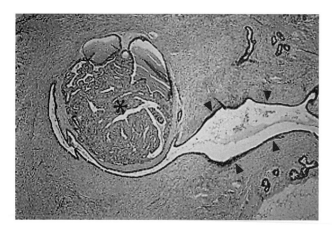

FIGURE 1.1. Histologic section of a benign papilloma (asterisk) within a mammary duct (arrowheads). There is material within the duct that represents the remnants of a serosanguineous discharge.

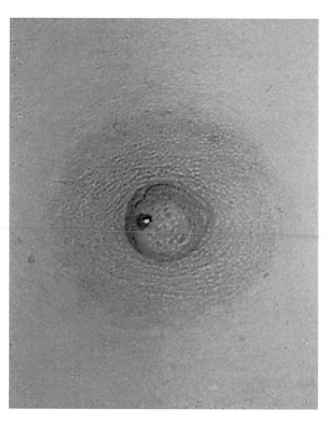

FIGURE 1.3. Serosanguineous nipple discharge originating from a single duct orifice. The discharge was unilateral, spontaneous, and persistent.

clothes. Discharges that accompany cancer usually contain gross or occult blood.[12] Therefore, a positive Hemoccult test for blood is another indication that a nipple discharge merits ductography. The one exception to these indications is bloody nipple discharge late in pregnancy. This has been attributed to hyperplasia of ductal tissue or vascular engorgement and only requires clinical follow-up to ensure resolution.[18] On the other hand, some authors have advocated ductography for the evaluation of spontaneous unilateral nipple discharge, regardless of its character.[19] In our practice, we usually perform ductography in cases with unilateral, spontaneous, persistent bloody, serous, or serosanguineous discharge.

CONTRAINDICATIONS TO DUCTOGRAPHY

The only reported contraindication to ductography is mastitis or breast abscess.[10,13] This is because it is thought that the retrograde injection of contrast medium into a duct could cause the infection to spread to other areas in the breast.

PREPROCEDURE EVALUATION

Physical examination and appropriate imaging workup are recommended prior to any interventional procedure, including ductography. In the majority of cases physical examination and imaging workup will not disclose the source of a nipple discharge, and ductography is the recommended next step. In one series of 204 patients who underwent ductography for nipple discharge, only 29 (14%) had a palpable abnormality.[13] Of the 18 women in that series with carcinoma as the cause of the nipple discharge, only 9 had a mammographically evident tumor. Occasionally, mammography or ultrasonography identifies the source of a nipple discharge (Figures 1.4–1.6).

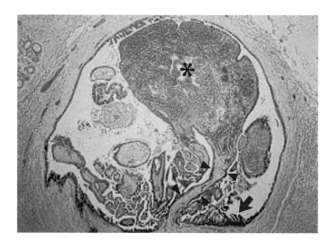

FIGURE 1.2. Histologic section of an infarcted papillary carcinoma (asterisk). Note the fronds of neoplastic cells (arrow) within the duct near the base of the stalk (arrowheads).

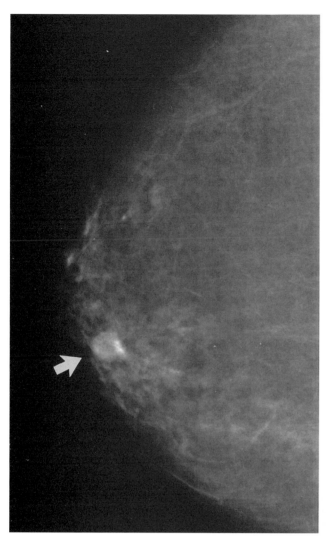

A

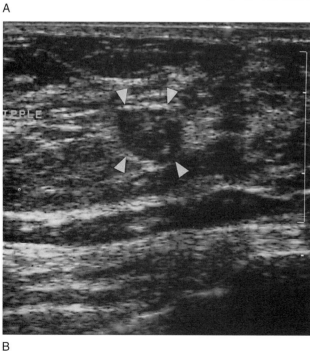

B

FIGURE 1.4. Routine mammography (**A**) in a patient with bloody nipple discharge demonstrates a round, circumscribed, retroareolar nodule (arrow). Correlative ultrasonography (**B**) confirms the presence of a circumscribed hypoechoic nodule (arrowheads) within normal breast parenchyma. Excisional biopsy revealed intraductal papilloma.

←

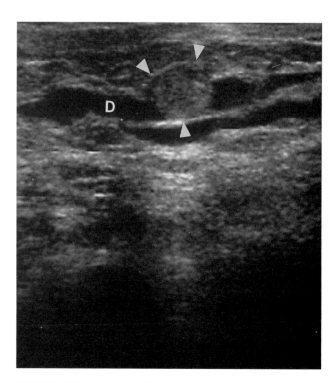

FIGURE 1.5. A slightly different sonographic appearance of intraductal papilloma causing nipple discharge. In this case the circumscribed solid nodule (arrowheads) is identified within a dilated duct (D).

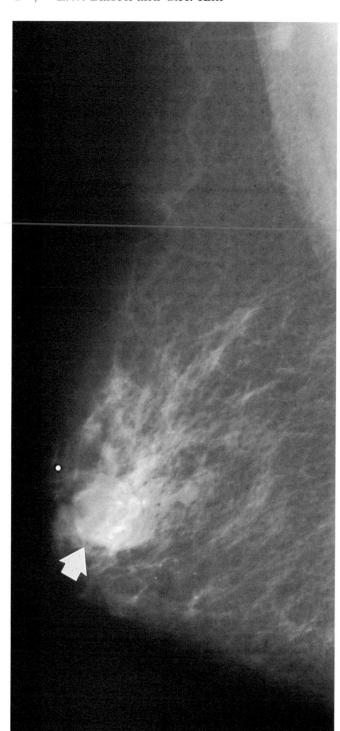

A

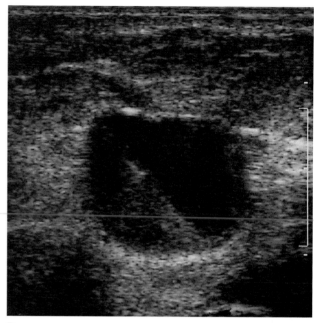

B

FIGURE 1.6. Palpable mass associated with bloody nipple discharge. (**A**) Mediolateral oblique mammogram reveals a circumscribed, lobulated mass in the subareolar region adjacent to a metallic BB placed over the palpable mass. (**B**) Ultrasonography reveals a lobulated mass with both solid and cystic components corresponding to the palpable findings. Ultrasound-guided core needle biopsy revealed intracystic papillary carcinoma.

Even so, ductography may be helpful in confirming that a mammographic or sonographic finding is truly related to the nipple discharge (Figure 1.7).

Cytologic evaluation of the discharge is not considered reliable and is not recommended as part of the diagnostic workup because of a high false negative rate.[16,17,20]

TECHNIQUE FOR PERFORMING DUCTOGRAPHY

Nipple discharge should be present at the time of ductography. Therefore, if a discharge is not currently present, the examination may have to be rescheduled.

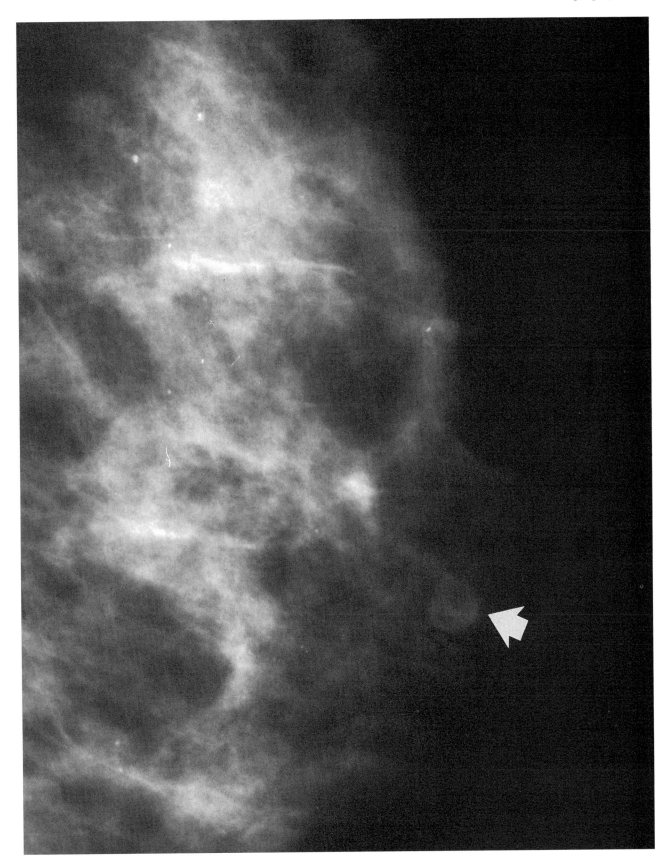

FIGURE 1.7. Mammography and ductography of an intraductal papilloma responsible for bloody nipple discharge. (**A**) Close-up of mediolateral oblique mammogram shows a circumscribed, round nodule (arrow) in the subareolar area.

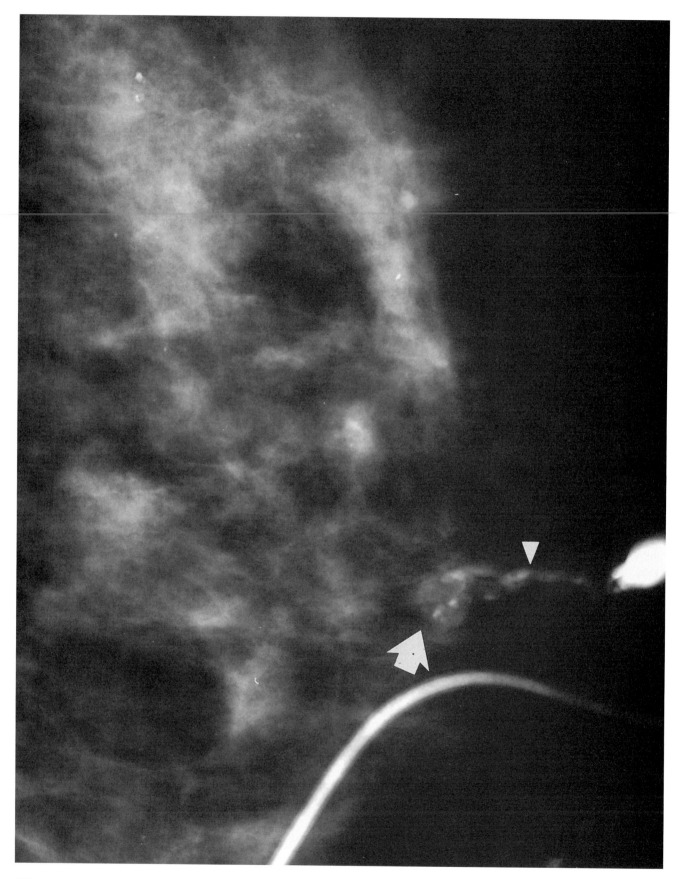

FIGURE 1.7. (B) Contrast injection confirms that the circumscribed nodule (arrow) is located within the discharging duct (arrowhead). Surgical excision guided by methylene blue injection into the discharging duct revealed an intraductal papilloma.

The materials and equipment needed for ductography are listed in Table 1.1 and illustrated in Figure 1.8. Performance of ductography requires optimal visibility in order to identify the small orifice of the discharging duct. A high-intensity lamp allows better visibility of the duct, and some believe the warmth of the lamp relaxes the musculature around the orifice of the duct allowing easier cannulation. Most radiologists use a binocular magnifier to better visualize the ductal orifice. The nipple is first cleansed with a sterilizing solution to remove keratin plugs or clotted blood and to disinfect the skin. Some radiologists use sterile soap or Betadine for this purpose, whereas others use only alcohol.

A 27- or 30-gauge straight or curved blunt needle-catheter system is connected to a 3- or 5-cc syringe filled with water-soluble contrast agent such as iothalamate meglumine (Conray). Nonionic contrast can be used to reduce the possibility of a contrast reaction secondary to extravasation of contrast material outside the ductal system. However, there have been no documented cases of water-soluble contrast reactions related to ductography, and most experienced radiologists do not believe that nonionic agents are necessary.[21] Special care should be taken to remove all air from the needle and tubing prior to injecting the contrast agent into the duct, since air bubbles result in filling defects that can be confused with intraluminal lesions.

The patient may be supine or seated upright for the procedure. The supine position is usually preferred for patient comfort. The first step is to locate the appropriate duct for cannulation. The duct is usually identified by the presence of a small amount of spontaneous discharge (Figure 1.3). In addition to the fluid, the orifice may be slightly dilated or erythematous.[19] If the discharge is not evident, the areola can be gently squeezed to attempt to elicit the discharge. Sometimes there is a "trigger point" farther away from the nipple upon which gentle pressure reproducibly elicits the discharge.[19] The patient can often identify the location of the trigger point, if asked.

TABLE 1.1. *Ductography materials and equipment*

High-intensity light source
Binocular magnification lenses
Sterile gloves
Sterile gauze pads
3- to 5-cc syringe
18-gauge needle (for drawing up contrast solution)
Alcohol wipes
60% iothalamate meglumine (Conray, Mallinkrodt, St. Louis, MO)
27–30-gauge ductogram cannula
Dressing tape for securing cannula to breast
Methylene blue dye (optional, for preoperative localization)
Collodion solution (optional, for preoperative localization)

See also Figure 1.8

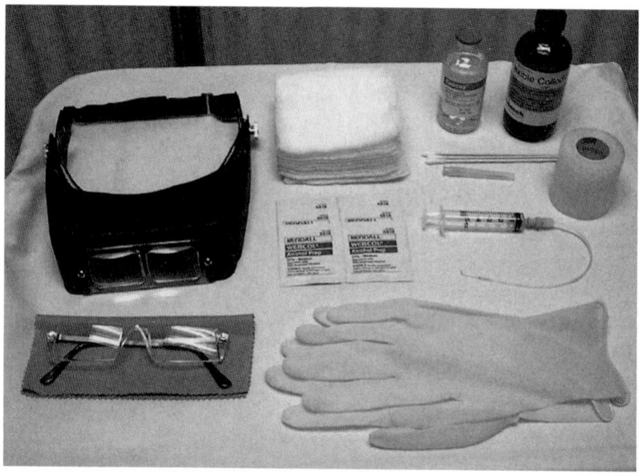

FIGURE 1.8. Materials and equipment used in performing ductography.

Once the discharging duct is identified, the tip of the cannula is carefully and gently guided into the orifice. This may require gentle probing of the duct orifice with twirling or angling of the tip to facilitate entry.[22] In other cases, circumferential traction around the areola may help to "spread out" the nipple surface and expose the orifice. Some authors advocate the use of a flexible guidewire or filament as well as a topical lubricant to facilitate painless cannulation of the duct,[23,24] but most believe that this is unnecessary. The cannula should not be forced or it may perforate the duct. In most cases, insertion of the tip a few millimeters into the duct is sufficient for the injection of the contrast agent. If there is any resistance to advancing the cannula once the needle tip has entered the duct, the nipple may be pulled out slightly in order to straighten the course of the main (proximal) duct. The contrast should be injected slowly because of the small size of the cannula and the viscosity of the contrast agent. The patient is asked to report any feeling of fullness, discomfort or pain immediately. It is best to inject small amounts of contrast agent initially, as too much contrast may obscure a small lesion or cause extravasation, especially if there is a duct obstruction more distally. If necessary, additional contrast may be injected after the initial images are obtained. In most cases, less than 1 cc of contrast agent is needed to obtain adequate opacification of the ductal system of interest.

Following contrast injection, the needle-catheter can either be taped in place with the needle in the duct or it can be removed. Magnification craniocaudal and 90° lateral mammograms are promptly obtained with mild to moderate compression. Since some of the ductal branches may overlap, additional mammographic images, including rolled views, may be required to visualize a filling defect that is obscured by overlying opacified ducts on standard projections.

8 / L.W. Bassett and C.H. Kim

RADIOGRAPHIC FINDINGS

Normal Ductogram

Normal ducts are smooth in contour and free of fixed intraluminal filling defects (Figure 1.9A). However, there is great variability in the appearance of normal duct systems (Figures 1.10–1.12). For example, the caliber of normal ducts can vary greatly. The progressive orderly arborization of ducts retrograde from the nipple may begin just posterior to the nipple (Figure 1.10) or at varying distances from the nipple (Figures 1.11 and 1.12), and a main

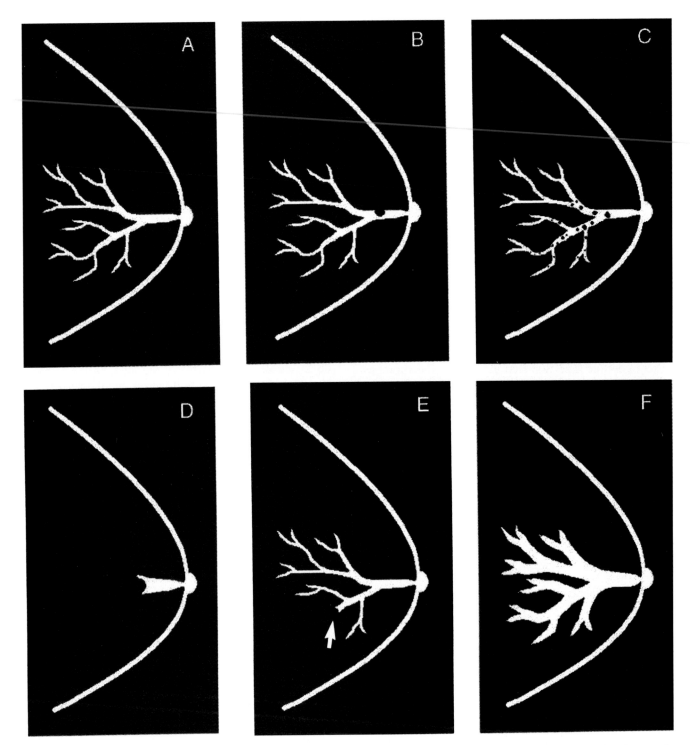

FIGURE 1.9. Schematic representation of normal and abnormal ductograms. **(A)** Normal. **(B)** Solitary filling defect in a main duct. **(C)** Multiple filling defects in several ducts. **(D)** Abrupt cutoff in a main duct. **(E)** Abrupt cutoff (arrow) in a secondary duct. **(F)** Ductal ectasia.

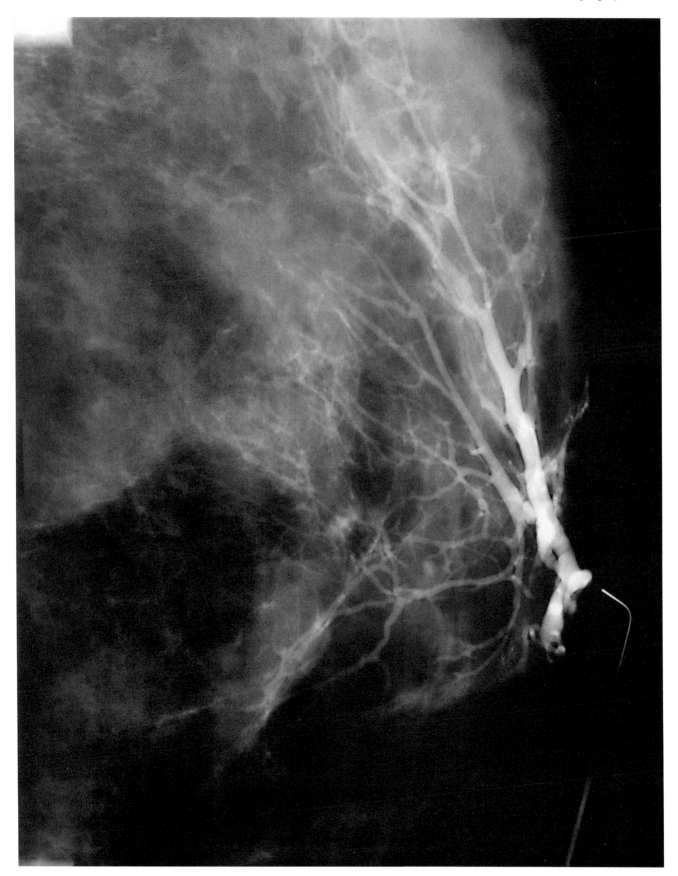

FIGURE 1.10. Normal ductogram. The opacified duct lumens are relatively large near the nipple, vary in size, have smooth contours, and taper distally. There are no intraluminal filling defects.

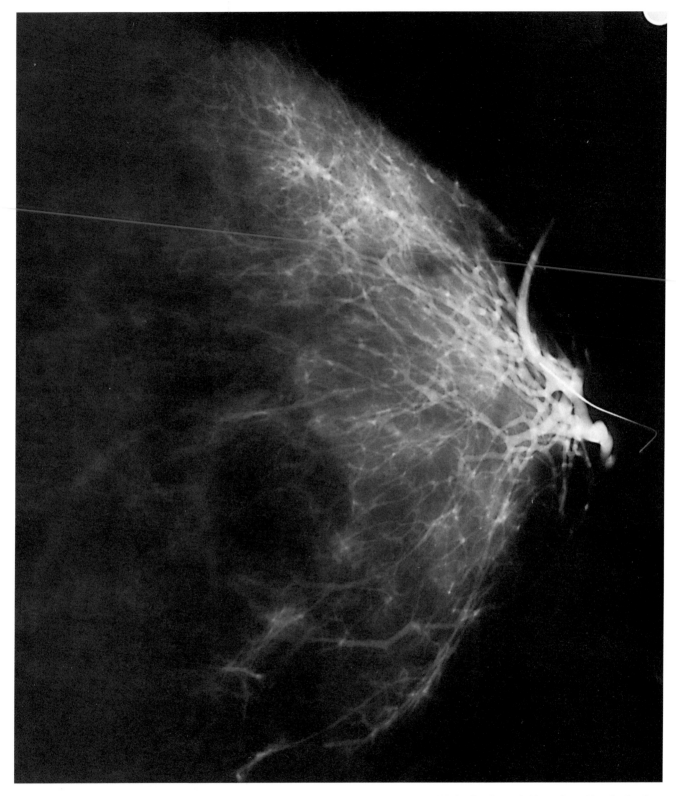

FIGURE 1.11. Normal ductogram. The ducts taper more rapidly and are more widely distributed. Note that this single duct system extends over a large portion of the breast.

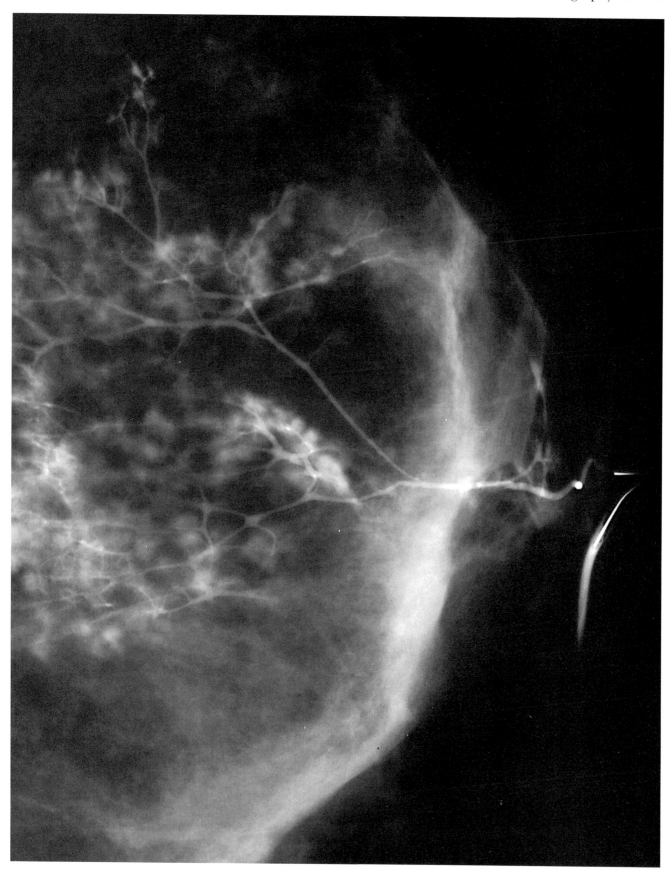

FIGURE 1.12. Normal ductogram. The ducts are small in caliber and begin branching farther from the nipple. Note the "lobular blush" associated with contrast entering the lobules.

duct can have numerous secondary branches or only a few. Furthermore, the overall volume occupied by a single duct system may be limited or expansive, sometimes extending into multiple quadrants. There are other variations in the appearance of normal duct systems. In some cases the contrast material may extend to the lobules resulting in a contrast "blush" surrounding the adjacent ducts (Figure 1.12).[19] Leborgne found that the duct system tended to vary among age groups.[5] He noted that the ducts were more numerous and fine in young women with abundant lobular development during lactation. After menopause, there tends to be progressive involution starting at the periphery of the lobe and progressing toward the center.

Abnormal Ductogram

An abnormal ductogram may demonstrate the following radiographic features: single or multiple filling defects

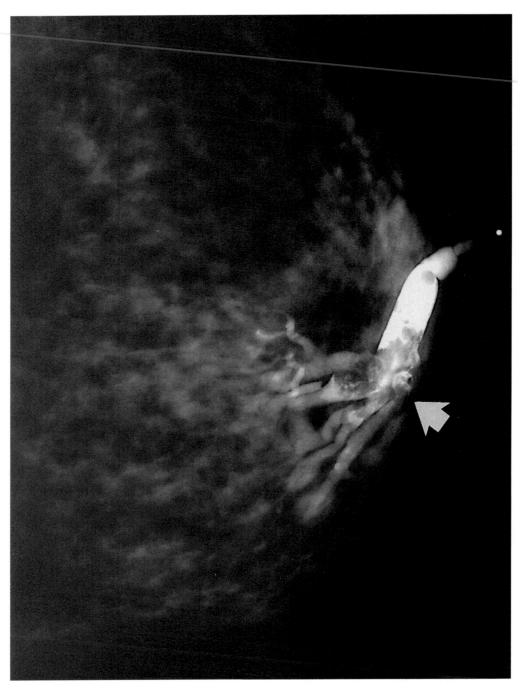

FIGURE 1.13. Filling defect. The patient had a bloody nipple discharge. The duct is dilated proximal to a large lobulated filling defect (arrow) that extends into multiple branches of the duct. Excisional biopsy revealed intraductal papilloma.

within one or more ducts, abrupt cutoff of contrast within a main or secondary duct, irregularity of the duct wall or duct contour, and abnormal (enlarged) caliber of a single duct or an entire ductal system (Figure 1.9B–F). In general, a ductogram can identify the site of an intraluminal lesion but not the specific pathology. Because of the non-specific nature of abnormalities detected on ductography, excisional biopsy is usually recommended whenever there is a localized abnormality.

The most common cause of an intraductal filling defect in a woman with spontaneous bloody or serous nipple discharge is a benign papilloma (Figure 1.1).[13] Ducts containing papillomas are usually dilated from the nipple to the lesion (Figures 1.13–1.15). Fibrocystic changes are the second most common cause of intraluminal filling defects.[13] Filling defects due to fibrocystic changes may be identical to those due to papillomas or may show more diffuse wall irregularities. Filling defects that are multi-

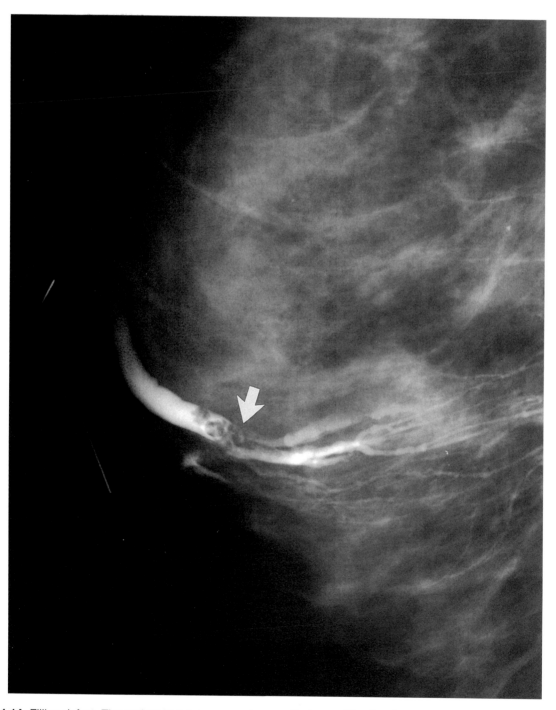

FIGURE 1.14. Filling defect. The patient had a serosanguineous discharge. The duct is dilated proximal to a filling defect (arrow) at the site of duct branching. Excisional biopsy revealed intraductal papilloma.

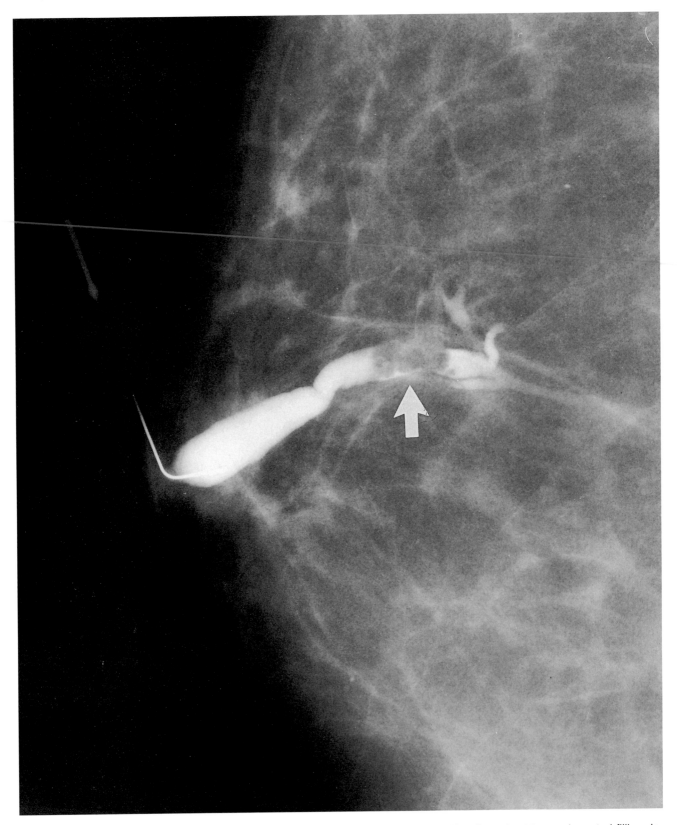

FIGURE 1.15. Filling defect. The patient had bloody nipple discharge. The duct is dilated proximal to an elongated filling defect (arrow). Excisional biopsy revealed intraductal papilloma.

ple can be due to papillomatosis, fibrocystic change or intraductal carcinoma (Figure 1.16). Other causes of intraductal filling defects include blood clots, air bubbles (Figure 1.17) and debris, especially when seen in conjunction with ductal ectasia.

An abrupt cutoff in a main or secondary duct is another abnormal finding that identifies a lesion on ductography. If an intraluminal lesion completely obstructs the duct, the result is an abrupt cutoff of contrast material in the ductogram. Again, papillomas are the most com-

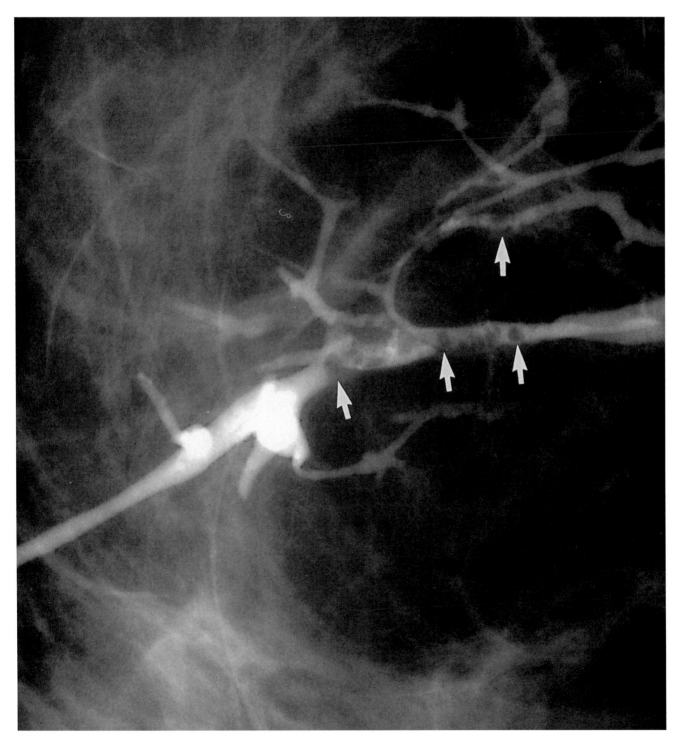

FIGURE 1.16. Multiple filling defects. The patient complained of intermittent bloody discharge. Mammography and physical examination were negative. Ductography revealed numerous filling defects in the ductal system distal to the branching of the main duct. Surgery revealed extensive ductal carcinoma in situ.

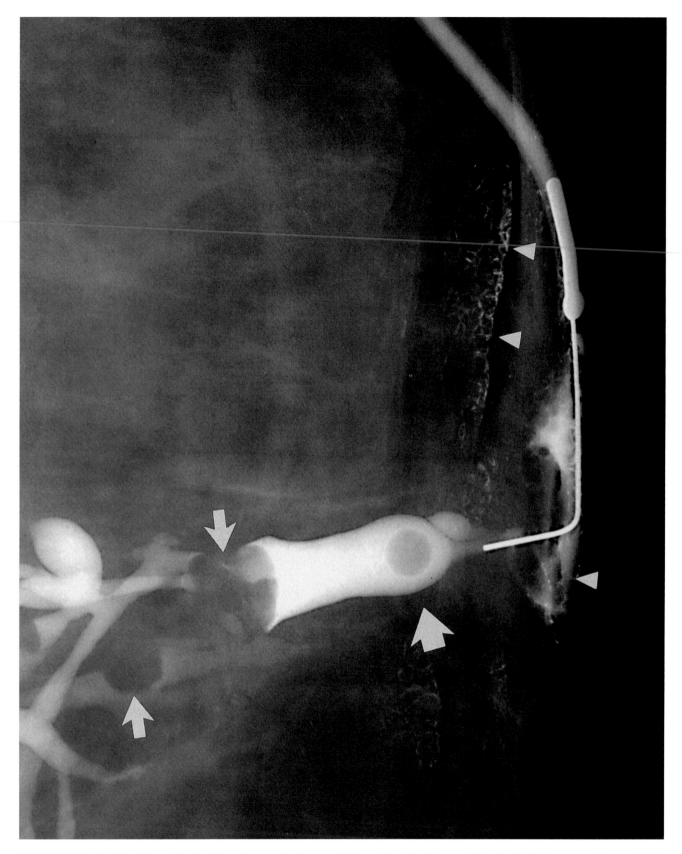

FIGURE 1.17. Multiple filling defects. There is a perfectly round filling defect just beyond the nipple that represents an air bubble (large arrow). Other filling defects noted distally (small arrows) represent actual lesions. The mottled densities (arrowheads) along the interior surface of the breast are due to contrast that has leaked out of the duct orifice. Excisional biopsy of the lesions revealed multiple papillomas.

mon cause of this finding (Figure 1.18). Other intraluminal lesions, including fibrocystic changes (Figure 1.19) and carcinoma (Figure 1.20), can result in a similar appearance. An abrupt cutoff of a duct can also be due to previous surgery in that area.

Irregularity in the wall of the duct is also considered abnormal and may result in an undulating or "beaded" appearance of the contrast within the duct (Figure 1.21). This is often related to fibrocystic changes in the adjacent parenchyma. Another abnormal finding on ductog-

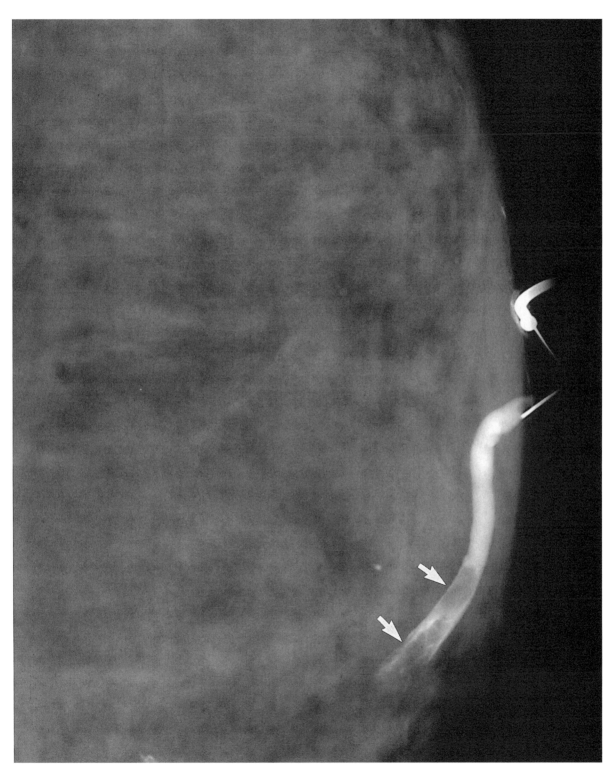

FIGURE 1.18. Cutoff of main duct. In this case, the intraluminal filling defect (arrows) completely obstructs the passage of contrast material distally. Excisional biopsy revealed an intraductal papilloma.

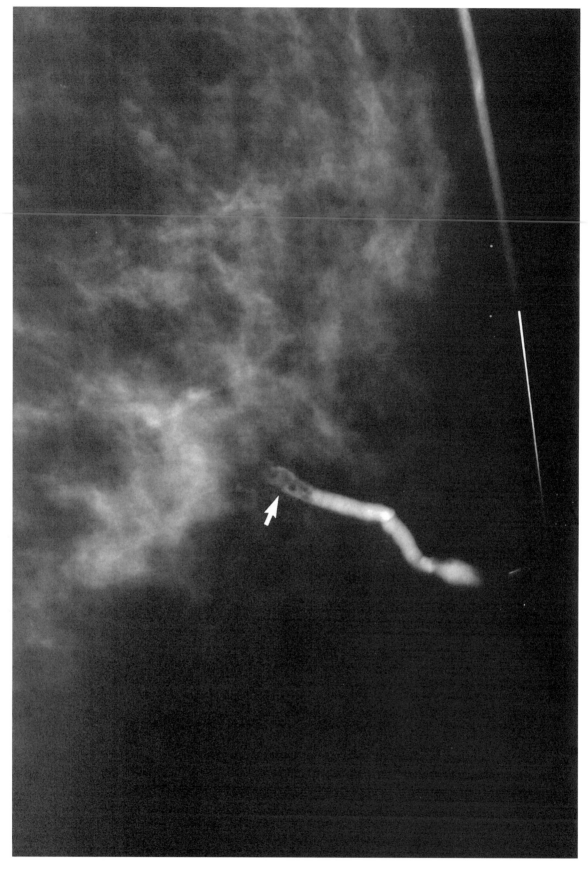

FIGURE 1.19. A lobulated filling defect (arrow) with a cutoff sign. The patient had a bloody discharge. Excisional biopsy revealed microglandular adenosis as the cause of the ductogram findings.

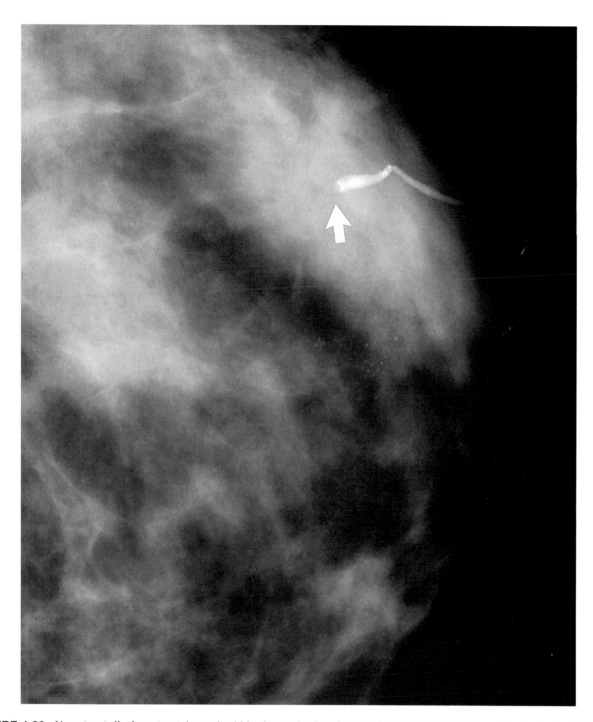

FIGURE 1.20. Abrupt cutoff of contrast (arrow) within the main duct in a patient with spontaneous bloody nipple discharge. Both mammography and physical examination were negative. Surgical biopsy revealed ductal carcinoma in situ.

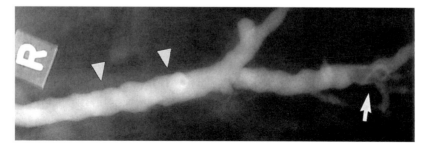

FIGURE 1.21. Irregularity of the wall of the duct (arrowheads) and localized filling defect (arrow) in a patient with recurrent nipple discharge. Pathology revealed fibrocystic changes.

19

raphy that can be seen with fibrocystic changes is the presence of cysts which become opacified with contrast material due to their communication with the ductal system (Figure 1.22). In addition, irregularity of duct contour, such as narrowing or angular displacement of the duct, may result from mass effect or cicatrization associated with a neighboring carcinoma.

Ductal ectasia can also be associated with nipple discharge, which is usually white or brown but occasionally bloody. The ductogram findings of ductal ectasia include

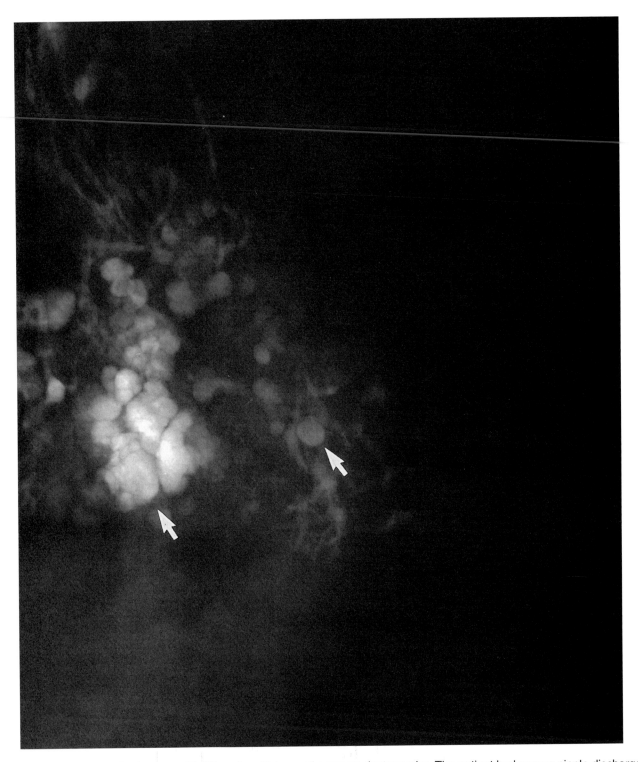

FIGURE 1.22. Fibrocystic changes with filling of multiple small cysts on ductography. The patient had serous nipple discharge. (**A**) On the craniocaudal projection, the contrast agent is pooled in numerous small cysts (arrows) that communicate with the ductal system.

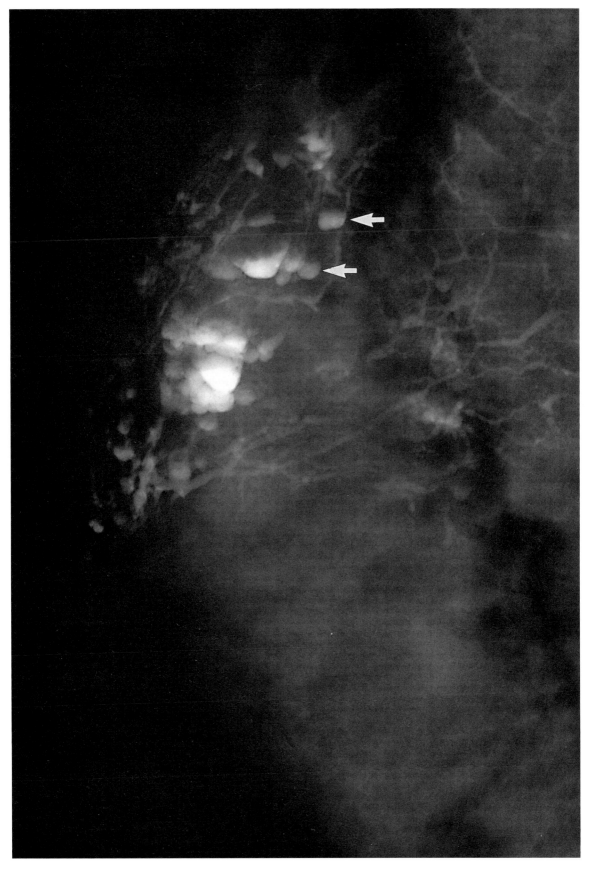

FIGURE 1.22. (B) The 90° lateral view shows layering of the contrast agent (arrows) at the bottom of the fluid-filled cysts. No localized filling defects were identified. The discharge resolved spontaneously.

irregular dilatation of the involved duct and abrupt tapering of the distal branches (Figures 1.23 and 1.24).

"Pseudolesions" are filling defects or other abnormal findings encountered during ductography that are not found at surgical exploration.[19] It is unclear whether they represent transient lesions such as blood clots or debris or these areas were excluded from the surgical specimen. The exact cause of these lesions has yet to be determined.

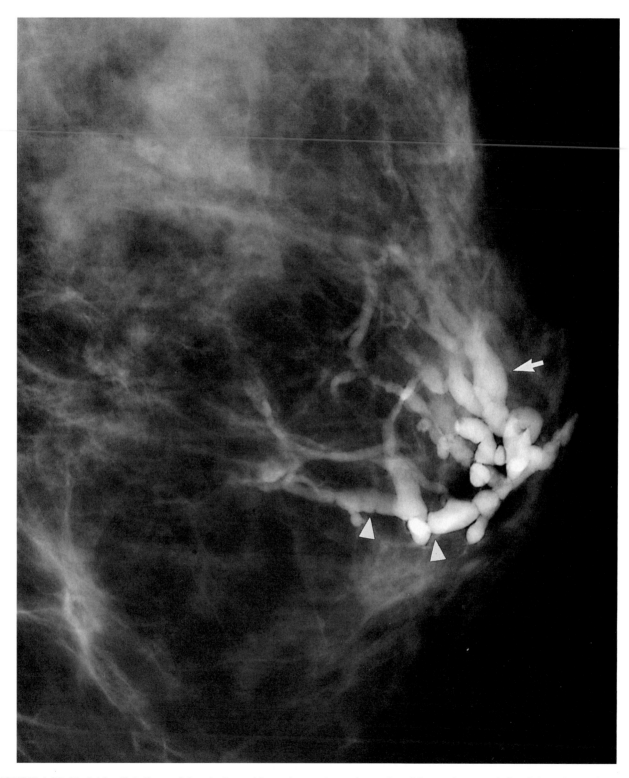

FIGURE 1.23. Variable dilatations of the ducts and irregular contours (arrowheads) are characteristic of ductal ectasia in this patient with spontaneous brown nipple discharge. Note the areas of diffuse enlargement, as well as ducts that are more bulbous in appearance (arrow). There were no localized filling defects.

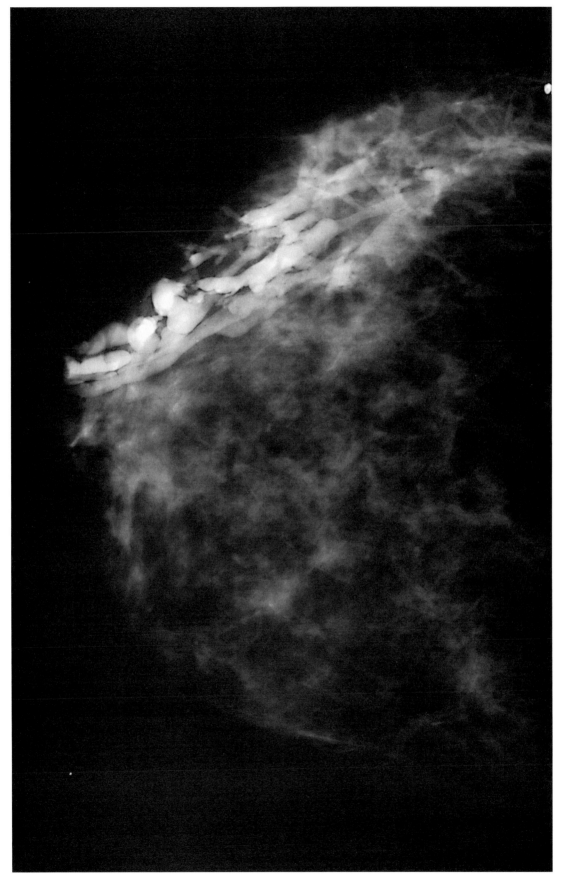

FIGURE 1.24. Another example of ductal ectasia showing dilatation of the ducts extending more distally.

PREOPERATIVE DUCTOGRAPHY

If a filling defect or cutoff is proximal to the initial branching of the major duct, it is usually possible to localize the lesion for the surgeon simply by identifying the involved duct at the nipple orifice. This is accomplished by cannulating the discharging ductal orifice and injecting a mixture of contrast material and methylene blue due in approximately equal amounts. The contrast material in the mixture makes it possible to visualize the duct mammographically.

After mammography confirms that the appropriate duct with the abnormality has been selected, the cannula can be removed and the patient may proceed to surgery. A small amount of collodium applied topically at the duct orifice prevents the dye-contrast mixture from escaping from the duct. In the operating room, the surgeon can then spot the abnormal duct by identifying the methylene blue at the orifice and within the duct. Since the intraluminal lesion is proximal to ductal branching, the surgeon can follow the methylene blue-stained duct distally to the lesion.

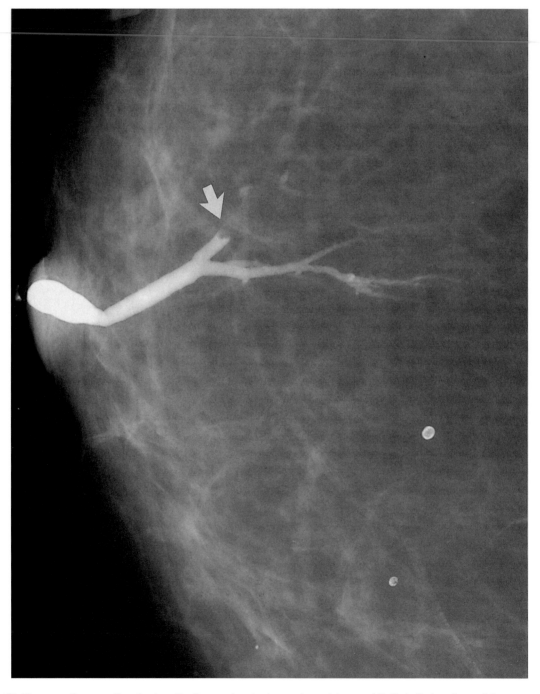

FIGURE 1.25. Preoperative needle-wire localization under ductography guidance. (**A**) Cutoff sign (arrow) in a secondary duct branch in a patient with bloody nipple discharge. The mammogram was negative.

In some circumstances needle/wire localization of the intraductal lesion may be useful or preferred. Particularly if single or multiple lesions are located beyond the initial branching point of the main duct, it may be very difficult for the surgeon to find the lesion with only methylene blue dye for guidance. This is because it would not be possible to determine which of the methylene blue-stained branches of the duct actually contained the lesion. This would be even more problematic if the lesion were in a secondary branch farther away from the main duct. In such cases, needle/wire localization with ductography guidance can be performed to pinpoint the lesion for the surgeon preoperatively. First, the duct is cannulated and contrast material is injected in the usual manner. Mammograms are then obtained as for diagnostic ductography. After identifying the lesion on ductography, the preoperative needle/wire localization can be performed using mammographic guidance (Figure 1.25). In the operating room, the surgeon uses the

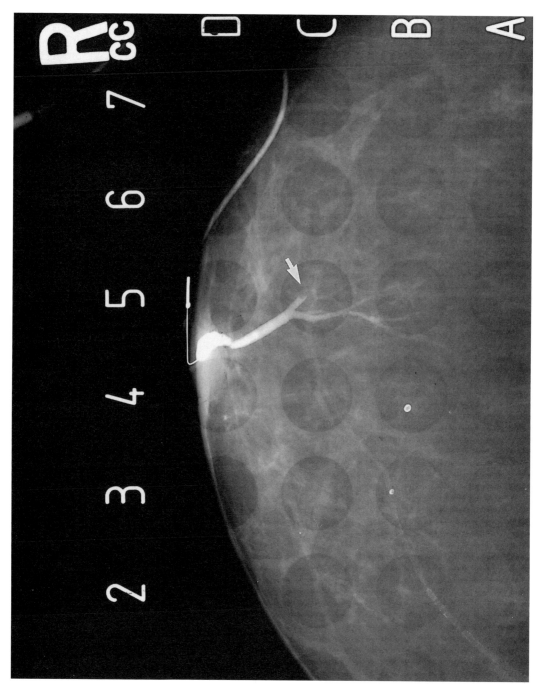

FIGURE 1.25. (B) Initial scout view of the breast with a compression hole plate was obtained immediately after ductography. The alphanumeric grid is used to identify the correct hole for needle insertion. In this case, the lesion (arrow) is located within hole C-5.

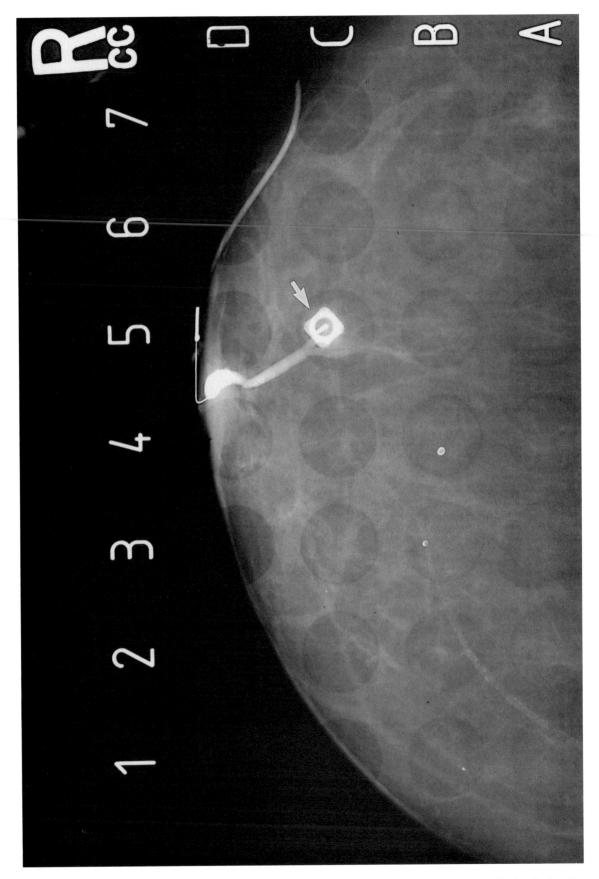

FIGURE 1.25. (C) Without releasing compression or changing position, a second mammogram is obtained after the needle (arrow) is inserted. The x-ray beam is directed down the shaft of the needle, which appears as a point within the needle hub.

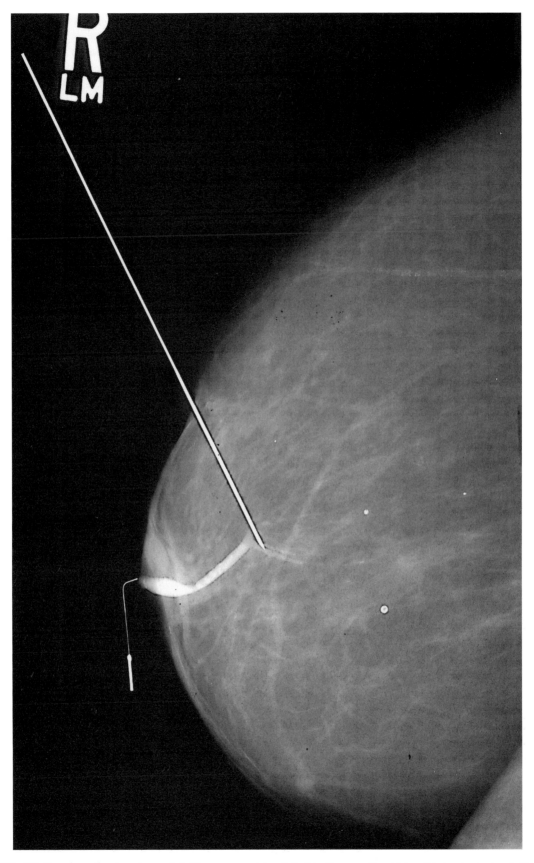

FIGURE 1.25. (**D**) Compression is released, taking care not to dislodge the needle, and a third mammogram is obtained in the orthogonal projection in order to view the depth of the needle tip within the breast. Once the tip is adjusted to the appropriate position, a wire is then pushed out the tip of the needle, and a final mammogram is obtained.

localization wire as a guide to the site of the filling defect in the same way as for a preoperative needle/wire localization of a nonpalpable mammographic abnormality.

COMPLICATIONS

There are only a few complications associated with ductography. The most common is perforation of a duct with extravasation of contrast medium into the surrounding breast parenchyma. While the contrast agent is being injected, the patient may experience a sudden sharp pain followed by a burning sensation. This usually indicates contrast extravasation, and mammography should be performed (Figures 1.26 and 1.27). If there is evidence of extravasation, the procedure should be terminated. There are no serious consequences from extravasated contrast agents, but the ductogram usually has to be repeated a few days later after the contrast agent has been resorbed. Rarely, contrast medium may be visualized within lym-

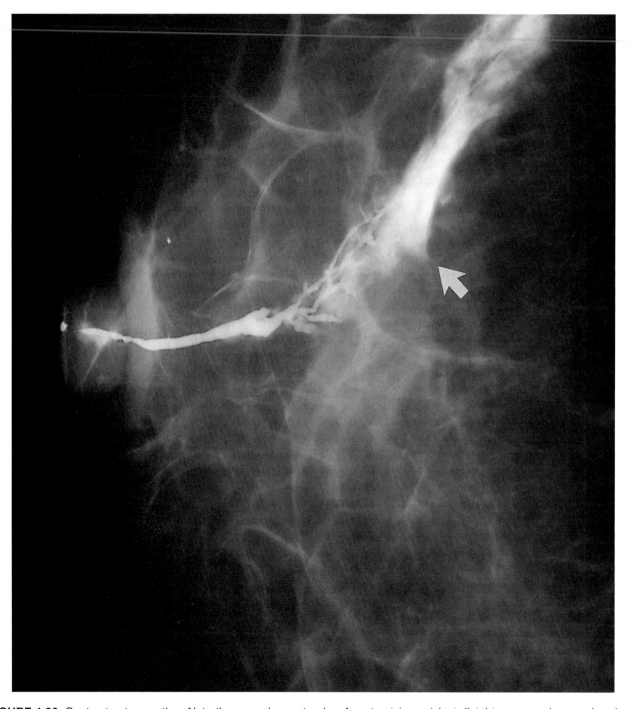

FIGURE 1.26. Contrast extravasation. Note the amorphous streaks of contrast (arrow) just distal to a normal-appearing duct.

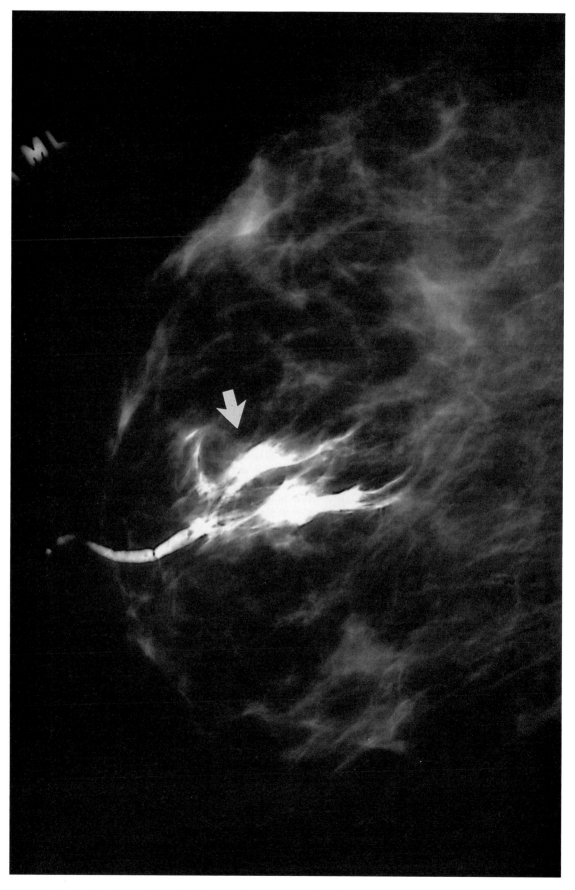

FIGURE 1.27. Contrast extravasation. In this case the extravasation (arrow) originates from the ducts more proximally.

phatic vessels in the breast even in the absence of obvious perforation. This is only a problem if the lymphatic opacification obscures the ductal system.

Vasovagal reaction is another potential risk associated with the procedure. Therefore, a patient should not be left alone during the procedure and, if she complains of faintness or lightheadedness or begins to show signs of sweating or skin flushing, she should immediately be placed in the supine position and treated accordingly. While there is a hypothetical risk of a hypersensitivity reaction to the contrast agent, there are no reports of this in the literature. Theoretically, the risk may be reduced by the use of nonionic rather than ionic contrast agents, but most experts believe this is not necessary.

Finally, inflammation or mastitis, although uncommon, is another complication associated with ductography. The patient is instructed to contact the breast imaging center or referring physician if symptoms of redness, pain or swelling develop during the days following the procedure.

REFERENCES

1. Ries E. Diagnostic lipiodol injection into milk ducts followed by abscess formation. Am J Obstet Gynecol 1930;20:414–416.
2. Hicken NF, Best RR, Hunt BB. The roentgen visualization and diagnosis of breast lesions by means of contrast media. AJR 1938;39:321–343.
3. Reis RA, Mesirow SD. Studies in the evaluation of mammography. JAMA 1938;110:1900–1905.
4. Romano SA, McFetridge EM. Limitations and dangers of mammography by contrast medium. JAMA 1938;110:1905–1910.
5. Leborgne RA. The Breast in Roentgen Diagnosis. Montevideo: Impresora Uruguay, 1953.
6. Björn-Hansen R. Contrast mammography. Br J Radiol 1965;38:947–951.
7. Funderburk WW, Syphax B. Evaluation of nipple discharge in benign and malignant diseases. Cancer 1969;24:1290–1296.
8. Threatt B, Appleman HD. Mammary duct injection. Radiology 1973;108:71–76.
9. Ouimet-Oliva D, Herbert G. Galactography: a method of detection of unsuspected cancers. AJR 1974;120:55–61.
10. Sartorius OW, Smith HS. Contrast ductography for the recognition and localization of benign and malignant breast lesions: an improved technique. In Logan W (ed) Breast Carcinoma. New York: Wiley, 1977;281–300.
11. Reynolds HE, Jackson VP, Musick BS. A survey of interventional mammography practices. Radiology 1993;187:71–73.
12. Donegan WL. Diagnosis. In Donegan Wl, Spratt JS (eds) Cancer of the Breast. Philadelphia: Saunders, 1995;158–162.
13. Tabár L, Dean PB, Péntek Z. Galactography: the diagnosic procedure of choice for nipple discharge. Radiology 1983;149:31–38.
14. Love SM, Schnitt SJ, Connolly JL, Shirley RL. Benign breast diseases. In Harris JR, Hellman S, Henderson IC, Kinne DW (eds) Breast Diseases. Philadelphia: Lippincott, 1987;22.
15. Threatt B. Ductography. In Bassett LW, Gold RH (eds) Breast Cancer Detection: Mammography and Other Methods in Breast Imaging, 2nd ed. Orlando: Grune & Stratton, 1987;119–129.
16. Jones MK. Galactography: procedure of choice for evaluation of nipple discharge. Semin Interv Radiol 1992;9:112–119.
17. Leis HP, Cammarata A, LaRaja RD. Nipple discharge: significance and treatment. Breast 1985;11:6–12.
18. Haagenson CD. Diseases of the Breast. Philadelphia: Saunders, 1971;276–291.
19. Cardenosa G, Doudna C, Eklund GW. Ductography of the breast: technique and findings. AJR 1994;162:1081–1087.
20. Ciatto S, Bravetti P, Berni D, et al. The role of galactography in the detection of breast cancer. Tumori 1988;74:177–181.
21. Fajardo JJ, Jackson VP, Hunter TB. Interventional procedures in diseases of the breast: needle biopsy, pneumocystography, and galactography. AJR 1992;158:1231–1238.
22. Jackson VP. Galactography. In Bassett LW, Jackson VP (eds) Diagnosis of Diseases of the Breast. Philadelphia: Saunders, 1997;283–289.
23. Berna JD, Guirao J, Garcia V. A coaxial technique for performing galactography. AJR 1989;153:273–274.
24. Hou MF, Huang TJ, Huang YS, et al. A simple method of duct cannulation and localization for galactography before excision in patients with nipple discharge. Radiology 1995;195:568–569.

CHAPTER 2

Needle Localization for Surgical Procedures

Liane E. Philpotts

Needle localization and open surgical biopsy has for years been the gold standard for diagnosis of nonpalpable lesions of the breast. Needle localization was first described in 1965.[1] Early localization procedures were performed with a freehand method, which involved estimating the lesion location from measurements made from the films.[2–6] The needle was inserted while the breast was held manually. For increased accuracy, mammographic-guided needle localization was then developed, whereby the needle was inserted under guidance from mammographic images obtained while the breast was maintained in compression.[7] This had the advantage of improving the proximity of the needle to the lesion and resulted in needle insertions that were always parallel to the chest wall. Further developments resulted in needle localizations performed by sonographic guidance as well.[8] Needle localizations performed by these methods have for many years proved to be safe and highly accurate for the diagnosis of nonpalpable breast lesions.

With the introduction of core biopsy in the management of lesions found by imaging, the role of needle localization and open surgical biopsy has changed.[9] While not used solely for the diagnosis of all imaging-detected breast lesions, needle localization with open surgical biopsy is often now reserved for removal of core biopsy-proven malignant or other suspicious lesions and for patients in whom surgical biopsy is preferred over core biopsy. While the spectrum of lesions and indications for needle localization have evolved, this procedure remains an integral part of the diagnosis and treatment of imaging-detected breast lesions.

INDICATIONS FOR NEEDLE LOCALIZATION

Needle localization prior to surgery is generally indicated for lesions that are nonpalpable and visualized by imaging, either sonographically or mammographically. It is necessary for lesions that require removal for either diagnostic or therapeutic reasons. Sometimes palpable lesions will require localization if the clinical findings are vague or if there is uncertainty whether the palpable finding corresponds to an imaging abnormality. For diagnostic biopsy, accurate needle localization allows sampling of an abnormality with a minimum of surrounding tissue. For lesions already known to be malignant, accurate localization facilitates complete removal of the cancer with clear margins.

For facilities where core biopsy is not available, needle localization and open surgical biopsy will be used for diagnosis of all nonpalpable suspicious lesions found by imaging. In many facilities, however, diagnosis of imaging-detected lesions will be achieved primarily with core biopsy. The role for needle localization and open surgical biopsy is for those lesions that are proven to be malignant or those that require excision for complete diagnosis. Histologic diagnoses of atypia, radial scars, and lobular carcinoma in situ found on core biopsy are examples of histologic entities for which surgical removal is often performed.[10,11] In addition, cases of imaging–histologic discordance or insufficient sampling with core biopsy may also require excision.[12]

Besides needle localization and open surgical biopsy subsequent to core biopsy, other indications are for pa-

31

tients in whom a single surgical procedure may be therapeutic. Small lesions suspicious of ductal carcinoma in situ (DCIS) or small invasive carcinomas in patients in whom axillary node sampling may not be necessary may be better suited to primary surgical excision.[13] This practice has been found to be effective as a single surgical procedure and can often be therapeutic with no further intervention necessary.

Needle localization and open surgical biopsy are also indicated for patients who are not able to successfully undergo core biopsy. Stereotactic biopsy with a prone table has limitations in terms of patient tolerance and lesion location. Ultrasound-guided core biopsy is limited by lesion visibility. Most calcifications and some mass lesions may not be sonographically detected. Other cases that may be better suited to needle localization and open surgical biopsy are lesions presenting as architectural distortion. As these lesions may represent radial scars, surgical excision may be preferred.

With the utilization of core biopsy for the diagnosis of many imaging-detected lesions, the spectrum of lesions for which needle localization and open surgical biopsy are performed has changed. This shift has led to a change in the positive predictive rate for needle localization procedures. With appropriate selection of cases for core biopsy, the positive predictive rate (i.e., the percentage of cases resulting in a diagnosis of malignancy) for needle localization procedures has been shown to double.[9] Rates as high as 55% have been reported. However, the positive predictive rate for needle localization depends not only on the utilization of core biopsy, but also on the sizes and stages of the cancers detected. Audits of individual practices should include assessment of these factors.

EQUIPMENT USED FOR LOCALIZATION

Needle localization procedures can be performed with equipment found in all breast-imaging departments. Mammographically guided needle localization can be performed on standard mammography units. A fenestrated compression paddle to accommodate insertion of the needle is necessary. Sonographic-guided localizations are optimally performed with a linear, high resolution, handheld transducer, 7.5 MHz or higher.

Film Versus Digital Imaging

Imaging can be performed with film or digital systems. While film has been used for many years, digital systems are now being used more commonly. Digital spot mammography (DSM) has the advantage of allowing more rapid acquisition of images (in seconds rather than minutes) with less radiation dose, resulting in completion of the needle localization procedure in approximately half the time of using film.[14] This results in less discomfort

for the patient and less chance of vasovagal reactions; it also increases the number of procedures potentially performed in a given time.

There are differences in performing needle localization with digital spot systems compared with film. Digital spot images show only a relatively small portion of the breast, 5×5 cm, while film images allow visualiza-

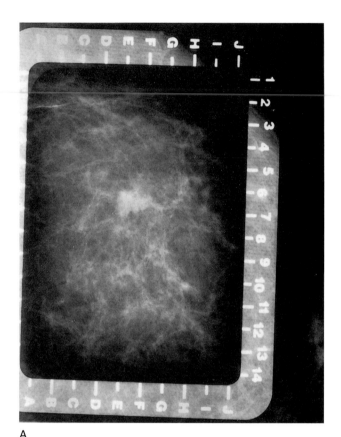

A

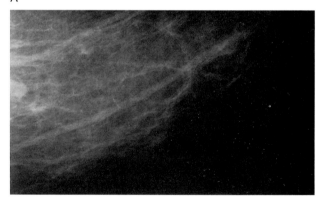

B

FIGURE 2.1. (A) A film-screen image obtained for needle localization shows a lesion located within the fenestrated paddle. The remainder of the breast outside the paddle can also be visualized. This aids in localizing the lesion with respect to other landmarks in the breast. (B) A digital image for needle localization shows a spiculated mass within the 5×5 cm opening of the paddle. Only that portion of the breast within the imaging window can be visualized.

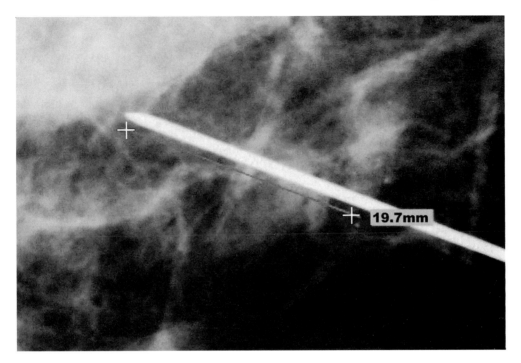

FIGURE 2.2. A digital image shows an ill-defined mass located approximately 2 cm from the tip of the needle. Digital tools such as calipers can determine the exact location of a lesion from the distal tip of the needle prior to wire deployment.

tion of a larger area of the breast, facilitating lesion detection with respect to adjacent landmarks (Figure 2.1). With the increased speed of image acquisition with DSM, additional imaging to localize the abnormality can be performed easily. Despite the ease of obtaining digital images, however, it has been shown that the number of images obtained by needle localizations performed with digital imaging was actually similar to that obtained with conventional film.[14] Other differences are the amount of magnification inherent in the images. Digital images have greater magnification, making the relation of the needle or wire to the lesion more intuitively difficult to determine. Software available for digital systems include tools, such as calipers and rulers, which allow accurate measurement of the needle in relation to the lesion (Figure 2.2).

Wire Localization

Needle localization is most commonly performed with a needle and wire system. There are two needle/wire systems commonly in use. Both require accurate placement of a needle in the breast, after which either a hook-wire or a retractable curved-end, or J-wire is inserted.[15–19] The hook-wire system involves withdrawing the needle, resulting in release of the hook to anchor the wire in the breast. In contrast, the localizing needle can remain in place in the breast with the J-wire (Figure 2.3). There are advantages and disadvantages to both methods.

The hook-wire system has the advantages of being a relatively stable marker that provides a tactile guide to the surgeon to indicate lesion location. The wire has a thickened segment near the distal end of the wire that can be detected during surgical dissection. A lesion located at the thickened portion of the wire is optimally localized

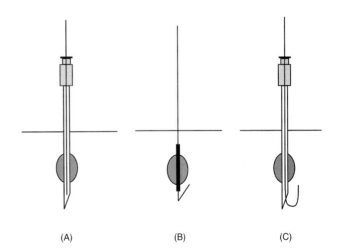

(A)   (B)   (C)

FIGURE 2.3. (**A**) Accurate placement of a needle with respect to a lesion is required before deployment of a wire. (**B**) For hook-wire systems, the needle is withdrawn over the wire, resulting in engagement of the wire. (**C**) For retractable, J-wire systems, the wire is deployed through the needle, which can remain in place with the wire. The distal end of the wire forms a J shape to anchor the system in place.

for surgical removal. The hook, or barb, prevents movement out of the breast. However, the hook of the wire, if improperly placed or pushed into the breast, can be displaced away from the targeted area. The hook permits one-way, forward movement, a ratchet-like effect. Also, the hookwire is thin, and care must be taken intraoperatively to avoid surgical transection. The retractable J-wire that remains with the needle in place in the breast has the advantage of providing a stiffer guide for surgical dissection, which can be performed from remote incision sites. After deployment, the retractable wire can be withdrawn into the needle, if repositioning is necessary. The disadvantage is that this system does not have a more precise localizing feature, such as the thickened area of the hook-wire, to identify the exact lesion location. The choice of needle localizing system is largely a matter of surgeon preference, as both have been shown to be effective in localizing breast lesions.

Needles used for localization are 20 gauge. There are several lengths of needle/wire combinations available. The hookwire system is available in 5 cm and 9 cm needle sizes with corresponding 15 cm and 25 cm wires. A monofilament hook-wire and a braided hook-wire are available. The retractable, J-shaped needle/wire system comes in four sizes (3, 5, 7, and 9 cm), with corresponding wires. The choice of needle size depends on the depth of the lesion and the size of the breast. The majority of lesions can be localized with a 5 cm needle. For very deep lesions or large breasts, or if the exact location of a lesion in one view is not known with certainty, a larger needle can be chosen. It is preferable to use a longer needle than a short one if there is any doubt, as needle position deep to a lesion is preferable to one that is too short. To determine adequate needle length, the skin-to-lesion distance in the view orthogonal to the one used for insertion of the needle should be measured. This represents the maximum skin-to-lesion distance that may be required.

TECHNIQUE OF NEEDLE LOCALIZATION

Review of all imaging studies prior to the time of needle localization is recommended. This is particularly important for patients who have had films at another facility. If adequate mammographic or sonographic studies have not been obtained, the patient should be scheduled to have such a workup, preferably before the day of the needle localization procedure. In some cases such a review or workup will negate the need for surgery, and needle localization can be canceled.[20] Recognizing skin calcifications or diagnosing a mass as a cyst are examples of cases for which biopsy would not be necessary. Furthermore, the approach to localization (i.e., mammographic or sonographic guidance) can be decided on and properly scheduled. This practice decreases the chance of cancellation on the day of the procedure, resulting in less anxiety for

the patient and better use of breast imaging department facilities.

Informed consent is not routinely obtained by the physician performing the needle localization. A survey of practicing radiologists determined that fewer than half obtained informed consent from the patient before proceeding with the localization.[21] Many times, consent is obtained by the surgeon and is inclusive of the localization and surgical procedures. Regardless of whether written or verbal consent is obtained, the procedure should be clearly explained to the patient before beginning.

Mammographic-Guided Needle Localization

The approach chosen for needle insertion is generally the shortest from the skin surface to the lesion. This minimizes the distance the needle must travel in the breast, decreasing the chance for deviation of the needle from the target. Generally, approaches are from either the medial or lateral or the superior or inferior direction, but any approach is possible. In some cases, the approach with the shortest distance may not be chosen. Lesions in the inferior aspect of the breast are sometimes more easily localized from either the medial or lateral side. Inferior approaches require somewhat uncomfortable positioning for the patient, having to straddle the mammography machine, which must be rotated 180°. It can also be awkward for the radiologist performing the procedure, who must insert the needle from below, often from a kneeling position. Other circumstances when the shortest approach may not be chosen include cases where the lesion is visualized more clearly in one projection or when reproducing the track from a preceding core biopsy. Concern over malignant seeding of the needle track during core biopsy has led some to recommend excision of the track, particularly in cases of mucinous carcinomas.[22]

Needle localization is generally performed with the patient in the sitting position. A chair that can be reclined is beneficial for expeditious treatment of vasovagal reactions. After deciding on the approach to be used, the patient's breast is placed under firm, but tolerable, compression with a fenestrated paddle to allow insertion of the needle (Figure 2.4). Most mammography units have a

FIGURE 2.4. (A) Mediolateral oblique and (B) craniocaudal views (arrows) demonstrate a new, 8 mm lobulated mass in the upper outer quadrant of the left breast of a 95-year-old woman. Because of the small size of the lesion and advanced age of the patient, surgical excision was chosen instead of core biopsy. (C) A superior approach was elected, and the breast was compressed in the craniocaudal direction. An image was obtained that shows the lesion within the opening of the compression paddle. (D) The alphanumeric coordinates on the fenestrated paddle allow positioning of crosshairs to mark the site of needle insertion.

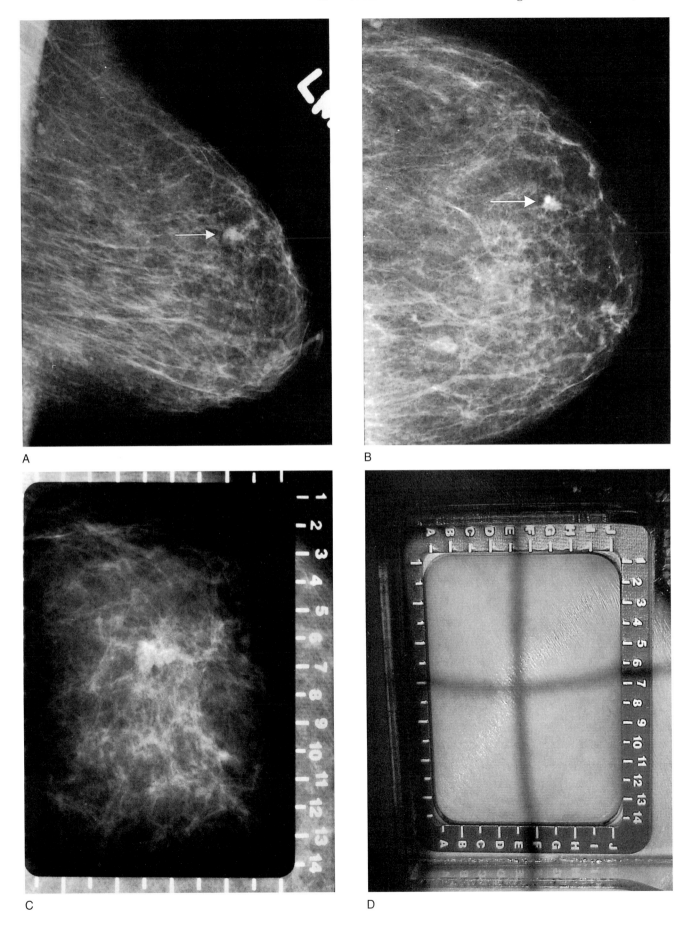

A

B

C

D

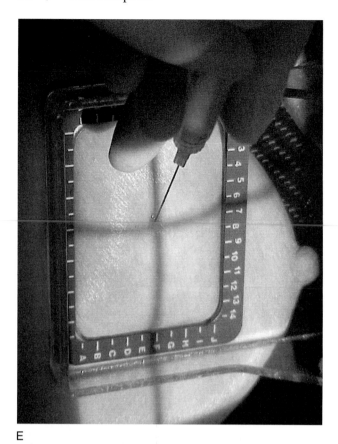

E

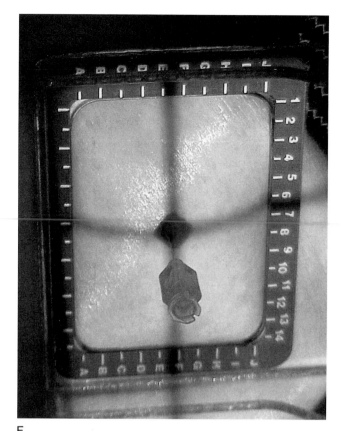

F

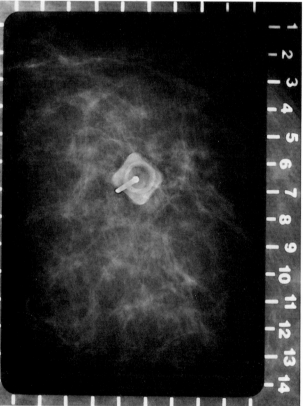

G

FIGURE 2.4. (E) After sterile preparation of the skin with Betadine and alcohol, local anesthetic was administered with a 25-gauge needle as a skin wheal. **(F)** The localizing needle was then inserted with the shadow of the hub superimposed over the junction of the crosshairs. **(G)** The image obtained shows that the hub of the needle obscures the small mass, indicating that the needle is in good position.

needle localization paddle that has an alphanumeric grid around the opening to indicate the site of needle insertion.

With the abnormality located within the opening of the paddle, the coordinates of the lesion can be determined from the alphanumeric grid, and the skin entry site is indicated by the two crossbars. This represents the x- and y-axis coordinates of the lesion. The skin is prepped with Betadine and alcohol. Local anesthetic, consisting of 9 parts lidocaine (lidocaine hydrochloride 1% solution) and 1 part sodium bicarbonate, can be injected intradermally. Addition of a small amount of sodium bicarbonate to the lidocaine alters the pH, lessening the burning sensation experienced by the patient. Administration of too much local anesthetic can obscure a mammographic abnormality. While local anesthetic does not significantly change the amount of discomfort experienced by the patient, many physicians and patients prefer it.[23]

The needle should be inserted in a single, steady motion, with the hub of the needle superimposed over the crossbars of the grid. The divergence of the light beam on the mammography unit is similar to that of the x-ray beam, so the shadow of the hub of the needle should lie directly over the skin entry site for the needle to traverse the lesion as determined from the initial image. Holding the needle hub delicately on alternate sides with the thumb and index finger allows visualization of the shadow of the hub. The hand otherwise obscures the shadow of the needle hub, which may result in incorrect positioning of the needle in the breast.

The length of needle to be inserted can only be roughly gauged from the mammographic images and the thickness of the compressed breast. Generally, the needle should be inserted as far as possible without penetrating the opposite skin surface. Needle depth will change upon release of compression and recompression in the orthogonal direction. A needle tip position deep to a lesion is preferable to one that is short of the target.

An image is obtained with the needle at its final position. The needle should be visualized in the short axis superimposed on the lesion. If the needle is not in such a position, it should be withdrawn and reinserted. Generally, the needle should be superimposed, adjacent to, or within 5 mm of a lesion. A space between the needle/wire and the lesion that is greater than 1 cm has a greater chance of failure to remove the abnormality surgically, or it may require that larger amounts of tissue be resected surgically.[24,25]

After satisfactory positioning of the needle, the breast can be released from compression to obtain an image in the orthogonal projection. During release of compression, mild pressure should be exerted on the needle to prevent the needle tip from withdrawing from the lesion in the breast. The distal tip of the needle should stay immobilized within the breast while the skin climbs outward toward the hub of the needle. If this does not happen, the needle tip could end up short of the desired point (Figure 2.5).

The orthogonal image is preferably performed with a small spot compression paddle centered over the estimated course of the needle within the breast (Figure 2.6). This allows greater access to the hub of the needle for exchange of the wire than a larger compression paddle. The orthogonal view is performed to check the relation of the needle to the lesion along the z-axis. Ideally, for hook-wire systems, the needle should extend 1–2 cm beyond the epicenter of the lesion. Exchange of the wire and removal of the needle at this point results in positioning the lesion at the thick portion of the wire. The barb, or hook, of the wire measures 1 cm and the thick portion 2 cm. Lesion location anywhere along the thick or barbed portions is acceptable. Lesion location proximal to this point, however, is problematic, as the surgeon has no tactile landmark and may dissect beyond the lesion. If the needle tip extends more than 3 cm beyond the lesion, the needle can be withdrawn the necessary amount. Centimeter markings on the needle facilitate withdrawal of the correct amount of needle length.

If the needle tip is short of a lesion, it is best to return to the original projection in which the needle was inserted and obtain another image. If the needle is aligned with the lesion, it can be advanced. If not, it should removed and reinserted. Advancing a needle that is short of its target while in the orthogonal projection can lead to an incorrect position in relation to the lesion in the x- or y-axis, as the needle and lesion are no longer in the same plane.

For the retractable, curved J-wire system, the wire is inserted into the needle. The wire has a memory and thus forms a curve, or J shape, when extended outside the needle. If repositioning is necessary, the wire may be re-

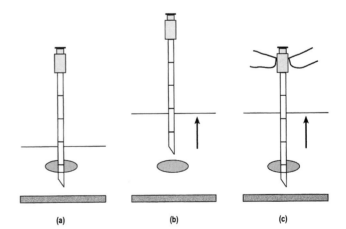

FIGURE 2.5. (A) A needle is placed into a lesion while the breast is in compression. **(B)** If the hub of the needle is not held firmly while compression is released, the needle tip may withdraw from the lesion within the breast. **(C)** If gentle pressure is exerted on the needle, release of compression should result in the distal end of the needle remaining in appropriate relation to the lesion while the skin moves toward the hub of the needle.

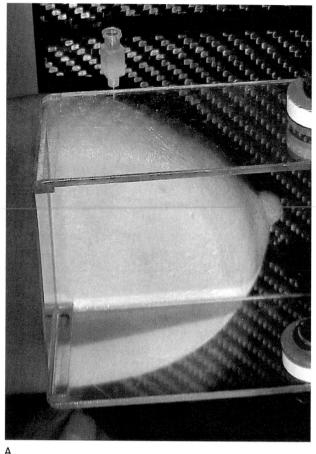

A

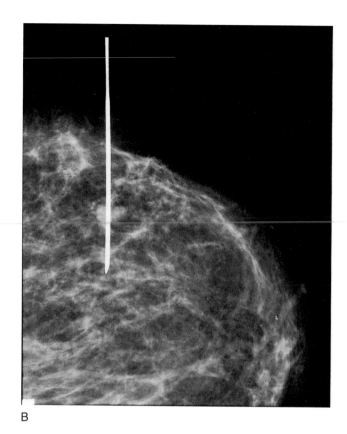

B

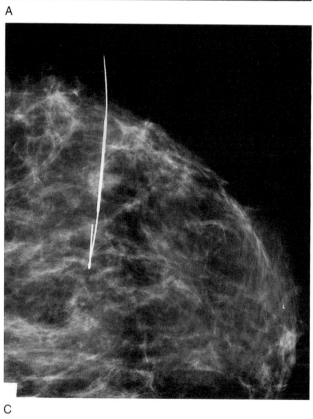

C

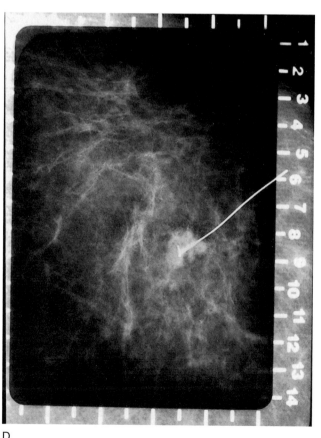

D

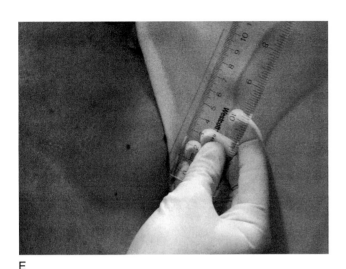

E

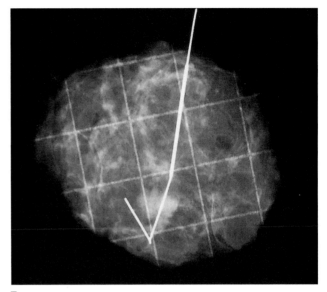

F

FIGURE 2.6. This is a continuation of the case shown in Figure 2.4. (**A**) After insertion of a needle in the craniocaudal projection, the breast was compressed in the orthogonal projection with a smaller, nonfenestrated compression paddle. (**B**) The lateral image shows the needle extending through and beyond the lesion. (**C**) After insertion of the wire and removal of the needle, the mass is appropriately positioned at the thickened segment of the wire. (**D**) Recompression in the craniocaudal projection with the wire protruding through the opening of the fenestrated paddle shows the wire in short axis superimposed on the lesion. (**E**) After the final images with the wire are obtained and the breast is released from compression, the length of wire extending outside of the breast is measured. (**F**) The specimen radiograph documents the presence of the mass in the surgical specimen. The distal portion of the hook-wire is also present. A benign papilloma was diagnosed at histology.

tracted into the needle, the needle position corrected, and the wire replaced. To exchange the needle for the wire in hook-wire systems, the wire is inserted into the hollow needle to the point where a burnished mark on the wire reaches the hub of the needle. A slight resistance can usually be felt when this point is reached. At this stage, the end of the wire extending out of the needle is held securely while the needle is pulled over the wire and out of the breast. This action results in deployment of the barb of the wire at the site of the tip of the needle, anchoring the wire in place. If a forward force is applied to the wire during exchange, the thin, flexible wire can extend deep into the breast beyond the lesion. In fatty breasts this can end up in a location remote from the lesion.

After placement of the needle/wire, images should be obtained to demonstrate the relation of the needle/wire to the lesion for the surgeon. These should be either two orthogonal views or one view in the projection parallel to the wire. The orthogonal images determine whether the lesion is traversed by the wire or is superior, inferior, medial, or lateral to it. To obtain an image perpendicular to the wire, an open paddle must be utilized that allows the wire extending out of the breast to be free. While some believe that it is not advisable to compress the breast with the wire in place in this direction for fear of displacing of the wire, it can be performed without significant prob-

lem or wire movement if desired. After the final images are obtained, the length of the wire extending outside the breast should be measured. Repeat measurement in the operating room will determine whether there has been significant wire movement. The wire extending outside of the breast should be covered by gauze, which is lightly taped to the skin. The wire should not be tightly affixed, as some mobility with patient motion is desirable, to prevent displacement of the wire tip inside the breast.

The images should be printed on hard copy and the lesion and wire clearly marked. In addition, either verbal or written comments should be conveyed to the surgeon as to the length of wire used, the length of wire extending outside of the breast, and the relation of the lesion to the wire, particularly to the thick portion or barb. Communication is an essential component to successful needle localization procedures. The patient is given her films and released from the department to the operating room.

Special Techniques for Needle/Wire Localization

Occasionally two or more needles/wires will be required to localize multiple lesions or to bracket a large area in an attempt to completely excise a suspicious lesion (Figures 2.7 and 2.8). When more than one needle is to be used, careful planning of the approach is necessary. When

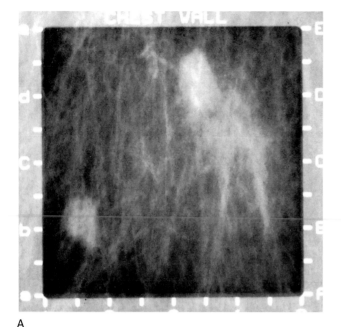

A

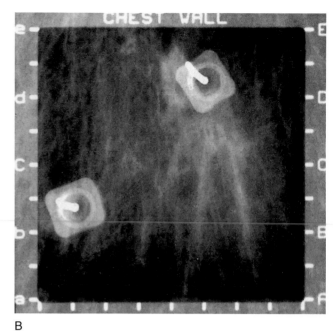

B

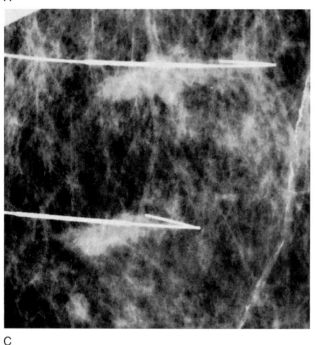

C

FIGURE 2.7. Patient with two masses that were both previously diagnosed as invasive ductal carcinoma by core biopsy required needle localization for surgery. (**A**) Both masses were positioned within the opening of the fenestrated paddle. (**B**) Two needles were inserted in the same direction from the lateral projection. (**C**) The orthogonal, craniocaudal image after deployment of both wires shows the masses appropriately positioned along the thickened segments of the wires.

feasible, the needles should be inserted in the same direction and both within the fenestration of the paddle. When different directions of insertion are necessary or if both needles cannot be included together, needles must be inserted sequentially. Attention to avoiding displacement of already engaged wire(s) is necessary.

When very faint calcifications require excision, needle localization can be performed with magnification technique. While the technique is similar to standard localizations, estimations of distances are not as direct. The distance of the needle to the lesion will appear amplified on the images. This must be taken into account when deploying the wire and relayed to the surgeon, who may not appreciate the different imaging technique. Other differences with using magnification technique include positioning of the patient, who must straddle the mammography unit to accommodate the geometric magnification device.

While freehand insertions of needles are not frequently used for routine localizations, unusual circumstances may necessitate their use. A freehand technique for needle localization after stereotactic biopsy in which the mammo-

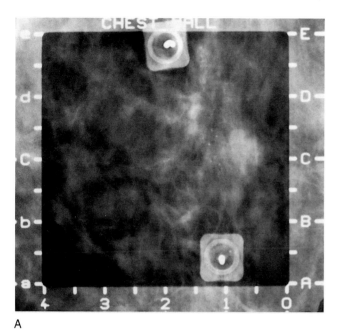

A

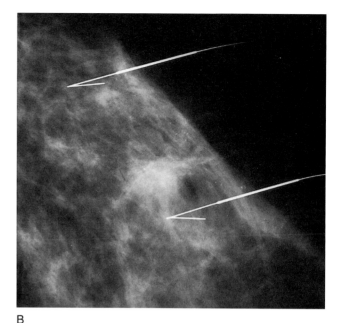

B

FIGURE 2.8. Needle localization was performed of a linear area of calcifications previously diagnosed as ductal carcinoma in situ by core biopsy. (A) To attempt to achieve complete excision of the tumor, the area of calcifications was bracketed by placing needles at either end of the lesion. (B) The area of calcifications is noted extending between the thickened segments of the two wires. (C) The specimen radiograph demonstrates the calcifications within the excised tissue. Only one hook-wire was included with the surgical specimen.

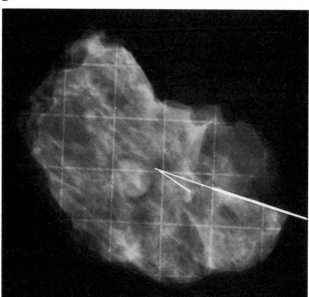

C

graphic lesion has been entirely removed has been described.[26] Using mammographic landmarks, such as the parenchymal pattern, calcifications, and vessels, the needle can be inserted and the area successfully removed.

Some surgeons may prefer a more anterior approach for dissection, and thus needle placement. This is particularly important for lesions in the superior aspect of the breast, where a greater thickness of tissue may have to be traversed to reach a lesion. By rolling the breast in an anteroposterior (AP) direction, with the nipple rolled superiorly before compression, the needle will ultimately assume a more AP course in the breast when released, and thus have a shorter skin-to-lesion distance (Figure 2.9).

Needle localization can be performed under stereotactic guidance. This method may be preferred for lesions seen predominantly in one mammographic view. With adequate workup this is an unusual occurrence, however, as most true lesions can be identified on two orthogonal views. Stereotactic needle localization is approached from the direction in which the lesion is best identified. The x, y, and z coordinates are determined in a similar method to core biopsy by identifying the epicenter of the lesion on the two stereotactic images. The localizing needle is then inserted to approximately 1 cm beyond the $z = 0$ point. For standard mammographic needle localizations the wire is deployed while the breast is com-

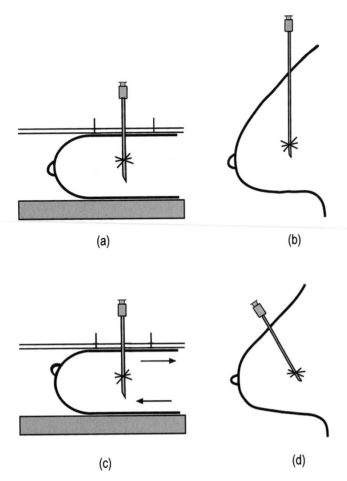

(a)   (b)

(c)   (d)

FIGURE 2.9. (A, B) For a centrally located lesion, insertion of the needle perpendicular to the chest wall with the breast compressed in the craniocaudal projection may require the needle to traverse a large amount of breast tissue when the breast is released. (C, D) If the breast is rolled in an anteroposterior (AP) direction, with the nipple rolled superiorly before compression, the site of insertion of the needle will be at a more anterior skin surface. Upon release of compression, the breast will "unroll," and the needle will assume a more AP course in the breast. This results in a shorter skin-to-lesion distance.

pressed in the orthogonal direction to insertion. For stereotactic localization, particularly with hook-wires, if the wire is inserted while the breast is still in compression, the wire may hook onto tissue deep to the lesion in the z-direction. Release of compression will result in pulling in of the wire deep to the targeted area (the "accordion effect"). It is preferable, thus, to gently release the breast from compression and then insert the wire. An alternative approach for stereotactic needle localization is use of a lateral arm attachment, available for prone stereotactic units. Because the needle is inserted in a direction opposite to the direction of compression, the inaccuracy in the z-direction found with standard stereotactic localization is avoided.

Ultrasound-Guided Needle Localization

Needle localizations can be performed quickly and accurately with US guidance. This method may be more comfortable than mammographically guided localization as the patient is positioned supine and the breast is not compressed. The only requirement is that the lesion be visible with ultrasound. Thus most calcification lesions and some mass lesions are not amenable to this technique.

With real-time imaging, the needle can be inserted adjacent to the transducer and into or just beyond the lesion in a relatively direct course from the skin surface (Figure 2.10). The needles used for needle localization can be difficult to perceive with ultrasound unless inserted parallel to the transducer face, which is usually not desired as it results in a larger skin to lesion distance. The wires can be even more difficult to visualize sonographically. However, most needles and wires can be visualized sufficiently with real-time imaging to allow confident placement of the needle in the desired location (Figure 2.11). Once the needle is in place, wire insertion is then performed, completing the procedure in less time than mammographically guided localizations. A mammogram can be obtained after ultrasound localization but is not essential, particularly in cases where the lesion is mammographically occult. Hard copy ultrasound and/or mammographic images should be sent with the patient to the operating room to demonstrate the relation of the wire to the lesion.

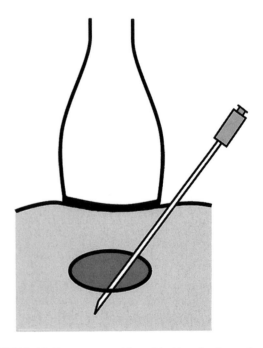

FIGURE 2.10. For sonographic-guided localizations, the needle can be inserted adjacent to the transducer, in either the short or long axis, toward and through the lesion. This results in a relatively direct course of the needle/wire from the skin to the lesion.

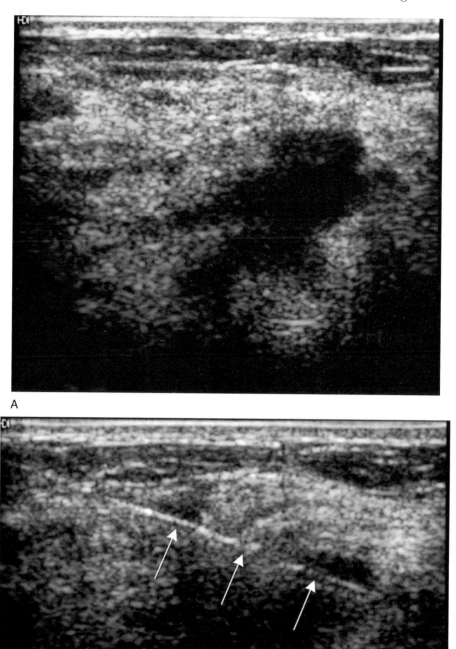

A

B

FIGURE 2.11. (A) An irregular, hypoechoic mass was found in the left breast of a 51-year-old woman. Core biopsy diagnosed a radial scar and fibrocystic changes. **(B)** Needle localization was performed with ultrasound guidance. The needle (arrows) can be seen traversing the lesion.

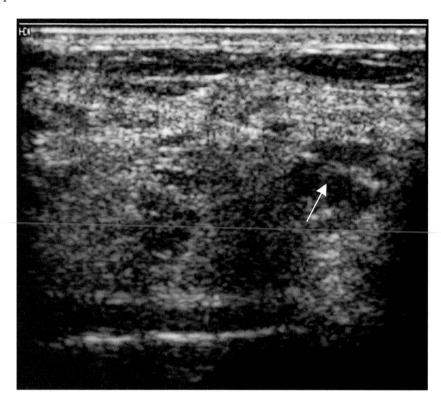

FIGURE 2.11. (C) After deployment of the wire and removal of the needle, the hook-wire can be seen in good position, with the barb of the hook (arrow) within the lesion. Histology of the surgical specimen showed benign fibrocystic changes with no evidence of malignancy.

Unlike mammographically guided localizations, the needle is often inserted in an anteroposterior direction rather than parallel to the chest wall. Care must be taken to visualize the needle tip at all times and not to advance the needle or wire too deeply, thereby risking penetrating the chest wall. This can lead to serious complications including pnemothorax or migration of the wire.

Other Methods of Localization

Very superficial lesions can be difficult to localize with a needle/wire system, as accurate localization results in very little of the wire being inside the breast and most protruding outside. In such cases, a marker such as a metallic BB can simply be placed on the skin surface directly over the lesion with mammographic or sonographic guidance. The surgeon can then remove the tissue from the subcutaneous region to a variable depth determined from the images.

Various dyes have been utilized as a method to localize an abnormality for surgery. This method still requires the accurate insertion of a needle to the lesion, after which the dye is injected and the needle is withdrawn. Radiographic contrast material can be added with the dye or air can be injected to document the site on the mammographic images. Dyes that have been utilized include methylene blue, isosulfan blue, Evans blue, toluidine blue, and isocyanide green. Success of dye localization depends on avoiding overinjection and minimizing the time between injection and surgery. Too large a volume of dye injected or too long a delay before surgery can result in diffusion of the dye in the breast and imprecise localization of the area to be excised. This can result in surgical misses or excision of an abnormally large specimen. Other disadvantages of this method include the possible interference of methylene blue in estrogen receptor analysis of the excised tissue.[27] Dye alone is rarely utilized today, but some may use it in combination with needle/wire localization.

Recently success with carbon marking for the purpose of localization of core biopsy sites has been reported.[28] Injection of an aqueous suspension of carbon at the termination of a core biopsy is an alternative to metallic clips or other devices to mark the site of biopsy. Localization of a biopsy site is particularly important for small malignant lesions that may have been completely removed by the core biopsy procedure. The technique for carbon marking involves insertion of an 18-gauge needle through the needle track after 14- or 11-gauge stereotactic biopsy. Less than 0.3 ml of 4% weight/weight aqueous suspension of activated charcoal powder is injected along the entire needle track to the point of skin entry. The advantage of this method is that it obviates the need

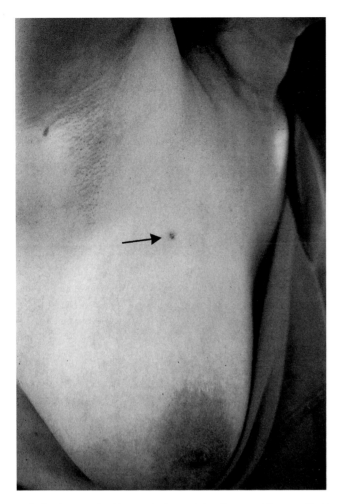

FIGURE 2.12. A skin mark (arrow) is observed in a patient who had previously undergone carbon marking during stereotactic core biopsy. Surgical dissection is performed by tracing the carbon trail to the distal end, which represents the site of biopsy. (From Mullen et al.,[28] with permission.)

for needle localization prior to surgery. Unlike dyes, carbon is permanent and does not diffuse with time. The carbon mark is seen as a tattoo on the skin surface (Figure 2.12). Surgical dissection is accomplished by dissecting the carbon trail to the distal end, which represents the site of the core biopsy. The disadvantage of carbon marking is that it leaves a permanent visible mark on the skin which may not be acceptable for some patients with benign results who do not require surgery.

DIFFICULT CASES

With the increasing use of core biopsy for initial diagnosis of many breast lesions, the case selection referred for needle localization has changed. Cases not amenable to core biopsy, such as extremely posterior lesions, will be referred for needle localization. Such cases can also prove to be challenging for needle localization.

Lesions that are in the posterior aspect of the breast, near the chest wall or axillary regions, can be difficult to localize. If lesions are visible by ultrasound, then sonographic localization should be the method of choice. If mammographic localization is necessary, then there are techniques that can be of aid in accomplishing the task. Use of a small spot compression paddle with a fenestrated window may allow imaging of more posterior tissue than a regular full compression paddle (Figure 2.13). A paddle with an eccentrically located window may also prove beneficial. Exaggerating the breast in the medial or lateral directions in the craniocaudal projection can allow access to posteriorly located lesions. A Cleopatra view may also help in approaching lesions in the axillary tail. Other techniques that have been described for lesions located posteriorly and superiorly on the chest wall include compression of only the superior portion of the breast, rather than the entire breast, with a small compression paddle.[29] The breast must be sufficiently thick to have success with this technique.

Needle localization of lesions seen in only one mammographic view can prove to be difficult. Several different approaches for successful needle localization in these cases have been proposed. Adequate imaging workup with mammography, ultrasound, and even MRI will usually clarify the three-dimensional location of a lesion in the breast. On the rare occasion that a suspicious lesion is seen predominantly in one mammographic projection only, nonstandard localization methods may be necessary. The simplest technique to use, if possible, is to perform localization with the mammographic views in which the lesion can be identified. The projection in which the lesion is best identified, as well as an angled projection less than the usual 90°, can be used to achieve fairly accurate localization. Other proposed methods include slight angulation of the needle in the breast in the same projection as insertion, with calculation of the geometric foreshortening effect of the needle, to determine the location of the lesion along the shaft of the needle.[30] Orthogonal oblique views, nonstandard mammographic images, have also been suggested.[31] Currently, the easiest method for needle localization of lesions seen in only one view is probably stereotactic localization, as described above.

Needle localization of lesions in patients who have undergone augmentation mammoplasty with prosthetic implants is achieved similarly to that in patients with unaugmented breasts. Mammographic-guided localization parallel to the chest wall with posterior displacement of the implant should allow accurate needle placement with avoidance of the implant. If the lesion is located in close proximity to the implant, then needle placement adjacent to rather than within the lesion is acceptable (Figure 2.14). Alternatively, sonographic localization could be performed as real-time visualization of the needle allows avoidance of the implant. Needle insertion parallel to the implant is

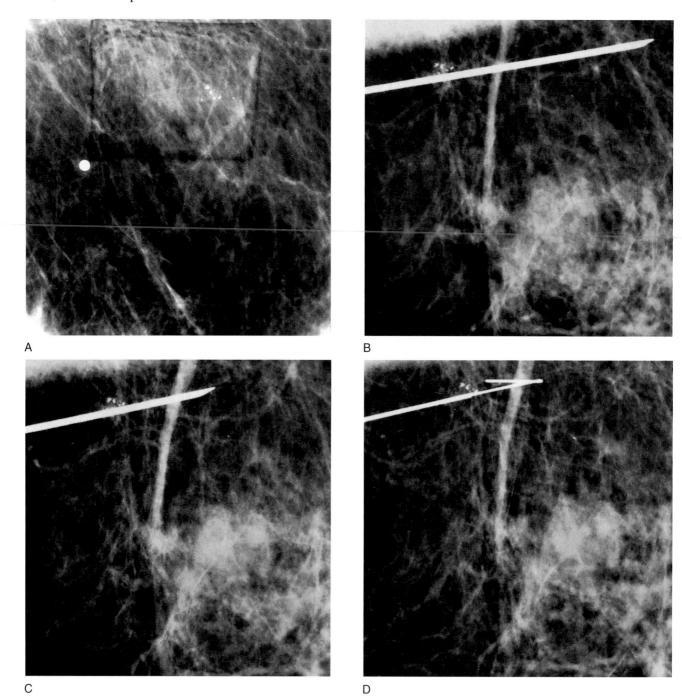

A

B

C

D

FIGURE 2.13. Needle localization was recommended for a new cluster of pleomorphic calcifications located in the far posterior aspect of the right breast of a 78-year-old woman. (**A**) A small fenestrated compression paddle was used to image the posteriorly located lesion. A BB is placed in one corner of the opening to facilitate orientation of the digital image. (**B**) After needle insertion, the orthogonal image shows the needle positioned parallel to the pectoralis muscle and extending beyond the lesion. (**C**) The needle is withdrawn to the appropriate position. (**D**) After deployment of the wire, the calcifications are noted at the hook segment of the wire. Successful surgical excision resulted in a diagnosis of calcifications associated with fibrocystic changes.

advisable, however, as more direct insertion adjacent to the transducer will result in the needle being directed toward the implant. Despite careful needle positioning, rupture of an implant is still possible, and the patient should be informed of this risk before beginning the procedure.

Occasionally, during needle localization, it will become apparent that abnormalities seen on the mammographic images are not the same lesion or not a true lesion at all. If multiple lesions are present, accurate identification of the same lesion in all projections can be

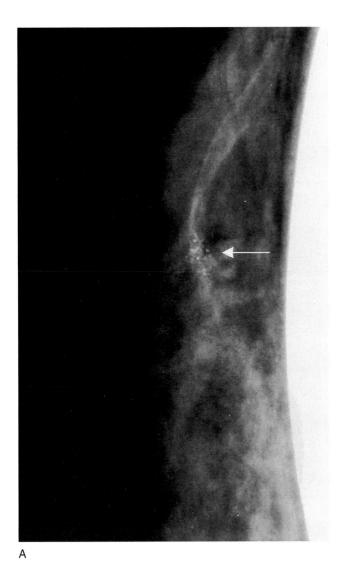

A

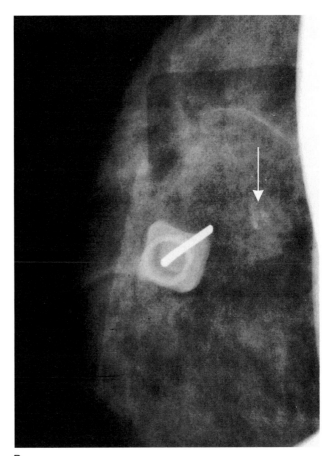

B

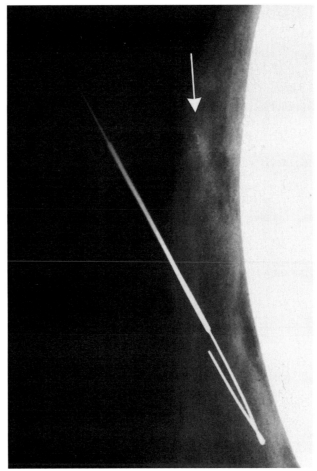

C

FIGURE 2.14. (**A**) A new cluster of amorphous calcifications (arrow) was noted in a 50-year-old patient with silicone implants. (**B**) Needle localization was performed by inserting the needle just anterior to the lesion to avoid rupturing the implant. (**C**) A magnified image shows the calcifications posterior to the proximal thickened segment of the wire. The calcifications were successfully removed without damage to the implant. The histology was benign.

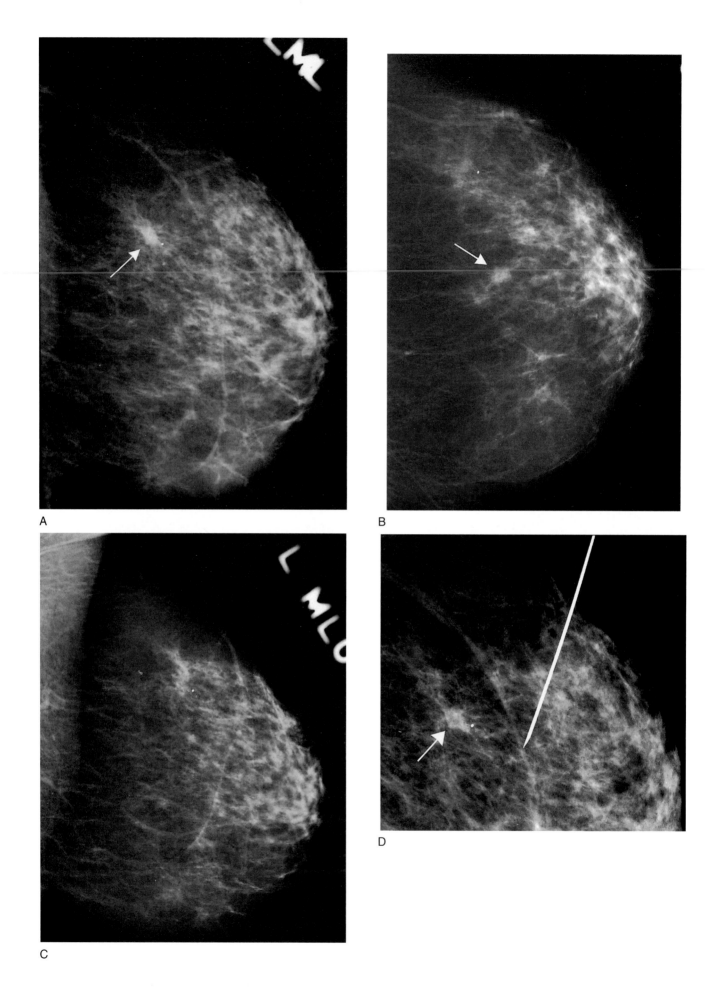

A

B

C

D

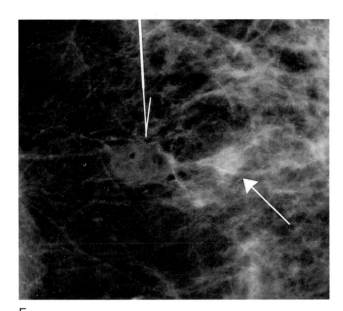

E

FIGURE 2.15. Needle localization was recommended for a "lesion" in the left breast of a 51-year-old woman. (**A**) Mediolateral and (**B**) craniocaudal images show the area of concern (arrows). (**C**) Of note is that no corresponding abnormality was identified in the mediolateral oblique view. (**D**) When the needle was first inserted in the craniocaudal direction, the orthogonal (lateral) image showed the needle located anterior to the density (arrow). (**E**) Subsequently, when the needle was inserted from the lateral direction, the orthogonal (craniocaudal) image showed the needle posterior to the lesion. This indicated that the two densities were not in the same plane and therefore were not the same "lesion." Surgery was canceled, and the wire was removed from the breast. Mammographic follow-up for 2 years has been unremarkable with no recurrent area of concern.

difficult. Also, despite adequate imaging workup, it is possible that abnormalities identified in different projections are not true lesions. When needle insertion in one projection results in the needle being positioned in a different plane from the "lesion" in the orthogonal projection, this possibility must be questioned (Figure 2.15). Failure to recognize this would lead to erroneous wire placement and unnecessary surgery.

Needle localization of lesions that have previously undergone core biopsy that resulted in complete removal of the imaging finding is a recent challenge to the breast imager. With the increasing use of vacuum-assisted devices that obtain large core specimens, complete removal of a lesion occurs in a substantial number of cases.[32,33] If no marking device, such as a clip, was deployed at the time of core biopsy, localization of the biopsy site can be difficult. In such cases, needle localization and surgery should be expedited to increase the chances of identifying the biopsy site by residual hematoma. Ultrasound may prove to be useful for some lesions that can no longer be visualized by mammography, such as those in dense

breasts. Sonography may identify a residual lesion, hematoma, or even needle track from the core biopsy that can facilitate needle placement (Figure 2.16). Also, a freehand approach for needle localization of lesions completely removed by core biopsy using landmarks in the breast has been performed.[26]

Needle localization with computed tomography (CT) guidance has been described.[34] The most common reason for CT guidance was the inability to image an abnormality on two orthogonal views. CT localization is used with the patient in the supine position. Scanning is used to localize the abnormality, after which thinner slices through the area can be obtained. A metallic marker can be placed on the skin above the lesion as a reference guide. The angle of insertion can be determined and the needle inserted. The needle position is verified with ad-

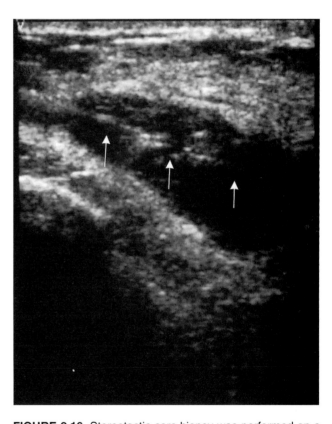

FIGURE 2.16. Stereotactic core biopsy was performed on a 2 mm cluster of calcifications in a 56-year-old woman. The patient refused to have a biopsy-marking clip placed at the time of biopsy. Histology revealed ductal carcinoma in situ necessitating surgery. As the parenchymal tissue was extremely dense, the biopsy site could not be identified at the time of surgery 1 week later. Ultrasound was utilized for needle localization by placing the needle (arrows) through the needle track, which was still visible due to hematoma. The wire was deployed at the distal end of the track. No residual carcinoma was found but the original biopsy site was confirmed. (From Philpotts LE. The potential complications and pitfalls of stereotactic biopsy. *MammoMatters*, Spring 2001;8:7–17, with permission.)

ditional images through the area, and the wire deployed. Needle localization with CT is more expensive than with mammography or ultrasound guidance, and the radiation dose is greater. CT localization is rarely utilized, as other techniques are usually favored.

COMPLICATIONS

Complications with needle localization procedures are uncommon. The procedure is extremely safe when performed correctly with well-established standard techniques. While serious complications are rare, minor complications can occasionally occur, and recognition and preparation for rapid treatment is necessary for all personnel involved.

Vasovagal reactions are the most common complication, reported in 7% of cases.[35] Actual syncope is less common, occurring in only 1%. While anxiety and pain contribute to this phenomenon, the fact that the patient is upright is a main factor; vasovagal reactions are extremely uncommon when the patient is supine. Because of the possibility of these types of reactions, the patient should never be left alone during the procedure. Distracting the patient with light conversation may avert some reactions. When vasovagal reactions occur, patients should be transferred to a recumbent or Trendelenburg position. Cold towels applied to the forehead can be beneficial. Other interventions are rarely necessary. These reactions, especially when recurrent, can severely disrupt and delay the needle localization procedure.

Other minor complications of needle localization include prolonged bleeding and pain.[35] Bleeding lasting 5 minutes or longer has been reported in 1% of cases. Severe pain has also been reported in 1%. These minor complications did not adversely affect the outcome of the procedures.

More serious complications of needle localization have been reported but are infrequent occurrences with the techniques currently utilized. Insertion of the needle or wire into the chest wall may result in pneumothorax. Placement of a hook-wire into the pectoralis muscle can result in migration to remote locations.[36–40] The likely mechanism for this is forward propelling of the wire with muscular contraction. Migration of the wire into the pleural cavity and cervical region by this mechanism has been reported. Techniques for needle insertions parallel to the chest wall can avert this serious complication. However, freehand techniques as well as ultrasound-guided localizations, in which needle insertion can be in an anteroposterior direction, risk this complication. Wire movement is also a risk in large, fatty breasts, resulting not only in inaccurate localization, but possible disappearance of the external portion of the wire into the breast. Wires have been found migrated within the breast, the axillary area, and even the buttocks. Surgeons should not use the wire as a retraction device during surgery, as the distal end can likewise be displaced from the targeted lesion. Using adequate length wires and attention to the external wire both pre- and intraoperatively can avoid such "lost wires." Another potential complication is transection of the wire intraoperatively, with resultant retraction of the distal portion into the breast.[36,41] This complication is a concern with hook-wires that can be cut with surgical scissors. Careful dissection with scalpels will avoid this complication.

Another possible complication with the hook-wire is intraoperative breakage of the wire. If the wire is pulled on, the deep portion can break, usually at the elbow of the barb, leaving the 1 cm barb of the wire in the breast. If unidentified, these wire fragments may be left in the breast. Studies have shown stability of such fragments over time, causing no serious symptoms or sequelae on subsequent mammography (Figure 2.17).[42]

An unusual occurrence after needle localization and surgical biopsy is the finding of metallic particles on subsequent mammograms.[43–45] The precise etiology of this phenomenon is unknown but may represent shavings produced during the needle and wire exchange or during surgery. Use of a braided hook-wire resulted in wire fragments in the breast after intraoperative cutting of the wire.[45] Awareness of this possibility is important, as the small metallic particles can simulate microcalcifications.

ACCURACY OF NEEDLE LOCALIZATION

With adequate prebiopsy imaging evaluation, proper localization technique, specimen radiography, and good communication between the radiologist and surgeon, needle localization is successful in the majority of cases. The failure rate for needle localization and open surgical biopsy has been reported to range from 0% to 17%, with a mean of 2.6%.[25] With modern techniques and equipment, failure rates of 1% to 3% should be possible.[25,46] The precise reasons for failed cases are difficult to ascertain from the literature. The possible reasons for misses include poor needle placement, movement of the needle/wire, and poor communication between the radiologist and surgeon.[25,47]

Some of the factors related to the success or failure of the needle localization and surgical biopsy procedures have been described.[25] The distance of the needle to the lesion has an important role. Actual penetration of the lesion by the needle, rather than close proximity, was required for statistical significance. The size of the lesion was also found to be important, with significantly more misses in small (<1 cm) lesions than in larger ones. The volume of the surgical specimen (>10 cm^3), not surprisingly, was also related to success. Interestingly, the number of lesions localized in the breast was found to be a factor, with more failures in patients with more than one lesion localized. The precise reason for this is unknown, but awareness of this possibility may avert failures. Lesions consisting of

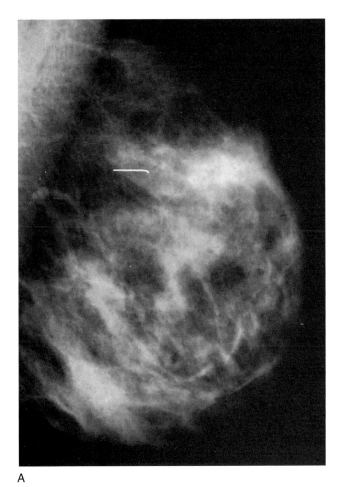
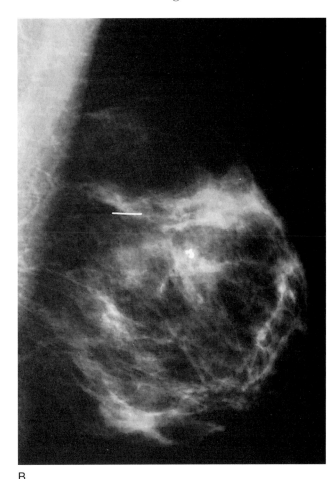

A

B

FIGURE 2.17. (**A**) Intraoperative breakage of a hook-wire occurred during biopsy of a lesion that proved to be benign. (**B**) Subsequent mammograms have showed no change in the location of the wire fragment over an interval of more than 13 years.

calcifications have also been suggested to have an increased chance of failure.[25] While intradermal calcifications likely represent some needle localization failures, the fact that some masses become palpable during surgery may also account for the difference in failure rates.

With specimen radiography, failure to excise the targeted lesion should be immediately recognized. If the procedure appears unsuccessful (e.g., specimen radiographs do not show the lesion to have been removed), the surgical procedure should be terminated and imaging should be repeated after the patient has sufficiently healed. If the lesion is shown to persist, repeat localization can be attempted. Specimen radiography will be discussed in detail in Chapter 9.

CONCLUSION

Needle localization with open surgical biopsy is an accurate, safe, and effective technique for diagnosis of lesions of the breast found by imaging. Current equipment and techniques of imaging and needle placement allow localization and excision of lesions with a low failure rate. Complications are very rare, and the procedure can be

successfully performed in most patients. As many cases of lesions detected by imaging are currently diagnosed by core biopsy, the case selection for needle localization has changed. Many cases will be more challenging because of lesion location, failure to successfully perform core biopsy, and lesion visualization secondary to removal by core biopsy. Thorough understanding of the techniques of needle localization will aid in successful completion of these difficult cases. Although the role of needle localization and open surgical biopsy is changing, as alternative techniques for diagnosis become available, it remains an integral part of breast imaging.

REFERENCES

1. Dodd GD, Greening RR, Wallace S. The radiologic diagnosis of cancer. *In* Nealon TF Jr (ed). Management of the Patient with Cancer. Philadelphia: Saunders, 1965;88.
2. Libshitz HI, Feig SA, Fetouh S. Needle localization of nonpalpable breast lesions. Radiology 1976;121:557–560.
3. Hall FM, Frank HA. Preoperative localization of nonpalpable breast lesions. AJR 1979;132:101–105.

4. Homer MJ. Localization of nonpalpable breast lesions: technical aspects and analysis of 80 cases. AJR 1983;140:807–811.

5. Gisvold JJ, Martin JK. Prebiopsy localization of nonpalpable breast lesions. AJR 1984;143:477–481.

6. Loh CK, Perlman H, Harris JH, et al. An improved method for localization of nonpalpable breast lesions. Radiology 1979; 130:244–245.

7. Kopans DB, Lindfors K, McCarthy KA, et al. Spring hook-wire breast lesion localizer: use with rigid-compression mammographic systems. Radiology 1985;157:537–538.

8. Kopans DB, Meyer JE, Lindfors KK, et al. Breast sonography to guide cyst aspiration and wire localization of occult solid lesions. AJR 1984;143:489–492.

9. Rubin E, Dempsey PJ, Pile NS, et al. Needle-localization biopsy of the breast: impact of a selective core needle biopsy program on yield. Radiology 1995;195:627–631.

10. Dershaw DD, Morris EA, Liberman L, et al. Nondiagnostic stereotaxic core breast biopsy: results of rebiopsy. Radiology 1996;198:323–325.

11. Philpotts LE, Shaheen NA, Carter D, et al. Comparison of rebiopsy rates after stereotactic core needle biopsy of the breast with 11–gauge vacuum suction probe versus 14–gauge needle and automatic gun. AJR 1998;172:683–687.

12. Liberman L. Clinical management issues in percutaneous core breast biopsy. Radiol Clin Noth Am 2000;38:791–807.

13. Gundry KR, Berg WA. Treatment issues and core needle breast biopsy: clinical context. AJR 1998;171:41–49.

14. Dershaw DD, Fleischman RC, Liberman L, et al. Use of digital mammography in needle localization procedures. AJR 1993;161:559–562.

15. Kopans DB, DeLuca SA. A modified needle hookwire technique to simplify preoperative localization of occult breast lesions. Radiology 1980;134:781.

16. Kopans DB, Meyer JE. Versatile spring hookwire breast lesion localizer. AJR 1982;138:586–587.

17. Homer MJ. Nonpalpable breast lesion localization using a curved-end retractable wire. Radiology 1985;157:259–260.

18. Homer MJ, Pile-Spellman ER. Needle localization of occult breast lesions with a curved-end retractable wire: technique and pitfalls. Radiology 1986;161:547–548.

19. Homer MJ. Localization of nonpalpable breast lesions with the curved-end retractable wire: leaving the needle in vivo. AJR 1988;151:919–920.

20. Meyer JE, Sonnenfeld MR, Greenes RS, et al. Cancellation of preoperative breast localization procedures: analysis of 53 cases. Radiology 1988;169:629–630.

21. Reynolds HE, Jackson VP, Musick BS. A survey of interventional mammography practices. Radiology 1993;187:71–73.

22. Reynolds HE, Jackson VP, Musick BS. Preoperative needle localization in the breast: utility of local anesthesia. Radiology 1993;187:503–505.

23. Harter LP, Curtis, JS, Ponto G, et al. Malignant seeding of the needle track during stereotaxic core needle breast biopsy. Radiology 1992;185:713–714.

24. Chatwick DR, Shorthouse AJ. Wire-localization biopsy of the breast: an audit of results and analysis of factors influencing therapeutic value in the treatment of breast cancer. Eur J Surg Oncol 1997;23:128–133.

25. Jackman RJ, Marzoni FA. Needle-localized breast biopsy: why do we fail? Radiology 1997;204:677–684.

26. Brenner RJ. Lesions entirely removed during stereotactic biopsy: preoperative localization on the basis of mammographic landmarks and feasibility of freehand technique—initial experience. Radiology 2000;214:585–590.

27. Hirsch JI, Banks WL, Sullivan JS, et al. Effect of methylene blue on estrogen receptor activity. Radiology 1989;171:105–107.

28. Mullen DJ, Eisen RN, Newman RD, et al. The use of carbon marking after stereotactic large-core-needle breast biopsy. Radiology 2001;218:255–260.

29. Sickles EA. Practical solutions to common mammographic problems: tailoring the examination. AJR 1988;151:31–39.

30. Kopans DB, Waitzkin ED, Linetsky L, et al. Localization of breast lesions identified on only one mammographic view. AJR 1987;149:39–41.

31. Vyborny CJ, Merrill TN, Geurkink RE. Difficult mammographic needle localization: use of alternate orthogonal projections. Radiology 1986;161:839–841.

32. Burbank F, Parker SH, Fogarty TJ. Stereotactic breast biopsy: improved tissue harvesting with the Mammotome. Am Surg 1996;62:738–744.

33. Liberman L, Zakowski MF, Avery S, et al. Complete percutaneous excision of infiltrating carcinoma at stereotactic breast biopsy: how can tumor size be assessed? AJR 1999;173:1315–1322.

34. Spillane RM, Whitman GJ, McCarthy KA, et al. Computed tomography-guided needle localization of nonpalpable breast lesions: review of 24 cases. Acad Radiol 1996;3:115–120.

35. Helvie MA, Ikeda DM, Adler DD. Localization and needle aspiration of breast lesions: complications in 370 cases. AJR 1991;157:711–714.

36. Bronstein AD, Kilcoyne RF, Moe RE. Complications of needle localization of foreign bodies and nonpalpable breast lesions. Arch Surg 1988;123:775–779.

37. Van Susante JL, Barendregt WB, Bruggink EDM. Migration of the guide-wire into the pleural cavity after needle localization of breast lesions. Eur J Surg Oncol 1998;24:446–448.

38. Bristol JB, Jones PA. Transgression of localization wire into the pleural cavity prior to mammography. Br J Radiol 1981;54: 139–140.

39. Owen AW, Kumar EN. Migration of localizing wires used in guided biopsy of the breast. Clin Radiol 1991;43:251.

40. Davis PS, Wechsler RJ, Feig A, et al. Migration of breast biopsy localization wire. AJR 1988;150:787–788.

41. Homer MJ. Transection of the localization hooked wire during breast biopsy. AJR 1983;929–930.

42. Montrey JS, Levy JA, Brenner RJ. Wire fragments after needle localization. AJR 1996;167:1267–1269.

43. Korbin CD, Denison CM, Lester S. Metallic particles on mammography after wire localization. AJR 1997;169:1637–1638.

44. Katz JF, Homer MJ, Graham RA, et al. Metallic fragments on mammography after intraoperative deployment of radiopaque clips. AJR 2000;175:1591–1593.

45. D'Orsi CJ, Swanson RS, Moss LJ, et al. A complication involving a braided hook-wire localization device. Radiology 1993;187:580–581.

46. Gallagher WJ, Cardenosa G, Rubens JR, et al. Minimal-volume excision of nonpalpable breast lesions. AJR 1989;153: 957–961.

47. Yankaskas BC, Knelson MH, Abernethy ML, et al. Needle localization biopsy of occult lesions of the breast: experience in 199 cases. Invest Radiol 1988;23:729–733.

CHAPTER 3

Patient Selection and Follow-Up for Biopsy

Ellen Shaw de Paredes

As the breast imager has evolved as a breast interventionalist, the clinical responsibility associated with breast imaging has increased. The radiologist not only performs the biopsy procedure but also is responsible for correctly selecting the best procedure for the patient preoperatively and for communicating the results afterwards. The breast interventionalist must understand the indications and techniques for performing procedures, the selection of the appropriate procedure for the patient, and the risks, contraindications, and limitations of each procedure.

Percutaneous breast biopsy developed in the late 1980s and 1990s to become a widely acceptable and utilized method for diagnosis of a nonpalpable breast lesion. The purpose of performing a percutaneous biopsy rather than an open or excisional biopsy is to obtain a diagnosis with a less invasive and less costly procedure. The roles of percutaneous breast biopsy are the following: (1) to confirm a benign diagnosis for lesions that are indeterminate by mammography and to avoid surgical biopsy of these lesions, and (2) to diagnose a highly suspicious lesion as malignant, thus avoiding a two-step surgical procedure for diagnosis and treatment. The technique is also utilized to sample palpable breast masses with or without imaging guidance.

Methods of guidance include, primarily, mammography with stereotactic guidance or sonographic direction. In many cases, either technique is acceptable for a particular lesion or patient, and it is the operator who decides the method of preference. In other cases the choice of technique is determined by the characteristics of the lesion or the patient that allows either visualization of or access to the lesion by only one method.

Clinical aspects of percutaneous breast biopsy relate to the proper assessment of the patient prior to the procedure to avoid unnecessary risk to her, and monitoring her during and after the procedure for any potential complication. Management of the patient after the procedure includes not only clinical follow-up but also obtaining the biopsy results and establishing a plan for patient management. Postprocedural assessment may involve a follow-up clinical visit with the patient for discussion of her results and for developing a management plan. The time spent by the breast imaging team before and after the procedure usually is greater than the time spent in the technical aspects of performing the biopsy. In this chapter the selection of patients and lesions for breast biopsy and the clinical parameters involved in pre- and postprocedure care of the patient are discussed.

DEVELOPMENT OF NEEDLE TECHNIQUES FOR BREAST BIOPSY

Percutaneous breast biopsies are performed for palpable or nonpalpable breast lesions that require further intervention for diagnosis. Historically, the method of management of a palpable breast mass was surgical excision, an approach still used by many surgeons. Later, 14-gauge Tru-Cut needles were utilized to diagnose a palpable breast mass. Although described many years earlier, fine needle aspiration biopsy (FNAB), the placement of a "thin" needle into a mass to retrieve cells for cytologic analysis, was developed in the1970s.[1] FNAB was preferable to nonautomated core needles for sampling palpable masses because it was less traumatic and allowed multiple passes in a fanning motion throughout a lesion.[2,3]

However, FNAB with palpation guidance of palpable breast masses has a false negative rate of 4–31%.[1] Palpation-guided core biopsy has a similar false negative rate. Liberman et al.[4] showed that imaging-guided core biopsy expedites the management of palpable breast masses, particularly in women with small, vague, deep, mobile or multiple lesions.

Nonpalpable lesions were traditionally managed by surgical excision following a needle localization procedure. As imaging techniques improved with new transducers for high-resolution ultrasound and with stereotaxis for mammographic imaging, percutaneous biopsy of nonpalpable lesions also developed.[5]

Initially, FNAB was used for biopsy of nonpalpable lesions with ultrasound or stereotactic guidance. FNAB requires accurate targeting of the lesions, greater skill in sampling technique than for core biopsy, and an expert cytopathologist. The specific diagnosis of cysts, many fibroadenomas, lymph nodes, and cancers can be achieved with FNAB.[6] However, many benign lesions do not yield specific cytologic diagnosis, and the sensitivity ranges from 78% to 100%.[1] In the RDOG-V multicenter trial of FNAB for nonpalpable lesions, the frequency of insufficient samples was 34%.[7] The rate of insufficiency was found to be higher when an on-site cytopathologist was not present; the rate was also higher for calcifications (46.1%) than for masses (26.6%).[7]

In 1990 Parker and colleagues[8] described the technique of large-gauge core biopsy using a biopsy gun, and with this the management of suspicious nonpalpable breast lesions changed considerably. Core biopsy affords tissue sampling with cellular morphologic as well as architectural evaluation. Specific benign or malignant diagnoses, even for lesions that are difficult to diagnose by FNAB (e.g., fibrocystic changes), are possible with core biopsy.[8,9]

The early use of 16- to 20-gauge core needles with automated guns provided for histologic diagnoses of breast lesions. However, smaller core needles were associated with a higher insufficiency rate and a lower concordance rate than for biopsies with 14-gauge needles. Parker and his group[10] reported a 100% concordance with surgical excision and a 0% insufficient rate when 4 or 5 passes were used with ultrasound guidance for percutaneous biopsy and a 96% concordance for stereotactic guidance.[9]

The evaluation of tissue sampling with core needles has extended to large-gauge histologic sampling with directional vacuum assistance. Two probes (Mammotome, Ethicon Endo Surgery, Cincinnati, OH, and Minimally Invasive Breast Biopsy, US Surgical, Norwalk, CT) have been developed for breast biopsy.

Directional vacuum assisted breast biopsy (VABB) has allowed improved biopsy of certain types of lesion that were challenging for gun-needle core sampling, such as large areas of microcalcifications or very small lesions.

In the case of loosely arranged microcalcifications, VABB is utilized to pull the tissue toward the needle trough, extending significantly the area that can be sampled with one needle puncture. Various authors[11–13] have demonstrated improved retrieval of calcifications using vacuum-assisted probes over 14-gauge automated core biopsy needles (100% versus 86–94% respectively).

In the case of microcalcifications, VABB provides a greater volume of tissue, thereby increasing the diagnostic accuracy for certain types of lesions. Burbank et al.[14] found mean core weights to be 17 mg with 14-gauge core needles versus 34 mg with the 14-gauge Mammotome versus 96 mg with the 11-gauge Mammotome probe. Berg and colleagues[15] found similar mean weights of samples in phantoms using these techniques.

The difference pathologically between atypical ductal hyperplasia (ADH) and ductal carcinoma in situ (DCIS) is in part related to the number of ducts involved. A single duct with morphologically atypical cells may be diagnosed as ADH, whereas multiple ducts with the same cellular pattern may be DCIS. The use of VABB has improved the diagnostic accuracy of diagnosing DCIS because of the greater volume of tissue sampling obtained during biopsy. The likelihood of upgrading a lesion diagnosed as ADH on a 14-gauge core biopsy to DCIS on excision ranges from 20% to 56%.[16–23] With vacuum-assisted biopsy, the percentage of cases upgraded to DCIS is reduced to 0% to 30%.[19–24] Among lesions showing DCIS on 14-gauge core needle biopsy, 16% to 35% actually represent invasive ductal carcinoma at excision.[16,19,25–27] With vacuum assisted biopsy, the likelihood of upgrading DCIS to invasive cancer decreases to 0% to 19%.[19,26,27] For these reasons, VABB has become the method of choice for the biopsy of microcalcifications.

Early reports of techniques[28,29] for core biopsy of the breast suggested that lesions less than 5 mm in diameter should not be biopsied by this method because of the possibility of removal of the visible lesion on mammography. If pathologic findings on core biopsy are atypical or malignant, excision is necessary. If the mammographic abnormality is removed, the patient's localization procedure for lumpectomy would be compromised. With VABB, the feasibility of placement of a radiopaque marker or clip at the biopsy site has resolved the lesion-removal dilemma.[30] Lesions as small as 1–2 mm can be successfully biopsied stereotactically, and a clip is placed to mark the area in case surgical excision is needed.

An additional biopsy device that has been developed for use with stereotactic guidance is the Advanced Breast Biopsy Instrumentation System (ABBI) (US Surgical, Norwalk, CT). The biopsy cannula size extends up to 2 cm in diameter. Numerous disadvantages are associated with this system, including the following: large tissue volume removed/impaired cosmesis, high failure to biopsy rate, high complication rate, and high cost.[31–33] Although the concept of ABBI is that the lesion may be removed via the cannula, assessment of tissue margins for cancers biopsied with ABBI showed positive margins in the vast majority,[33] making this an unreliable tool for excision. This technology is no longer widely available.

LESION SELECTION

Percutaneous breast biopsy is an alternative to excisional biopsy and is not generally considered a replacement for early follow-up of a probably benign lesion. Therefore, the positive predictive value of percutaneous biopsy should be similar to that of excisional biopsy series reported in the past (15% to 40% positivity for malignancy) if the same selection criteria are used as for needle localized biopsy.[34] At facilities where there is extensive utilization of percutaneous breast biopsy, this has increased the positive predictive value of preoperative needle localization. This has also resulted in an increase in excisional biopsies at these centers. This is due to the triaging of lesions for excision through percutaneous biopsy, and the selection of cases that are known cancers or high-risk lesions for excision. Currently, there are relatively few patients for whom excisional biopsy with needle localization for initial lesion diagnosis is necessary, and for whom percutaneous needle biopsy is not feasible.

Lesions classified as BIRADS 4 (suspicious) or BIRADS 5 (highly suspicious for malignancy)[35] are lesions for which percutaneous biopsy is appropriate. A benign diagnosis can be confirmed for BIRADS 4 lesions that are actually benign, saving the patient from unnecessary surgery. A malignant diagnosis is established for cancers, thereby providing important information for planning surgical management and therapy. The performance of core biopsy for the diagnosis of cancers can obviate a surgical procedure, where excisional biopsy for diagnosis would be performed first, followed by definitive surgery.

A BIRADS 3 lesion is probably benign, conveying a statistical likelihood of malignancy of 2% or less.[36] The standard recommendation for a BIRADS 3 lesion is early follow-up, usually at 6-month intervals. There are certain situations in which biopsy rather than follow-up of a BIRADS 3 lesion may be indicated.[37] They include the following: inability of the patient to obtain adequate follow-up mammography (e.g., travel), planned pregnancy, patient anxiety/wish, planned breast cosmetic surgery, and anticipated medical procedures that would not be performed with an undiagnosed breast lesion being present, such as transplant surgery, and unreliability about returning for follow-up. In addition, for patients with a BIRADS 5 lesion and in whom breast conservation is planned, percutaneous biopsy of an ipsilateral BIRADS

3 lesion may be indicated to exclude the possibility of multicentric disease. Also, in women in whom surgery is planned in the opposite breast, it may be appropriate to exclude the need for a surgical procedure on a probably benign BIRADS 3 lesion in the contralateral breast. In these limited situations, percutaneous needle biopsy may be offered as an alternative to early mammographic follow-up.

Lesions amenable to percutaneous biopsy include suspicious masses, calcifications, and focal asymmetric densities. Masses that are circumscribed and complex on ultrasound may be managed by FNAB first to determine if they are cystic; if they are not, core biopsy can then be performed. In non-cystic suspicious masses, core biopsy is performed with sonographic or stereotactic guidance.

Few BIRADS 4 or 5 lesions are not reliably evaluated by percutaneous biopsy, and most do not require surgical excision for diagnosis. Those lesions that are not seen on ultrasound and that occur in breasts measuring less than 25 mm in thickness when compressed usually require needle localization and excision rather than core biopsy. Lesions that are difficult to target may be better biopsied by excision because of the concern about undersampling. A dilated duct that is suspicious usually is excised, unless there are focal microcalcifications or a filling defect on galactography (Figure 3.1) that can be targeted for core biopsy.

Very fine, faint microcalcifications may be more difficult to visualize stereotactically because of the decreased compression of the tissue in the center of the biopsy aperture and the lack of a grid. However, with digital imaging and postprocessing tools such as magnification and inversion, these faint abnormalities can often be reliably visualized and biopsied. Indistinct densities or masses in dense parenchyma can also be difficult to visualize even with digital imaging. Displacing the breast tissue by rolling the breast slightly may be helpful to visualize such indistinct lesions.

In the past, lesions less than 5 mm in diameter were not considered to be well suited to stereotactic biopsy because of the possibility of removal of the entire mammographic abnormality.[28,29] However, with the advent of vacuum assisted biopsy and the capability of clip deployment, the limitation of biopsy of small lesions no longer exists[30] (Figure 3.2).

Areas of architectural distortion that may be radial scars are also generally not biopsied stereotactically but, instead, are excised. Because the pathologist relies on the distinctive spokewheel architecture and the cellular features to diagnose radial scar and because core sampling does not allow for observation of the architecture, radial scar is difficult to diagnose in this way[38,39] (Figure 3.3). Radial scar may be associated with carcinoma, particularly DCIS.[40] Therefore, if radial scar is diagnosed on core biopsy, excision is usually recommended.[23]

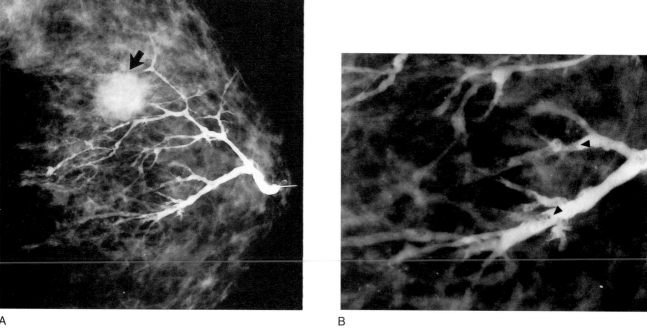

A   B

FIGURE 3.1. Galactogram (**A**, **B**) performed in a patient with a palpable mass (arrow) and bloody nipple discharge shows a high density mass with microlobulated margins. In the cannulated duct system (**B**) are multiple filling defects (arrowheads) that were targeted stereotactically and biopsied, showing ductal carcinoma in situ.

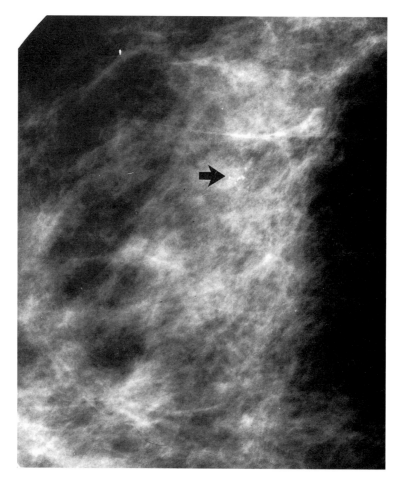

FIGURE 3.2. Right craniocaudal view (**A**).

FIGURE 3.2. Right craniocaudal magnified (**B**) view shows clustered pleomorphic microcalcifications (arrows), which represented ductal carcinoma in situ on core biopsy.

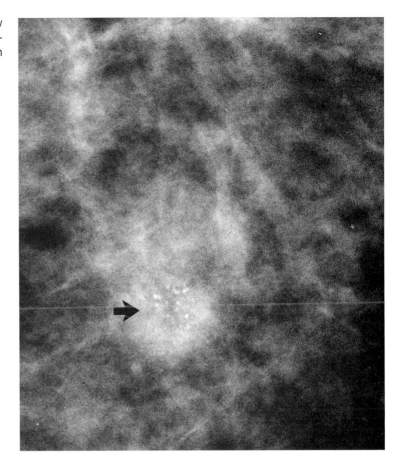

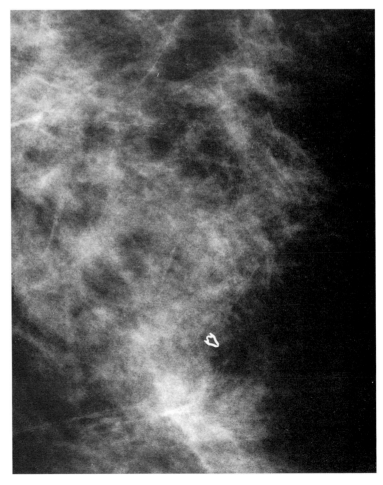

FIGURE 3.2. (**C**) A clip was deployed at the site, where the mammographic finding had been removed.

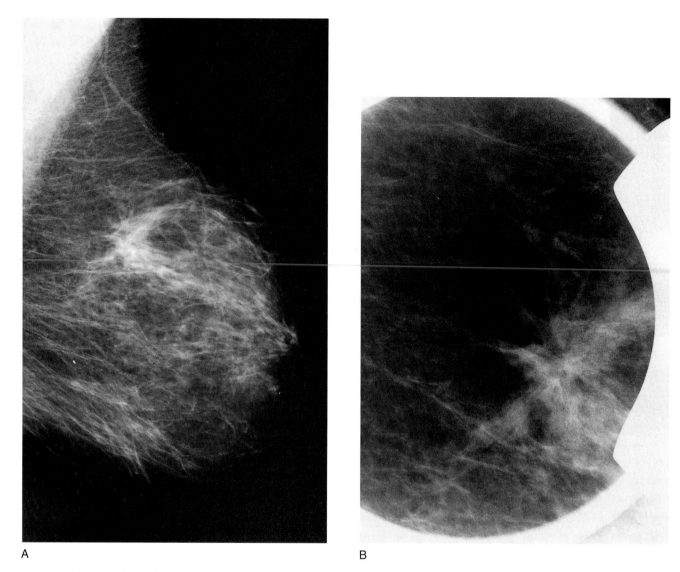

A

B

FIGURE 3.3. Right MLO (**A**) and spot MLO (**B**) views show a high density area of spiculation with a central density, considered a BIRADS 5 lesion. Core biopsy showed papillomatosis, and the excised specimen showed radial scar.

SELECTION OF EQUIPMENT AND APPROACH FOR PERCUTANEOUS BIOPSY

Three basic types of equipment currently exist for imaging-guided percutaneous biopsy: ultrasound, prone table stereotactic units, and add-on stereotactic devices to mammography units. As MRI advances and techniques are developed for MRI guided biopsy, an additional method of imaging guided biopsy will be available.

Ultrasound is an ideal method for biopsy of sonographically visible masses (Figure 3.4) and even, in some cases, areas of microcalcifications. Sonography offers particular advantages for the biopsy of masses that are located far posteriorly, because of the difficulty in positioning this area with stereotaxis. Also, because of positioning considerations, subareolar lesions are better suited to ultrasound-directed biopsy. In women in whom the

compressed breast thickness is less than 25 mm, and, therefore, in whom stereotactically guided biopsy is compromised or not possible, ultrasound also may offer a way to sample the lesion without the need for surgery. Sonography can be utilized for biopsy of patients with implants, of very obese patients who are heavier than the weight limit of the prone table, of pregnant patients, and of patients who are unable to lie prone.

Various advantages and disadvantages exist for prone versus upright stereotactic units. These factors are important in the selection of equipment for biopsy when the two options are available. Digital capability and vacuum assisted biopsy capability are now offered on both types of units. Differences exist primarily in the aspects of patient comfort and access to lesions.

Advantages of the prone table unit include the following: easier access to the inferior and medial aspects

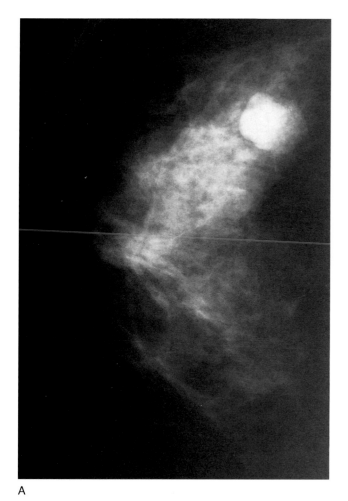

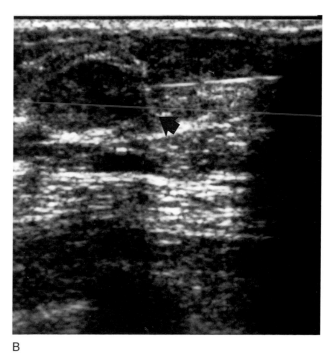

A   B

FIGURE 3.4. Right craniocaudal (**A**) and ultrasound (**B**) show a high density lobular circumscribed mass, which was solid on ultrasound. Core biopsy could be performed by either stereotactic or ultrasound guidance. In this case, ultrasound-guided biopsy demonstrated a fibroadenoma.

of the breast, lack of vasovagal reactions, and allowing for more space for biopsy equipment. Because of the necessity for a prone patient position, use of the table for breast biopsy may not be possible in women who cannot lie in this position (e.g., those with spine problems or those with recent abdominothoracic surgery). Women who weigh more than 300 pounds may exceed the table weight limit and therefore must have biopsy performed by alternate methods (i.e., sonographic guidance or upright stereotaxis). Lesions that are located far posteriorly near the chest wall or in the axillary tail may not be able to be positioned under the prone table compression plate aperture adequately (Figure 3.5). Another disadvantage of the prone position is that the patient may feel isolated from the biopsy team.

The add-on upright units can be used for stereotactic breast biopsy[41] with the patient in the seated or the decubitus position (Figure 3.5). If the patient is in the upright position, vasovagal reactions can occur. Other disadvantages are that the patient may have greater visibility

of the procedure. There is a shorter SID than with the prone table, so biopsy of very thick breasts with the vacuum assisted equipment may be more difficult. Access to the inferior aspect of the breast is accomplished with the patient in the decubitus position; however, it often more awkward than with the patient in the prone position.

One of the greatest advantages of the add-on unit over the prone table is the greater facility for imaging posteriorly located lesions and to biopsy a lesion at the chest wall[42] (Figure 3.6). Overall decreased cost of equipment as well as use of the unit for mammography, when it is not used for biopsy, are other advantages. The patient may feel more at ease because she is not so removed from the biopsy team as she is on the prone table. Patients who exceed the weight limit of the table and who do not have sonographically visible lesions can be biopsied with an upright unit. Patients with spinal problems or recent abdominal surgery are more comfortable in the upright or decubitus position. Patients with implants can be positioned in the implant-displaced position and maintained

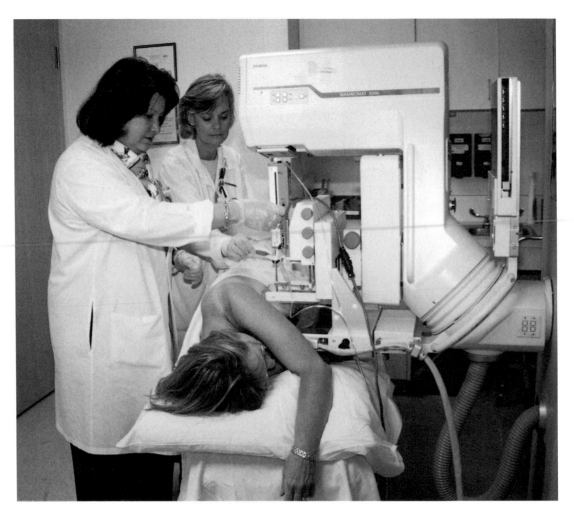

FIGURE 3.5. Patient in decubitus position for vacuum-assisted biopsy using an add-on stereotactic unit and a lateral approach.

in this position for stereotactic biopsy using an add-on unit.

Both the prone table and the upright units require a minimum breast thickness of about 2.5 cm, depending on lesion location. Options for a very thin breast include the use of ultrasound if the lesion is visible, adding a bolster to create a greater thickness, using a lateral arm attachment, use of a short throw needle or insertion of a Mammotome probe in a postfire position. Otherwise, needle localization and surgical excision may be the best choice for biopsy of a breast of this type.

PREPROCEDURAL ASSESSMENT

A prebiopsy review of the patient's imaging studies must be performed to determine the best type of biopsy for the patient and the type of lesion, the form of guidance, the equipment to be utilized, and the plan for approaching the lesion. Ideally, this imaging assessment should be conducted before the patient's arrival in the department so that procedure rooms are used most effectively, nec-

essary equipment is available, and the schedule is maintained. Complete imaging evaluation should have been completed prior to the biopsy appointment. If a 90° lateral view (mediolateral or lateromedial) has not been performed, it might be useful to obtain this on the patient's arrival in the department. This orthogonal view can be used to plan the approach for stereotactic biopsy and to serve as an aid to the technologist in positioning the patient for stereotactic biopsy.

The radiologist should also review pertinent breast-related medical history that might affect ultimate management decisions. Patients with known high risk factors, such as prior treated breast cancer or premalignant lesions in either breast, may have a higher level of suspicion attributed to an indeterminate lesion than normal risk women.

Clinical assessment of the patient prior to percutaneous biopsy includes an initial history taken at the time the biopsy is scheduled and physical assessment of the patient before, during, and after the procedure. The risk of significant complications requiring intervention is low (0.2%) with percutaneous large core biopsy.[43] However,

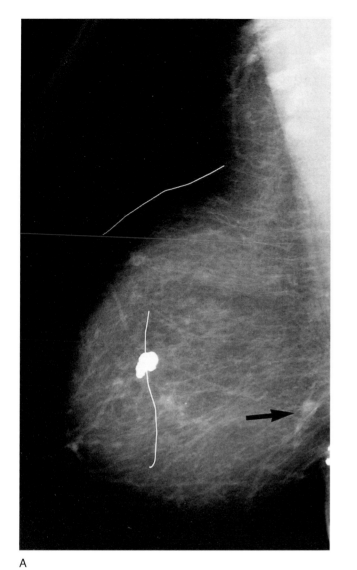
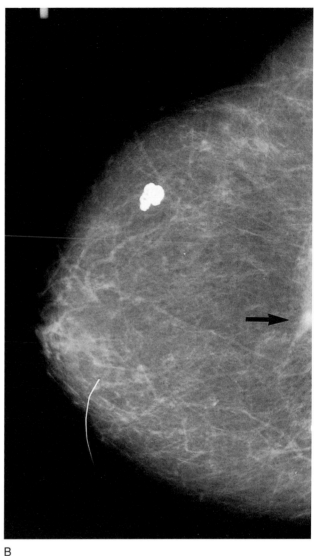

A   B

FIGURE 3.6. Left MLO (**A**) and craniocaudal (CC) (**B**) views. Multiple calcified fibroadenomas are present. There is also a small, indistinct mass (arrow) located far posteriorly at 6 o'clock. Options for biopsy of this lesion include ultrasound or stereotactic guidance. Because of the posterior location, the add-on stereotactic guidance unit was utilized. Pathology showed invasive ductal carcinoma.

clinical considerations for the selection of patients for percutaneous biopsy include a review of factors that might increase the risk of the infrequent but potential complications of bleeding or infection. A nurse or technologist may conduct a clinical interview of the patient at the time of scheduling and document this information in the patient's record (Figure 3.7). This interview also serves as an excellent opportunity for the assistant to provide instructions and information about the procedure and to address any concerns the patient has.

Routine preoperative blood work is usually not necessary but may be performed if there is a clinical indication of potential prolonged bleeding or if the patient has been on anticoagulant therapy. Possible causes of prolonged bleeding must be identified and either corrected

or considered as a potential contraindication to large-gauge core needle biopsy. Anticoagulant therapy[39] is generally considered a contraindication to large-gauge core biopsy. Patients who are on warfarin therapy should, under the care of their physician, discontinue use of the anticoagulant, and clotting studies should be performed prior to the biopsy. In patients who are at high risk for stroke or cardiac problems, and in whom discontinuation of warfarin is not considered safe, the Coumadin may be replaced with heparin until 12–24 hours before the procedure. Patients who take aspirin should discontinue its use at least 3 to 5 days before the scheduled biopsy. Aspirin prevents platelet aggregation[44] and inhibits platelet cyclooxygenase activity. Infrequently, non-steroidal antiinflammatory medications may cause thrombocytope-

62 / E. Shaw de Paredes

**Pre-Operative Patient Assesment
Precutaneous Breast Biopsy**

Name: _____ Med. Rec. #: _____

Date of Exam: _____

Phone: (_____) _____

Weight: _____

1) Do you have a history of the following: Yes ____   No ____

   Diabetes Mellitus?   Yes ____   No ____

   Liver Disease?   Yes ____   No ____

   Bleeding Problems?   Yes ____   No ____

   Rheumatic Fever?   Yes ____   No ____

   Artificial Heart Valve?   Yes ____   No ____

   Artificial Joints?   Yes ____   No ____

2) Do you take anticoagulants?   Yes ____   No ____

3) Do you take aspirin or nonsteroids daily?   Yes ____   No ____

   Advise patient not to take these medications for 5 days prior to procedure

4) Do you take prophylactic antibiotics before surgical or dental procedures?

                                                Yes ____   No ____

5) Do you have any allergies?   Yes ____   No ____
   If yes please describe: _____

   _____

FIGURE 3.7. Preoperative patient assessment form.

nia[45] and can affect clotting. Although anticoagulation is considered a contraindication to core biopsy, occasionally the patient is at great risk if anticoagulants are discontinued. Under these circumstances, biopsy can be performed while the patient is anticoagulated. Meloti et al.[46] found that in 11-gauge biopsies performed in patients who were not able to discontinue anticoagulants, 38% developed hematomas ranging from 13 to 40 mm; with 14-gauge needles, fewer hematomas occurred. The rates of hematomas in anticoagulated patients were similar to controls; however, their sizes were larger.

Medical causes of prolonged bleeding include clotting disorders, such as factor VIII or XI deficiency, uremia, myeloproliferative disorders, α-2 antiplasmin deficiency and lupus anticoagulant,[47] thrombocytopenia, and liver disease. If the patient is known to have such conditions, preoperative clotting studies or platelet counts may be necessary. The platelet counts should ideally be at least 50,000/dl[44] prior to performance of a large-gauge biopsy, as is normally required for surgical procedures. Depend-

ing on the lesion characteristics and skills of those involved in the performance and interpretation of the biopsy, FNAB may be an option in patients when potential bleeding problems cannot be corrected. Should bleeding occur during biopsy, compression must be applied until it is controlled. Use of lidocaine with epinephrine is also helpful. The breast can also be iced before the biopsy. If a palpable hematoma occurs, a pressure dressing may be applied, and the patient should be advised to utilize ice packs intermittently throughout the day.

Infections after percutaneous breast biopsy are relatively uncommon. In a multi-institutional study, Parker et al.[43] found a 0.1% incidence of breast abscesses. In comparison, data from needle localization and surgical excision series suggested a rate of postoperative infection of less than 10%,[48] mostly occurring in patients with surgical drains. Breast surgery is considered a clean/sterile procedure, and prophylactic antibiotics are not usually given. However, some authors[48,49] have suggested the use of prophylactic antibiotics for breast surgeries and have reported a decrease in postoperative infections. Platt and colleagues[49] reported 48% fewer postoperative infections in patients who had herniorrhaphy or breast surgery and who received preoperative antibiotic prophylaxis.

With stereotactic breast biopsy the operative field is quite small, and the compression device and biopsy gun are not sterile. Great care must be taken to maintain a sterile field. Although there have been no published data to recommend prophylactic antibiotics for core biopsy, many radiologists do prescribe prophylaxis for patients who are at high risk. Consultation with the patient's referring clinician may be appropriate to determine the necessity of antibiotic prophylaxis for some of these women.

Patients who are at higher risk to develop infections are those who are immunocompromised or who have insulin dependent diabetes. Patients who are at risk of complications if an infection should occur or from transient bacteremia are those with a history of an artificial heart valve, mitral valve prolapse, rheumatic heart disease, or joint replacements. In these situations, prophylactic antibiotics are administered to prevent bacterial endocarditis or joint infection respectively. Typically, patients with these histories are given prophylaxis when they undergo procedures in the mouth, upper respiratory tract, and gastrointestinal or genitourinary tracts. These may include radiologic procedures related to these organs.[50]

The Committee on Rheumatic Fever and Infection Endocarditis[51] has recognized that "practitioners must exercise their clinical judgment in determining the duration and choices of antibiotics when special circumstances apply." Antibiotic prophylaxis is not specifically recommended for biopsy through surgically scrubbed skin. Because the sterile field is so small and because the non-sterile components of the stereotactic equipment are near the field and are handled by the operator, one should consider the use of prophylactic antibiotics in high risk patients. Bacteremia is unlikely during the biopsy procedure, but this may occur intraprocedurally or later if cellulitis is present.[52] The need for and type of antibiotic in these patients has not been defined. Standard prophylaxis for prevention of bacterial endocarditis by the American Heart Association[52] includes the following: penicillin 2 g po, cephalosporin 2 g po, or clindamycin 600 mg po at 1 hour before the procedure.

Other aspects of the clinical assessment relate to the type of equipment and patient position for biopsy. Very obese patients (weighing more than 300 pounds) or those with spinal or orthopedic problems that prohibit a prone position are reasons for planning the biopsy procedure with ultrasound or stereotaxis using the add-on unit. An assessment of the patient's allergies is needed with particular attention to commonly used substances (i.e., Betadine, lidocaine, latex gloves, tape/adhesives). Reminders to patients to take regular medications, other than those that can cause anticoagulation, are important. Scheduling of diabetic patients with considerations regarding their schedule for insulin and meals is also an important clinical consideration.

Informed consent is obtained before the procedure. In situations where the patient is unable to give consent, her family member who is legally responsible must be available for consent. In addition to an explanation of the procedure and the potential risks, one should also explain to the patient the reason for the percutaneous procedure rather than surgical excision and the possible management plans based on the results. It is helpful for the patient to understand the reasons why she might need excision after the core biopsy. The patient should also understand that she may need a repeat biopsy or excision if the specimen is unsatisfactory.

POSTPROCEDURAL ASSESSMENT

After an FNAB, the skin should be cleaned with alcohol and a bandage applied to the puncture site. Ice may be applied to the breast if bleeding occurred during the biopsy. In most cases, however, no ice pack is necessary.

After core biopsy, manual compression is applied for at least 5 to 10 minutes to avoid a hematoma. The skin should be cleaned with sterile water or alcohol, and antibiotic ointment may be applied at the incision site. The skin incision is apposed with Steri-strips and a bandage or 4×4 gauge is placed over the Steri-strips, and the patient is advised to keep the Steri-strips in place for 48–72 hours. An ice pack is applied to the site for 30 minutes, and the patient is advised to reapply the ice pack after 2 hours and again later if necessary. Nonaspirin-containing analgesics may be used for pain.

The patient is instructed to observe the breast for any sign of bleeding or infection, and she is given information on whom to contact if this should occur. A small or moderate-sized hematoma is indicated by fullness at the puncture site with bruising. Small hematomas gradually resolve without intervention. A large hematoma may be a tender mass and may require surgical evacuation. Diffuse enlargement of the breast can also indicate extensive bleeding and should cause the patient to contact the designated physician.

Signs of mastitis include pain, erythema, purulent drainage from the biopsy site or nipple, skin thickening or swelling, increased skin temperature over the breast, and fever. If postbiopsy mastitis or abscess is suspected, culture and sensitivity testing of an aspirate or drainage can be performed. Most infections are produced by *Staphylococcus aureus* or anaerobes; a cephalosporin or a drug such as amoxicillin/clavulanate potassium (Augmentin)[53] can be used to treat mastitis.

The patient also is told how she will receive the biopsy results. The referring physician or radiologist may

---

Post Biopsy Instructions

Apply ice to the breast for 30 minutes three times on the day of your procedure to relieve swelling.

You may use Tylenol (two tablets) every four to six hours for pain as needed.

You may return to work after the procedure, but do not perform any strenuous activities for 24 to 48 hours.

You may remove the bandage tomorrow morning, but keep the thin strip of tape in place for two days. Keep the area dry for 2 days.

You may notice bruising in the area of the biopsy. This will usually clear in five to seven days.

If you notice any bleeding, drainage, excessive swelling, pain, redness, or heat around the biopsy area please call _____.

The final results of your biopsy are usually available in three to five working days. _____ will contact you with the results. If you have not heard your results within five working days, please call _____.

FIGURE 3.8. Postbiopsy patient instructions.

provide the results of the biopsy directly to the patient. In the case of positive results, the radiologist should be prepared to answer general questions regarding treatment options. If the radiologist does not provide the results directly to the patient, it is critical that he or she communicate to the referring physician the biopsy results and the overall recommendation based on the mammographic and cytologic or histologic findings. The radiologist also must inform the patient that the referring physician will provide the results if they are not directly provided to her.

If the radiologist provides the results to the patient, she may be asked to return for a wound check and to be given the results in person. This approach is especially worthwhile when the biopsy demonstrates a malignancy.

Regardless of who provides the biopsy results to the patient, postprocedural instructions should include the telephone number of the breast imaging facility to call if she has any problems or questions or if she has not received her biopsy results by an indicated period of time. If the results are benign and the radiologist recommends an early follow-up mammogram in 6 months, the patient may be scheduled for her follow-up appointment. Both written and verbal post-procedural instructions are helpful in clarifying the preceding points to the patient (Figure 3.8).

Reasons for excision or repeat biopsy after core biopsy include either an insufficient sample or nonconcordant results. Reasons for excision are the pathologic findings of a high risk lesion, a nonconcordant or indeterminate lesion, or a cancer, where lumpectomy will be performed for treatment.

The likelihood of an insufficient sample is decreased when multiple passes are made with a large-gauge core needle or even more so with VABB. Nonconcordant results occur when imaging and histologic findings are not explanatory of each other. For example, a BIRADS™ 5 lesion with a diagnosis of fibrofatty tissue is discordant. Liberman et al.[54] reported discordance of 3.1% in 1785 lesions that had undergone percutaneous biopsy, and of these, 24.4% were found to be cancer on excision.

A high risk lesion that necessitates excision is atypical ductal hyperplasia (ADH). The likelihood of underestimating of disease when DCIS is present but is called ADH on core biopsy ranges from 0% to 56%[16–24] depending on the type of needle and amount of sampling. Atypical lobular hyperplasia and lobular carcinoma in situ have been more debatable; however, several studies[55,56] have shown that these lesions may also be associated with finding malignancy on excision and should be removed after core biopsy.

Radial scar is both difficult to diagnosis on core biopsy and of concern when it is found. Radial scars may be associated with the areas of ADH or DCIS[40] in their periphery and should therefore be excised.

Most fibroadenomas are not problematic to pathologists for diagnosis from core specimens. However, the distinction between a cellular fibroadenoma and a phyllodes tumor can be difficult and may necessitate excision of the lesion.

Benign papillomas do not generally require excision. However, sometimes the fibrovascular core is not completely defined and the lesion is called an "indeterminate papillary lesion." In this case the possibility of papillary cancer exists, and the lesion should be excised. However, for some pathologists all benign papillomas are difficult to definitively diagnose as not malignant, and in this situation they will require surgical excision. Many also believe that all mucinous lesions should be surgically excised.

FOLLOW-UP AFTER PERCUTANEOUS BIOPSY

When carcinoma is found on core biopsy, definitive surgery can be planned. The patient can be scheduled for lumpectomy with sentinel node biopsy or axillary node dissection, if needed, or for mastectomy. Although core biopsy is a highly reliable method of diagnosis of breast abnormalities, a small percentage of cancers can be missed. Jackman and his co-investigators[57] reported a false-negative rate of 1.2% in 483 consecutive core biopsies. The malignancies were identified on repeat biopsy because of mammographic progression at 6 and 18 months after core biopsy. In comparison, others have reported a false negative rate of 2.9% to 6.7%.[10,58–60] However, it should be remembered that surgical excision, which is used as the gold standard for comparison of results with core biopsy, carries a similar false negative rate of 0 to 8%.[61]

There is no definite established standard for the frequency of mammographic follow-up after percutaneous needle biopsy. Many radiologists perform annual mammography following concordant, specific benign biopsies and 6-month follow-up after concordant but nonspecific biopsies.[62] Others, though, recommend the first follow-up for all biopsies to be at 6-months, with 6-month interval mammography twice more.[57]

Importantly, based on histology and mammography, the radiologist must define the presence of concordance or nonconcordance and render a decision regarding the need for rebiopsy, excision, or mammographic surveillance. Tracking patients who have had percutaneous biopsy can be challenging and time consuming, especially when follow-up activities are to be performed at other facilities. In addition, patient compliance with follow-up recommendations is variable.[63]

The responsibility of the radiologist who performs percutaneous biopsy has grown tremendously. At one time only a need for understanding of the procedures and technical parameters was necessary. Now these are best performed by those having a strong clinical knowledge of the medical issues that surround performing these procedures appropriately, safely, and effectively. Careful selection of the best procedure for the patient, her breast type, and the lesion requires knowledge of indications and risks of the various biopsy procedures, the technical considerations, and a rich understanding of mammography. The immediate care of the patient before and after the procedure is straightforward, but much thought and time are directed to the decision-making and communication processes that follow. The interventionalist must obtain the pathology results and then issue a final report with recommendations for follow-up mammography, rebiopsy or excision based on the findings. Communication with the patient about these recommendations is paramount and is probably best conducted by the interventionalist with a full knowledge of the procedural, mammographic, and histologic parameters. This communication then requires the radiologist to have the ability to address at least some of the clinical concerns and questions the patient may have.

The advancement of percutaneous biopsy during the last decade has been tremendous. Eliminating unnecessary surgeries for many benign breast lesions and improving the workup of cancers have improved the management of breast disease. However, a significant role still exists for surgical excision. Surgical intervention is appropriate not just for lumpectomy but also for biopsy of nonconcordant lesions, lesions in breasts too thin to biopsy stereotactically, or in the infrequent lesion best suited to excision.

REFERENCES

1. Rosen PP. Role of cytology and needle biopsy in the diagnosis of breast disease. *In* Breast Pathology. Philadelphia: Lippincott-Raven, 1997;817–834.
2. Donegan WL. Evaluation of a palpable breast mass. N Engl J Med 1992;327:937–942.
3. Shabot MM, Goldberg IM, Schick P, et al. Aspiration cytology is superior to tru-cut needle biopsy in establishing the diagnosis of clinically suspicious breast masses. Ann Surg 1982; 196:122–126.
4. Liberman L, Ernberg LA, Heerdt A, et al. Palpable breast masses: is there a role of percutaneous imaging-guided core biopsy? AJR 2000;175:774–787.
5. Svane G. Stereotactic needle biopsy of nonpalpable breast lesions. Acta Radiol 1983;24:284–288.
6. Shaw de Paredes E. Stereotactic needle biopsies: FNA. *In* Syllabus 26th National Conference on Breast Cancer. Washington, DC: American College of Radiology, 1994;14–15.
7. Pisano ED, Fajardo LL, Tsimikas J, et al. Rate of insufficient samples from fine needle aspiration for nonpalpable breast lesions in an multicenter clinical trial: the Radiologic Diagnostic Oncology Group 5 study. Cancer 1998;82:678–688.
8. Parker SH, Lovin JD, Jobe WE, et al. Stereotactic breast biopsy with a biopsy gun. Radiology 1990;176:741–747.
9. Parker SH, Lovin JD, Jobe WE, et al. Nonpalpable breast lesions: stereotactic automated large core biopsies. Radiology 1991;180:403–407.
10. Parker SH, Jobe WE, Dennis MA, et al. US guided automated large core breast biopsy. Radiology 1993;187:507–511.
11. Meyer JE, Smith DN, DiPiro PJ, et al. Stereotactic breast biopsy of clustered microcalcifications with a directional, vacuum assisted device. Radiology 1997;204:575–576.
12. Jackman RJ, Burbank FH, Parker SA, et al. Accuracy of sampling microcalcifications by three stereotactic breast biopsy methods (abstract). Radiology 1997;205P:325.

13. Reynolds HE, Poon CM, Goulet RJ, et al. Biopsy of breast microcalcifications using an 11 gauge directional vacuum assisted device. AJR 1998;171:611–613.

14. Burbank F, Parker SH, Fogarty TJ. Stereotactic breast biopsy: improved tissue harvesting with the mammotome. Am Surg 1996;62:738–744.

15. Berg WA, Kreb TL, Camposi C, et al. Evaluation of 14G and 11G directional vacuum assisted biopsy probes and 14G biopsy guns in a breast parenchymal model. Radiology 1997; 205:203–208.

16. Jackman RJ, Nowels KW, Shepard MJ, Finkelstein SI, Marzoni FA. Stereotactic large-core needle biopsy of 450 nonpalpable breast lesions with surgical correlation in lesions with cancer or atypical hyperplasia. Radiology 1994;193:91–95.

17. Liberman L, Dershaw DD, Glassman J, et al. Analysis of cancers not diagnosed at stereotaxic core breast biopsy. Radiology 1997;203:151–157.

18. Liberman L, Cohen MA, Dershaw DD, et al. Atypical ductal hyperplasia diagnosed at stereotaxic core biopsy of breast lesions: an indication for surgical biopsy. AJR 1995;164:1111–1113.

19. Burbank F. Stereotactic breast biopsy of atypical ductal hyperplasia and ductal carcinoma in situ lesions: improved accuracy with a directional vacuum assisted biopsy instrument. Radiology 1997;202:843–847.

20. Jackman RJ, Burbank F, Parker SH, et al. Atypical ductal hyperplasia diagnosed at stereotactic breast biopsy: improved reliability with a 14G directional vacuum-assisted biopsy. Radiology 1997;204:485–488.

21. Philpotts LE, Shaheen NA, Carter D, et al. Comparison of rebiopsy rates after stereotactic core needle biopsy of the breast with 11G vacuum suction probe versus 14G needle and automatic gun. AJR 1999;172:683–687.

22. Brem RF, Behrndt VS, Sanow L, Gatewood OMB. Atypical ductal hyperplasia: histologic underestimation of carcinoma in tissue harvested from impalpable breast lesions using 11G stereotactically guided directional vacuum assisted biopsy. AJR 1999;172:1405–1407.

23. Liberman L. Clinical management issues in percutaneous core breast biopsy. Radiol Clin North Am 2000;38:791–807.

24. Liberman L, Dershaw DD, Rosen PP, et al. Stereotaxic core biopsy of breast carcinoma: accuracy at predicting invasion. Radiology 1995;194:379–381.

25. Jackman RJ, Burbank FH, Parker SH, et al. Accuracy of sampling ductal carcinoma in situ by three stereotactic breast biopsy methods. Radiology 1998;209 (P):197–198.

26. Won B, Reynolds HE, Lazaridis CL, Jackson VP. Stereotactic biopsy of ductal carcinoma in situ of the breast using an 11G vacuum assisted device: persistent underestimation of disease. AJR 1999;173:227–229.

27. Liberman L, Vuoto M, Dershaw DD, et al. Epithelial displacement after stereotactic 11G directional vacuum-assisted breast biopsy. AJR 1999;172:677–681.

28. Dronkers DJ. Stereotaxic core biopsy of breast lesions. Radiology 1992;183:631–634.

29. Jackson VP, Reynolds HE. Stereotaxic needle-core biopsy and fine-needle aspiration cytologic evaluation of non-palpable breast lesions. Radiology 1991;181:633–634.

30. Liberman L, Dershaw DD, Morris EA, et al. Clip placement after stereotactic vacuum-assisted breast biopsy. Radiology 1997;205:417–422.

31. Ferzli GS, Puza T, Van Vorst–Bilotti S, et al. Breast biopsies with ABBI: experience with 183 attempted biopsies. Breast J 1999;5:26–28.

32. Baum JK, Raza S, Keller B, et al. ABBI breast biopsy: early experience using a combined radiological-surgical approach (abstract). AJR 1998;170:83.

33. Liberman L. Advanced breast biopsy instrumentation: analysis of published experience. AJR 1999;172:1413–1416.

34. Homer MJ, Smith TJ, Safaii H. Prebiopsy needle localization. Radiol Clin North Am 1992;30:139–153.

35. American College of Radiology. Breast Imaging Reporting and Data System (BIRADS™), 2nd ed. Reston, VA: American College of Radiology, 1995.

36. Sickles EA. Periodic mammographic follow-up of probably benign lesions: results of 3184 consecutive cases. Radiology 1991;179:463–468.

37. Sickles EA, Parker SH. Appropriate role of core biopsy in the management of probably benign lesions. Radiology 1993;188:315.

38. Evans P, Oberman H. Stereotactic needle biopsies: core and FNA. In Syllabus National Conference on Breast Cancer. Reston, VA: American College of Radiology, 1994;9–10.

39. Bird RE. Image guided needle biopsy of the breast. In Syllabus 26th National Conference on Breast Cancer. Reston, VA: American College of Radiology, 1994;25–27.

40. Rosen PP. Intraductal carcinoma. In Breast Pathology. Philadelphia: Lippincott-Raven, 1997;246–247.

41. Gaines JS, McPhee MD, Konok GP, Wright BA. Stereotactic needle core biopsy of breast lesions using a regular mammographic table with an adaptable stereotaxis device. AJR 1994; 163:317–321.

42. Cousins JF, Wayland AD, Shaw de Paredes E. Stereotactic breast biopsy units: pros and cons. Appl Radiol 1998;27:8–14.

43. Parker SH, Burbank F, Jackman RJ, et al. Percutaneous large core breast biopsy: a multi institutional study. Radiology 1994; 193:359–364.

44. Consensus Conference. Platelet transfusion therapy. JAMA 1987;257:1777.

45. Physician's Desk Reference. Montvale, NJ: Medical Economics, 2001.

46. Meloti MK, Berg WA. Core needle breast biopsy in patients undergoing anticoagulation therapy: preliminary results. AJR 2000;174:245–249.

47. Rapaport SI. Preoperative hemostatic evaluation, which tests if any? Blood 1983;61:229–231.

48. Platt R, Zaleznik DF, Hopkins CC, et al. Preoperative antibiotic prophylaxis for herniorrhaphy and breast surgery. N Engl J Med 1990;322:153–160.

49. Platt R, Zucker JR, Zaleznik DF, et al. Prophylaxis against wound infection herniorrhaphy or breast surgery. J Infect Dis 1992;166:556–560.

50. Chakraverty S, Baker EM, et al. Antibiotic prophylaxis in patients undergoing radiological procedures who are at risk of infectious endocarditis—do radiologists know what they are doing? Clin Radiol 1996;51:39–41.

51. Shulman ST, Amren DP, Bisno AL, et al. Prevention of bacterial endocarditis. Circulation 1984;70:1123A–1127A.

52. Dajani AS, Taubert KA, et al. Prevention of bacterial endocarditis: recommendations by the American Heart Association. Clin Infect Dis 1997;25:1448–1458.

53. Giamarellou H, Soulis M, Antoniadou A, Gogas J. Periareo-

lar nonpuerperal breast infection: treatment of 38 cases. Clin Infect Dis 1994;18:73–76.

54. Liberman L, Drotman M, Morris EA, et al. Imaging-histologic discordance at percutaneous breast biopsy: an indication of missed cancer. Cancer 2000;89:2538–2546.

55. Berg WA, Mrose HE, Ioffe OB. Atypical lobular hyperplasia or lobular carcinoma in situ at core needle breast biopsy. Radiology 2001;218:503–509.

56. Samardar P, Reddy SC, Shaw de Paredes E, et al. Significance of atypical lobular hyperplasia on core biopsy of the breast. *In* Scientific Program of RSNA, 86th Scientific Session. Oak Brook, IL: Radiological Society of North America, 2000.

57. Jackman RJ, Nowels KW, Roderiguez-Soto J, et al. Stereotactic, automated, large-core needle biopsy of nonpalpable breast lesions: false-negative and histologic underestimation rates after long-term follow-up. Radiology 1999;210:799–805.

58. Elvecrog EL, Lechner MC, Nelson MT. Nonpalpable breast lesions: correlation of stereotaxis large-core needle biopsy and surgical biopsy results. Radiology 1993;188:453–455.

59. Gisvold JJ, Goellner JR, Grant CS, et al. Breast biopsy: a comparative study of stereotaxically guided core and excisional techniques. AJR 1994;162:815–820.

60. Brenner J, Farjardo L, Fisher PR, et al. Percutaneous breast core biopsy of the breast: effect of operator experience in number of samples on diagnostic accuracy. AJR 1996;166:341–346.

61. Jackman RJ, Marzoni FA. Needle localized breast biopsy: why do we fail? Radiology 1997;204:676–684.

62. Lee CH, Philpotts LE, Horvath LJ, et al. Follow-up of breast lesions diagnosed as benign with stereotactic core needle biopsy: frequency of mammographic change and false negative rate. Radiology 1999;212:189–194.

63. Goodman KA, Birdwell RL, Ikeda DM. Compliance with recommended follow-up after percutaneous breast core biopsy. AJR 1998;170:89–92.

CHAPTER 4

Needles and Biopsy Probes

D. David Dershaw

When percutaneous tissue sampling of a breast lesion has been selected as an appropriate technique for the diagnosis of a suspicious area, a decision needs to be made about the technique that will be used to perform the biopsy. Issues of selecting the imaging guidance technique, sonography versus stereotaxis, are not addressed in this chapter. Considerations of core versus aspiration and types of tissue removal techniques that can be used for core biopsy are discussed.

The selection of the biopsy technique can be influenced by a variety of factors. These include characteristics of the target lesion and the breast, including lesion pattern, location of the lesion within the breast, and breast size, configuration, and compressibility. Factors that influence the selection of the needle or biopsy probe also include cost, size of the lesion, need for local anesthetic, volume of tissue needed for diagnosis, as well as availability of equipment and scheduling considerations.

ASPIRATION OR CORE BIOPSY?

Among the techniques available for tissue sampling, aspiration is the quickest and the least expensive. With this technique individual cells and clumps of cells are removed for analysis. A small gauge needle, a syringe and alcohol to cleanse the skin are required to perform the aspiration; these are readily available and inexpensive. Local anesthesia can be used but is not necessary. The aspiration can be performed without patient preparation, and results can be available at the time of the aspiration, if a cytologist is on site to interpret the specimen.

Despite these advantages, considerable disadvantages have resulted in the performance of core biopsy instead of aspiration in many situations. Limitations to the widespread use of aspiration cytology, especially in the United States, have included the high insufficient sampling rate that has particularly plagued those with less experience in this technique and those performing it in situations in which a cytologist or cytopathologist is not available to assess the adequacy of specimen retrieval. The inability to differentiate invasive from in situ cancer in most instances has also been a limiting factor. The nonspecificity of benign results, limiting the ability to correlate these results with the imaging pattern of the targeted lesion, has also been frustrating, as has been the classification of aspirates as atypical, requiring removal of larger volumes of tissue for a definitive assessment of possible malignancy.

Core biopsy makes available larger volumes of tissue that enable the pathologist to assess a portion of the targeted lesion and background architecture to make a diagnosis. When the lesion is accurately targeted, a final diagnosis can be made for most lesions based on the volume of tissue excised. A reliable diagnosis of invasive carcinoma can be made; definite histologies of benign entities can also be diagnosed, so that these can be correlated with the imaging pattern of the worrisome lesion. This makes it possible to determine if the lesion has been successfully biopsied.

While most would consider these to be significant advantages, core biopsy is more expensive to perform, requires the acquisition of special biopsy probes, often needs prescheduling, requires the use of local anesthetic, and cannot be done under stereotactic guidance in breasts that are too thin or areas of the breast that are too thin to accommodate the biopsy probe. Additionally, while cytologic results can be available within minutes of performing the tissue sampling, results from core biopsies can take a day or more before they are available.

This chapter reviews in detail the factors that may be considered when selecting a technique for imaging guided breast biopsy. In many situations, if all types of equipment are available and cost is not a consideration, most physicians would opt for the use of core biopsy because of the diagnostic advantages of larger amounts of tissue with intact architecture. However, there are certain situations in which the use of aspiration rather than core techniques may be advantageous. These include stereotactic biopsy of thin breasts or very thin areas of the breast that cannot accommodate a core biopsy probe. Core biopsies require the use of local anesthetic, whereas fine needle aspiration can be done without anesthesia. If the patient is allergic to anesthestic, tissue sampling by aspiration can eliminate the need for anesthesia. When a cyst aspiration has been attempted and the targeted lesion is found to be solid, performance of cytology aspiration with the needle in place in the lesion is appropriate. When a lymph node is targeted, cells are usually readily obtained, decreasing the likelihood of insufficient sampling. If epithelial cells are obtained from a lymph node, this invariably indicates metastatic carcinoma, so that staging is possible based on aspiration. When a targeted lesion is located within the axilla, the minimal needle motion required for aspiration and removal of smaller amounts of tissue may decrease the possibility of injury to large vascular structures and nerves in the axilla, diminishing the possibility of major complications.

SMALL-GAUGE NEEDLES FOR ASPIRATION

During aspiration procedures to obtain a specimen for cytologic analysis the needle needs to dislodge cellular material for analysis. The motion of the needle separates cells, and the diameter of the needle needs to be large enough to allow passage of cells into the syringe. Needles of 21–25 gauge are used, attached to a disposible syringe, usually with a 10 cc chamber. Some connect intravenous tubing between the syringe and the needle, making it possible to use one set of hands to create a vacuum to help harvest cells by applying negative pressure with the syringe while a second set of hands can manipulate the needle to dislodge cells (as well as hold the transducer, if the aspiration is being done under sonographic guidance) (Figure 4.1). The cost of this equipment is minimal, a few dollars at most.

The technique for aspiration is described in detail in Chapter 8 and is not discussed in detail here. In performing the aspiration, the needle tip only traverses the targeted lesion (Figure 4.2). No breast thickness greater than that of the target is needed. Therefore, issues of breast thickness that may limit the ability to obtain tissue with other biopsy techniques do not come into play during aspiration. The limited motion of the needle is advantageous in the axilla, where it is possible to cut through important vascular and neural structures that may be located near the targeted lesion.

GUN–NEEDLE COMBINATIONS

Core needle biopsy of the breast was first described using gun–needle combination biopsy devices. In these devices, a spring-loaded biopsy gun moves a cutting needle through the breast to obtain a core of tissue. Variables in available gun-needle combinations include disposable and nondisposable guns, needle gauge, size of the tissue collection chamber, and the distance the needle moves (i.e., the needle "throw").

The biopsy needle consists of an inner needle with a beveled leading edge and a tissue acquisition chamber. This fits inside an outer needle (Figure 4.3). The biopsy is performed by the consecutive movement of the inner and outer needles (Figure 4.4). Initially, the inner needle is fired into the breast. The bevel on the leading edge of the needle causes it to pass slightly downward (into the 6 o'clock axis) as it passes a distance into the breast, defined as the needle throw. After the inner needle has moved into the breast, the gun then fires the outer needle (Figure 4.5). This moves over the inner needle, forcing it slightly upward toward the 12 o'clock axis, compressing breast tissue into the tissue acquisition chamber of the inner needle and cutting it off from the rest of the breast. The gun causes the inner and outer needles to move within a fraction of a second. The individual components of the biopsy needle's movement are not perceptible. In order to remove the specimen, the needle must be removed from the breast. The outer needle is retracted over the inner needle, and the specimen is removed from the tissue acquisition chamber of the inner needle. Depending upon the design of the biopsy gun, the cutting needle may or may not need to be removed from the gun to expose the tissue acquisition chamber of the inner needle. To obtain the next core, the needle is reintroduced into the breast, and the procedure is repeated.

Gun–needle combinations are available in long-throw and short-throw combinations (Figure 4.6). Long-throw needles usually move 20–23 mm from their prefire to their post-fire position within the breast. Short-throw needles generally move 15–17 mm during the biopsy. The tissue acquisition chamber in long-throw needles is generally larger (about 17 mm) than that of the short-throw needle, which is about 11 mm.

Guns are available in both disposable and nondisposable forms (Figure 4.7). The cutting needles are all disposable. The decision of an individual facility to use disposable or nondisposable guns is based on the economics of these procedures. The nondisposable guns are about 100 times more expensive than the disposable ones. If a facility rarely performs these procedures, it is less expensive to use disposable guns. If a facility frequently does these biopsies, the cost per procedure is less using nondisposable guns.

The experience of a variety of investigators with cutting needles of gauges ranging from 18 up to 14 and larger has been reported.[1,2] These data indicate that regardless

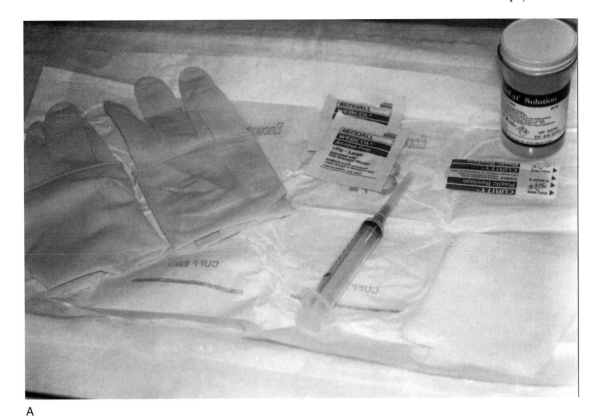

A

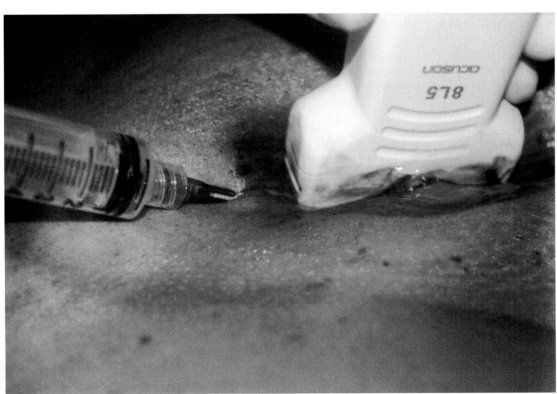

B

FIGURE 4.1. (A) Equipment needed for aspiration includes a small-gauge (21–25) needle, a 10 cc syringe, and an alcohol wipe. Gloves should be worn to protect the patient and physician. Some prefer to connect the syringe to the needle with tubing, making it possible for the physician to hold the transducer and manipulate the needle while an assistant creates negative pressure with the syringe, assisting in the harvesting of cells. **(B)** Aspiration is simply performed using a syringe, small needle, and sonographic guidance. The procedure is quick and inexpensive.

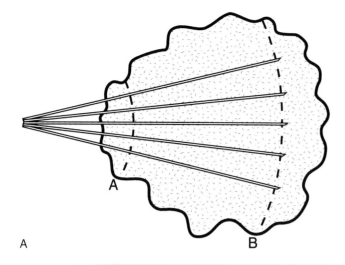

A

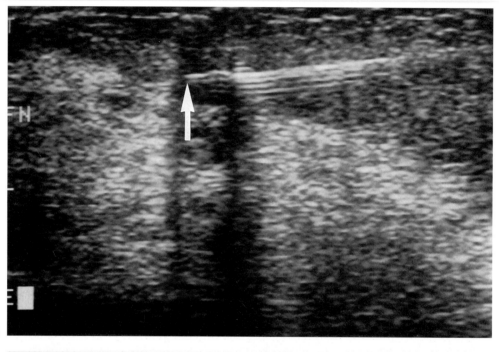

B

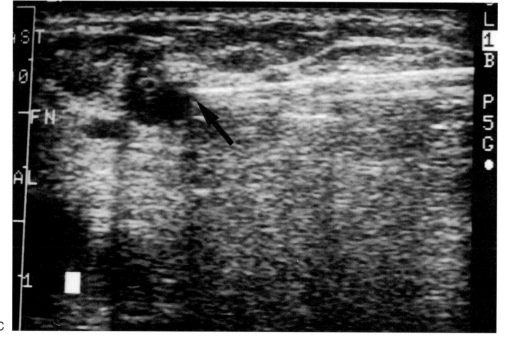

C

FIGURE 4.2. Movement of the needle during fine needle aspiration is confined to the borders of the target lesion. The needle is initially introduced to site "B," at the far edge of the target. Negative pressure is created, and the needle is fanned throughout the volume of the mass, being brought back to "A," angled slightly, and advanced to "B." This movement is repeated 5–10 times for each sampling, or until a sample is seen in the needle hub. Because of the limited motion of the needle, breast thickness is not a limiting factor when performing this tissue sampling. Also, because of the limited motion of the needle, this is a safe procedure to perform in the axilla, where firing a gun or introducing a large probe might hit a major vessel or nerve. (**B**, **C**) Movement of the needle tip within a mass during an aspiration is demonstrated with the farthest excursion (**B**, arrow) and nearest positioning (**C**, arrow) of the needle tip in the lesion while negative pressure is applied to the syringe.

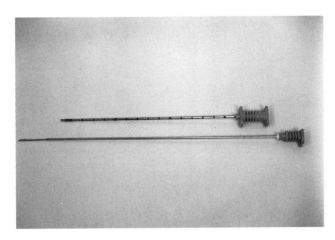

FIGURE 4.3. Components of a cutting needle. The upper needle is the outer component, which advances over the lower needle, cutting off tissue and capturing it in the chamber at the end of the inner needle.

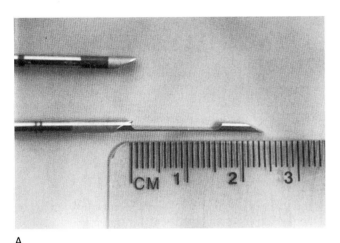

A

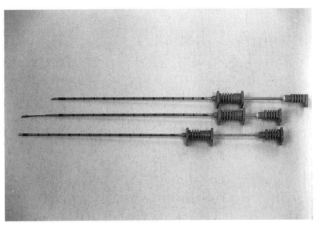

B

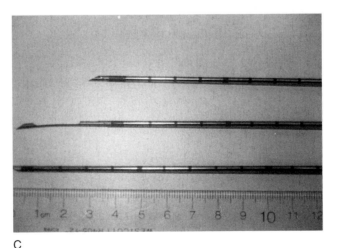

C

FIGURE 4.4. (A) The tip of this long-throw cutting needle is shown in the upper portion in the pre-fire position and in the lower portion with the inner needle fully advanced before the outer needle advances. The needle advances 23 mm to obtain tissue, and the tissue acquisition chamber can hold a specimen up to 17 mm long. **(B)** From top to bottom, the components of the cutting needle are shown in the prefire position, with the inner needle advanced, and in the final postfire position. **(C)** Close-up of the needle tips in the three positions shown in **B**. The downward angulation of the tip of the inner needle causes it to course somewhat downward when it fires into the breast. As the outer needle advances, the inner component is drawn upward, pushing tissue into the acquisition chamber before it is sliced off by the outer needle passing over the chamber.

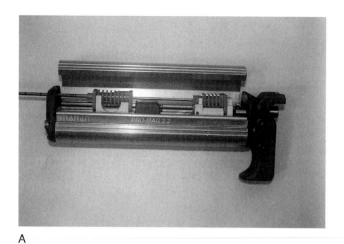
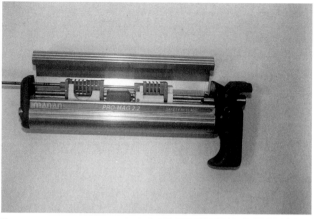

A   B

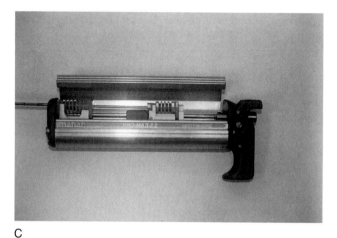

C

FIGURE 4.5. When positioned in the gun, the inner component of the cutting needle is held closer to the trigger, and the outer component is held nearer the needle exit site. These images show the three positions of the needle components in the gun during a biopsy. The gun is shown holding the cutting needle components in the prefire position (**A**), with the inner cutting needle advanced (**B**), and in the postfire position (**C**).

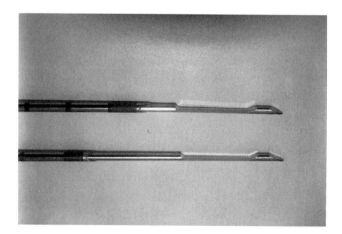

FIGURE 4.6. Tissue acquisition chambers of long- and short-throw needles are shown. Although the chamber of the long-throw needle is only a few millimeters larger than that of the short-throw needle, tissue sampling is better; and often the ability of the needle to pass through resistant tissue is improved with the long-throw needle.

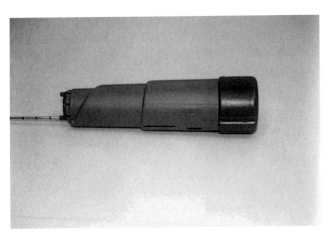

FIGURE 4.7. Disposable gun–needle combination can be more cost effective in facilities that perform few biopsies. The ability to obtain adequate tissue samples is comparable to that of nondisposable guns.

of the tissue sampled, 14-gauge biopsy needles provide better diagnostic results than 18- and 16-gauge needles. Larger volumes of tissue are harvested with the larger gauge needles, and the quality of the specimen is improved. Tissue fragmentation and crush artifact are considerably reduced with the use of 14-gauge needles. This may be particularly true when targeting fibroadenomas and areas of fibrocytic change. However, advantages in the diagnosis of malignant disease, both in situ and invasive, have also been shown with larger gauge needles.

Using 14-gauge needles, these authors have also reported better results with long-throw needles than with short-throw needles. Intra- and interstudy comparisons have demonstrated better diagnostic accuracy with long-throw 14-gauge needles than with short-throw 14-gauge needles. Therefore, when the breast is thick enough to accommodate the long-throw needle, it is generally recommended that this be used rather than the short-throw configuration (Figure 4.8). Whatever the size or the throw of these cutting needles, they all perform better when targeting lesions that are solid masses than clusters of calcifications. The inability of these types of biopsy probes to remove large, contiguous cores from the targeted lesion compromises their ability to obtain an accurate diagnosis in some of these cases.

In addition to needle size and throw, needles of identical gauge and throw from different manufacturers have been demonstrated to retrieve different volumes of tissue.[3] Performing biopsies on breast tissue from cadavers, it was demonstrated that tissue volumes from commercially available 14-gauge long-throw needles varied from 15–24 mm^3.

When performing core biopsies using these needles, it is advisable to obtain cores from throughout the volume of the lesion to optimize sampling. Generally, it is best to target the center of the lesion and sites near the margin at 12, 3, 6, and 9 o'clock. It is usually advised that during a stereotactic biopsy at least five cores should be

obtained when an uncalcified mass is being targeted, if this is possible. One investigator has shown that an accurate diagnosis was obtained in 91 of 92 (99%) biopsies of masses when five cores were obtained.[4] If only one specimen had been obtained, a diagnosis could have been made in 70%. Obtaining more than six specimens was not demonstrated to improve the ability to diagnose masses. When performing these biopsies under sonographic guidance, usually at least three cores through the lesion are obtained, if this is possible.

The ability to obtain a diagnosis when calcifications are targeted depends upon the presence of calcifications within the cores. Specimen radiography should be performed during the biopsy to ascertain if calcifications have been retrieved.[5] When calcifications are present in an individual core, the likelihood of making a diagnosis based on that core approximates 80% versus 40% if no calcification is present. The presence of calcification within the sampled tissue indicates that the correct site within the breast has been sampled. Accuracy of targeting cannot be guaranteed if calcification is not present within the retrieved cores. When calcification is the reason for biopsy, tissue should be removed until calcifications are found on specimen radiography of the cores or until the specimens become so hemorrhagic and fragmented that they do not appear to be of any diagnostic value.

These types of biopsy needles have the advantage of the lowest cost of biopsy probes that can be used to perform core biopsy procedures. Tissue is obtained from the targeted area in a piecemeal fashion, thrusting the needle through noncontiguous sites in the lesion. Because these needles slice off cores of tissue from various sites throughout the lesion, they are very effective in obtaining the diagnosis of lesions that are histologically homogeneous so that obtaining any tissue from the targeted lesion makes it possible for the pathologist to make a diagnosis. However, when the target is heterogeneous (e.g., ductal atypia mixed with ductal carcinoma in situ), this pattern of tissue sampling may decrease the likelihood of obtaining tissue from the most clinically important area of the lesion.

Because the needle dives into the 6 o'clock axis as it moves through the breast, pinpoint accuracy in targeting very small lesions, such as microcalcifications that are not tightly clustered, can be difficult with gun–needle combinations. The exact course of the needle as it travels through the breast can be altered by differing tissue density, slight needle angulation, and patient movement during the biopsy procedure. Therefore, when the target is extremely small, especially when it is microcalcifications, successful targeting can be difficult.

As has been described, the acquisition of tissue using gun–needle devices requires repetitive piercing of the target area with the needle. As the needle moves through a small volume of the breast, there is frequently progressive hemorrhage at the biopsy site and progressive disruption of the lesion by the repetitive skewering. Because

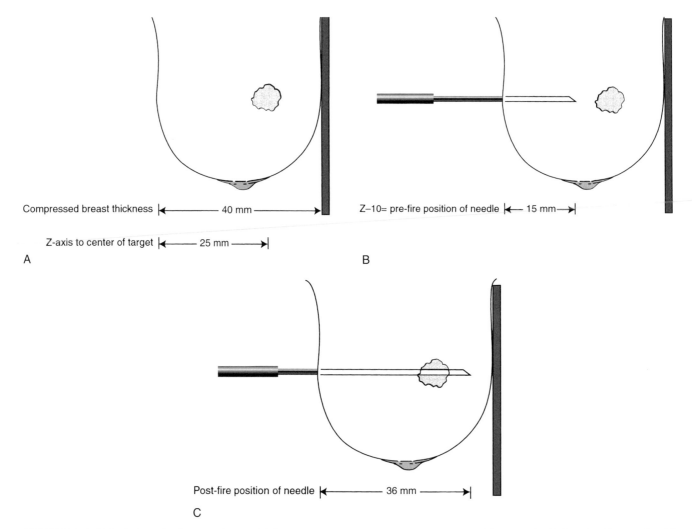

FIGURE 4.8. Calculation of adequate breast thickness to accommodate the movement of the needle during the biopsy should be done before a skin nick is made. Calculation requires knowledge of the compressed breast thickness, depth (*z*-axis) of the target, and distance traveled by the needle. (**A**) In this example, the compressed breast thickness is 40 mm, and the target depth from the skin is 25 mm. (**B**) In the prefire position, the needle is pulled back 10 mm from the target, so that it fires into the lesion. Therefore, the prefire position is 15 mm deep to the skin. (**C**) In this example the needle travels 21 mm during the biopsy. The postfire position of the needle tip is therefore 36 mm. There are 4 mm of breast between the needle tip and the Bucky, which is adequate. At least 2 mm of tissue should be between the needle tip and the Bucky. If adequate tissue is not available, the lesion should be approached from another angle. In some cases compression can be slightly decreased to increase breast thickness, so long as the compression is adequate to hold the breast stable during the biopsy.

of this effect, successful sampling of the lesion can sometimes be difficult after the first few cores have been obtained. As the retrieved tissue becomes increasingly hemorrhagic and disrupted by prior needling, its value for diagnosis is compromised.

DIRECTIONAL, VACUUM SUCTION BIOPSY PROBES

More recently introduced than gun–needle devices are directional, vacuum suction biopsy probes. These allow the removal of contiguous cores of tissue from a targeted site after a single insertion of the probe. The biopsy can be performed without firing the probe inside the breast, making it possible to perform biopsies on thinner breasts and thinner areas of the breast than might be possible when it is necessary to fire a needle within the breast.

These biopsy probes are connected to a vacuum source and its collection chamber for evacuation of blood from the biopsy site. The probe consists of an outer cutting needle, whose leading edge is pointed, with the point somewhat eccentric (Figure 4.9). This configuration cuts through tissue without the downward thrust given to the cutting needle of the gun–needle combinations by the beveled edge of the needle in those probes. Positioning

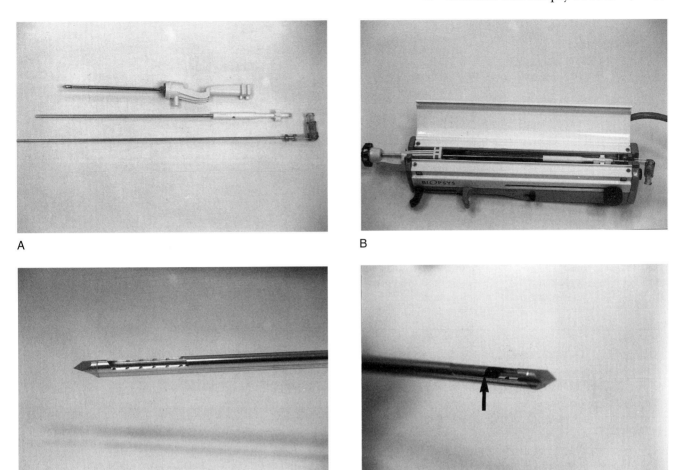

A

B

C

D

FIGURE 4.9. (A) Components of the vacuum suction biopsy probe include, from the top: the vacuum probe and tissue acquisition chamber; the cutting needle that advances into the tissue acquisition probe; and the solid probe that advances into the cutting probe after it is retracted from the breast, pushing the core out of the cutting needle. **(B)** These components are positioned within the biopsy/cutting probe motor, which is attached to a suction setup. **(C)** The tip of the tissue acquisition probe has a beveled end for cutting through the breast. A vacuum is exerted on breast tissue through small holes in the probe, drawing adjacent tissue into the tissue acquisition chamber. This probe can be rotated 360°, making it possible to remove any tissue near the needle tip. **(D)** The cutting probe (arrow) can be seen partially advanced into the tissue acquisition chamber. It has a rapidly rotating motion that cuts through tissue.

of tissue in the tissue acquisition chamber of the vacuum-suction devices does not depend upon the motion of the needle through the breast. Therefore, if it is desired, these probes can be fired within the breast (often improving the cutting action of the needle though the breast tissue) or they can be positioned at the site of the biopsy without firing the biopsy gun (the gun can be fired while the needle is outside of the breast).

When the probe is in proper position, the vacuum is activated, and tissue is pulled through a side hole in the needle into the cutting chamber of the probe. A cutter is then advanced over this tissue, freeing it from the rest of the breast. This core is then transported to an opening in the probe outside of the breast where it is retrieved (Figure 4.10). Multiple cores can be obtained without removing the probe from the breast. Also, it is possible to ro-

tate the probe 360°, facilitating removal of all of the tissue adjacent to the probe. Although the effectiveness of the vacuum to pull tissue into the cutting chamber varies with the resistance of different tissues, the vacuum is usually successful in retrieving tissue during three consecutive rotations of the probe. With gun–needle devices, the needle can only remove tissue located in the path of movement of the needle. Because the probe pulls tissue into the cutting chamber using suction and because contiguous cores of tissue can be obtained, entire volumes of breast tissue can be removed. The removal of larger volumes of tissue than can obtained through gun-needle combinations and the ability to remove a complete volume in the breast means that less accurate targeting is necessary to sample a lesion (Figure 4.11). This is particularly valuable when clusters of microcalcifications are targeted.

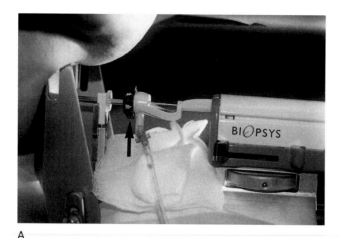 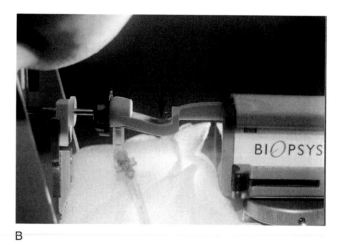

A   B

FIGURE 4.10. The vacuum suction biopsy probe is shown in place during a stereotactic biopsy. (**A**) The cutting needle has been advanced to obtain a core specimen from the breast. The dial (arrow) at the end of the probe is used to rotate it 360°. (**B**) The cutting needle has been retracted, and the core (arrow) is available to be placed in a preservative and sent for analysis.

Directional, vacuum suction probes are also available for use with sonographic guidance (Figure 4.12). Because lesions targeted under sonography are rarely microcalcifications but rather masses, the usefulness of the retrieval of larger volumes of contiguous tissue is somewhat controversial. However, they make it possible to completely remove targeted lesions and introduce localizing clips. These biopsy probes used under sonographic guidance may also be used on stereotactic units.

As with gun–needle combinations, the volume of tissue removed with directional vacuum-suction devices increases with increasing needle size. The probes are generally available in 14- and 11-gauge diameters. Increasingly, 11-gauge probes have been more widely used than the smaller 14-gauge instruments. In one study conducted on turkey breasts, it was found that the average weight of specimens obtained with a 14-gauge vacuum-suction device was 37 mg per core, with an 11-gauge vacuum suction device 94 mg per core, and with a 14-gauge gun–needle device 18 mg per core.[6] The same study found that there was less framentation of specimens when vacuum-suction devices were used than when gun–needle combinations were used (Figure 4.13).

For many lesions, particularly those that appear mammographically or sonographically as a solid mass, the lesion is histologically homogeneous; successful sampling of any portion of the lesion will make it possible for the diagnosis to be made in most of these cases. However,

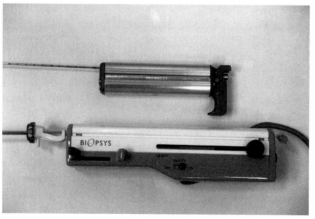 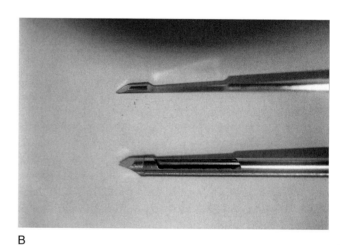

A   B

FIGURE 4.11. (**A**) A comparison of the size of the gun–needle device and the vacuum suction probe suggests the difference in the volumes of tissue removed by these two instruments. (**B**) Close comparison of the tissue acquisition chambers of these two probes demonstrates the capability of the 11-gauge vacuum probe (bottom) to extract larger amounts of tissue than the 14-gauge cutting needle (top). In some instances this difference can improve the ability to diagnose the target lesion accurately.

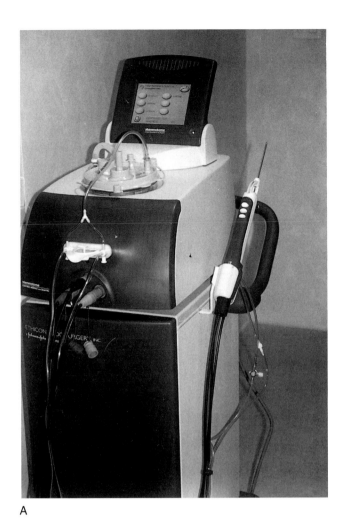

A

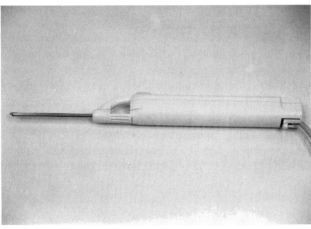

B

FIGURE 4.12. (A) Equipment for the sonographically guided vacuum suction probe. **(B)** Close-up view of the probe.

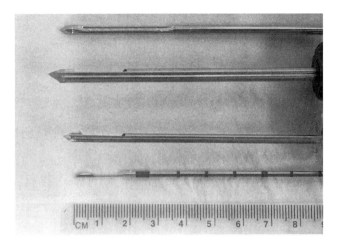

FIGURE 4.13. Tissue acquisition chambers of the most commonly used core biopsy probes. From the top: 11-gauge vacuum suction; 8-gauge vacuum suction; 14-gauge vacuum suction; 14- gauge, long-throw cutting needle.

ithelium has been transformed into atypical ductal hyperplasia (ADH), and some of the duct has undergone further transformation into ductal carcinoma in situ (DCIS). A similar problem exists when carcinoma is present throughout the sampled area of the duct wall, but some of the carcinoma is in situ and some is invasive. These types of lesions are usually characterized on imaging as microcalcifications.

As noted above, the successful retrieval of calcifications may be more difficult that the successful biopsy of a mass because the target is smaller. The ability to remove larger amounts of tissue increases the likelihood that calcium will be obtained during the biopsy procedure. Because of the heterogeneity of many lesions imaged as microcalcifications, the removal of larger volumes of tissue also makes it more likely that the most aggressive area of the lesion will be included in the biopsy specimen. Because of these issues, the use of directional vacuum-suction biopsy probes can considerably improve the validity of biopsy results obtained on lesions seen mammographically as microcalcifications.

Numerous studies have been published to support this conclusion. Of lesions found to be ADH at core biopsy using 14-gauge gun–needle combinations, 20–56% have been found to have carcinoma within the lesion at surgical excision.[7–14] Using vacuum-suction biopsy probes, this rate has been reduced to the 0% to 38% range. While there is some overlap in these values, it is probably reasonable to assume that the underestimation of DCIS as ADH is reduced from one half of core biopsies diagnosed as atypia with 14-gauge gun–needle devices to about one-fourth of biopsies yielding a diagnosis of atypia with 14- or 11-gauge directional vacuum-suction devices.

A similar improvement in diagnostic yield is found with invasive ductal carcinomas that have been underestimated as DCIS at core biopsy. Among lesions diagnosed

lesions that are histologically hetereogeneous are most accurately diagnosed by the removal of larger volumes of tissue. This increases the likelihood that the most aggressive area of the lesion will be sampled. These types of lesions are usually ducts in which some of the duct epas DCIS at core biopsies done with a 14-gauge gun-needle combination, 16% to 35% are found have coexistent invasive carcinoma at surgical biopsy.[7,10–18] Using directional, vacuum-suction probes this number can be reduced to 0–19%. Again, while there is some overlap in these ranges, it can generally be assumed that there is a 20% chance of the 14-gauge gun–needle biopsy diagnosis of DCIS being converted to invasive carcinoma at surgical biopsy. This likelihood can be reduce to about 10% when the core biopsy specimen is obtained using vacuum-suction probes.

Despite these advantages for directional, vacuum-suction probes, some disadvantages also exist. Perhaps the most important of these is the increased cost of using this technology. For 14-gauge vacuum-suction needles, the price is about 10 times higher for each needle than the 14-gauge cutting needle used in the gun–needle combination (the nondisposable gun). The cost of the biopsy gun and suction setup to perform these procedures is also about 10 times as expensive as the cost of a nondisposable gun for the cutting needle. If the 11-gauge directional, vacuum suction probe is used, this is approximately twice as expensive as the 14-gauge directional, vacuum-suction needle.

Because of the removal of larger volumes of tissue with the vacuum-suction probes, it is possible to completely excise lesions that are targeted for biopsy. Depending upon the results of the biopsy, rebiopsy of the area for definitive diagnosis or reexcision of the site for treatment might be necessary. Therefore, accurate localization of the site of the lesion will be necessary in some cases. If there is no adjacent landmark and if the lesion has been totally excised, accurate relocalization may be difficult or impossible. Acute biopsy changes can be seen during the procedure on mammographic or sonographic images. However, any evidence of biopsy is lacking on the mammograms of one-fourth of women taken immediately after the biopsy procedure.[19] When present, changes of hemorrhage and/or air at the biopsy site frequently resolve within a few days of the core biopsy procedure. When an automated gun–needle is used, these changes were reported to have totally resolved on mammograms of all women obtained 6 months after the original biopsy.[20] In a study of 14-gauge vacuum suction biopsy probes, post-core biopsy changes were found on 88% of mammograms obtained immediately following the biopsy procedure.[21] Among the 108 lesions included in this study, no residual mammographic evidence of the original lesion was seen in 13% of the cases. Of these women, 19 underwent needle localization procedures shortly after the core biopsy procedure (mean time to needle localization after core biopsy was 19 days). At the time of the needle localization, no mammographic changes due to the core biopsy were seen in 18 women (95%).

When selecting a lesion, particularly a small lesion, to undergo core biopsy, it is important to be able to mark the site for reexcision if the lesion is totally removed during the biopsy procedure and there is no nearby landmark. This makes it possible to localize the site if reexcision or repeat biopsy is necessary. In this situation, it is necessary to be able to mark the site of the lesion. This can be done by placing a localizing clip through the biopsy probe. (Figure 4.14) The cost of the clip is approximately equal to the cost of the 14-gauge vacuum-suction biopsy probe Additionally, positioning the clip can only be accomplished by using the more expensive 11-gauge vacuum-suction probe. It also requires that a mammogram be obtained at the completion of the biopsy to document the relation of the clip to the biopsy site. These factors considerably increase the cost of the biopsy procedure.

Fortunately, positioning a localizing clip also makes it possible to perform core biopsies of small lesions that might be totally excised, even through 14-gauge gun–needle devices. While some facilities do not perform core biopsies on small lesions (e.g., 5 mm in maximum diameter or smaller) because of the risk of not being able to relocalize the site for repeat biopsy or surgical reexcision, this is no longer a problem. Paradoxically, the largest biopsy probes, the 11-gauge vacuum-suction probes, must be used to remove the smallest lesions because they make it possible to deposit a localizing clip at the biopsy site.

Other, less expensive, localizing techniques have been described, but these are not in widespread use in the United States. The injection of pharmaceutical-grade charcoal is often performed outside of the United States.[22] However, this agent is not FDA approved for injection into the breast. Positioning an embolization clip has also been described, but this technique has not been widely adopted.

Some other disadvantages of vacuum-suction biopsy have been described. Mammographic alterations at long-term follow-up are, at most, extremely rare after the use of gun-needle combinations. One author has reported that mammography done 6–12 months after the core biopsy procedure showed no changes attributable to the biopsy in any of the 422 women biopsied with 14-gauge gun–needle probes.[23] No changes were seen in any of the 96 mammograms of women biopsied with a 14-gauge vacuum suction device. In 2% of the 266 women biopsied using an 11-gauge vacuum-suction device, mammographic changes persisted. However, these authors stated that all of the postbiopsy changes on the mammogram were categorized as BIRADS category 2 (benign; no biopsy or short-term follow-up required).

Because vacuum-suction probes remove larger volumes of tissue than gun–needle devices, there may be a greater chance of hemorrhage during the biopsy, but this risk is poorly documented. However, some physicians

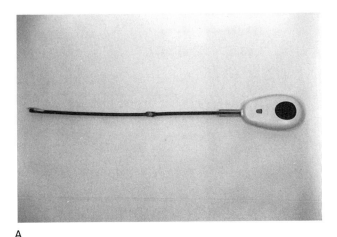

A

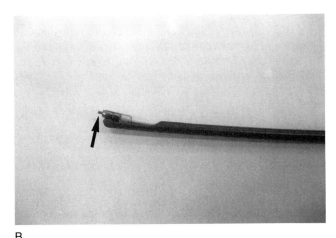

B

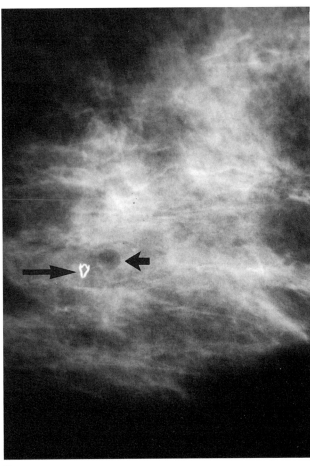

C

FIGURE 4.14. (A) The clip deployment device used for placement of a localization clip in the breast after core biopsy. The black circle on the white handle is depressed to release the clip into the breast. **(B)** The tip of the clip deployment device. The clip (arrow) is on the tip of the inner white catheter. It angles slightly upward when it is positioned. **(C)** Clip (long arrow) in place on a post-core-biopsy mammogram. Note that it is positioned just next to the small amount of air (short arrow) introduced into the breast during the biopsy.

consider it desirable to use epinephrine along with the injected local anesthetic for deep injection at the biopsy site. Epinephrine is useful for constricting local vasculature, decreasing bleeding, and prolonging the local anesthetic effect. In women with cardiac disease the use of epinephrine is not recommended.

ECONOMICS OF DIFFERENT BIOPSY PROBES

There are multiple advantages, both personal and societal, conveyed by the replacement of surgical breast biopsies with core needle biopsies. Diminished scarring, less time and risk to undergo the biopsy, and frequently faster determination of the presence or absence of malignancy are obvious advantages upon which a price cannot be placed. Additionally, there is a considerable diminution

in the cost of biopsy and the cost of mammographic screening that occurs by performance of these procedures percutaneously rather than surgically. Although cost calculations in dollars are variable from year to year and from venue to venue, a real reduction in cost has been demonstrated for these technologies.

It has been calculated that when the 14-gauge gun–needle biopsy technology with mammographic guidance, is used in place of surgical biopsy, the marginal cost of mammographic screening for women beginning at age 40 and ending at age 85 can be reduced by up to 23%.[24] In 1994 dollars, it was calculated that the cost per year of life saved could be reduced from $20,770 to $15,934. Numerous other studies have demonstrated a cost reduction of 40% to 58% using 14-gauge gun-needle percutaneous biopsy compared with the cost of a surgical diagnosis.[25–28] In these studies, the need for surgical biopsy was eliminated in 76% to 81% of women.

Although most of these studies were done using stereotactic guidance, sonographically guided biopsies have also been shown to be cost-effective. Using 14-gauge vacuum-suction devices with sonographic guidance, a 56% decrease in the cost of diagnosis has been demonstrated.[29] In that study, it was suggested that cost savings are maximized if lesions can be biopsied under sonographic rather than stereotactic guidance.

Despite its greater expense, vacuum-suction technology has also shown an ability to decrease cost of care. In a study of 11-gauge vacuum-suction breast biopsy, it was found that in 200 consecutive stereotactic biopsies, the need for surgical intervention was eliminated in 76% of cases.[30] The cost of surgical diagnosis was estimated at $1289. The cost of core biopsy diagnosis was $264 less, a 20% decrease. The authors concluded that even this more expensive technology results in a reduction in the cost of care compared to surgery. Also, despite its higher cost than other techniques for core biopsy, it was advantageous in making these procedures available to a larger number of women by increasing the number of lesions amenable to stereotactic biopsy.

ADDITIONAL EQUIPMENT

These procedures are performed using sterile technique. Sterile gloves should be used by the physician performing the biopsy. Assisting technologists or physicians should wear examining gloves if they come in contact with specimens or contaminated material and do not touch the sterile field. The skin at the biopsy site should be sterilized with povidone-iodine. At some facilities the breast is draped with sterile towels; others do not believe that this is necessary. Alcohol and 4 × 4 pads are useful for cleansing the skin after the procedure. If sonographic guidance is being used, the transducer can be cleaned with alcohol or covered with gel and then fitted with a sterile condom or examining glove. All equipment that comes in contact with the patient and is exposed to possible contamination should be soaked in a sterilizing agent between procedures (Figure 4.15).

A #11 scalpel is used to cut the skin and subcutaneous fibrous tissues, improving movement of the biopsy probe through these resistant tissues. Anesthesia is given for core biopsies and may also be used for aspiration procedures. Cutaneous anesthesia is given with a 3 cc syringe and 25-gauge 1.5 inch needle. For stereotactic biopsies done on a prone table, it can be useful to bend the needle almost 90° (Figure 4.16). A 10 cc syringe with a 21-gauge 1 inch needle can be used for deep anesthesia. One percent lidocaine with epinephrine or 2% carbocaine can be used as deep anesthesia. It is advisable not to inject epinephrine subcutaneously; it has been reported to cause skin necrosis.

For core biopsies a 10 cc syringe fitted with a needle

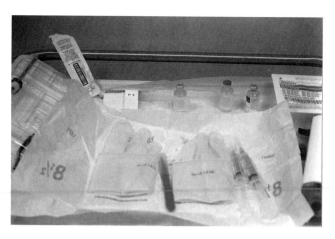

FIGURE 4.15. Equipment needed for a stereotactic core biopsy includes sterile gloves, scalpel for skin incision, anesthetic with needles for injection, sterile gauze, normal saline with syringe for assisting in removal of specimen from the cutting needle, agent for cleaning skin, biopsy probe, and gun. For sonographically guided procedures, a sterile contact agent (gel, alcohol, iodine soap) is also needed.

and filled with sterile normal saline should be available to help remove the specimen from the cutting needle or to keep specimens moist if they are kept outside of a preservative agent until specimen radiography is performed. The agent used to preserve the specimen should be selected by the laboratory that will be processing the specimen. Care should be taken throughout the biopsy or aspiration procedure not to contaminate the biopsy needle with preservative if it is being reintroduced into the breast.

At the end of the biopsy the wound should be bandaged. For aspirations, a simple bandage is usually adequate. After core biopsies, Steri-Strips can be used to close the skin wound. Sterile 4 × 4 gauze pads can then

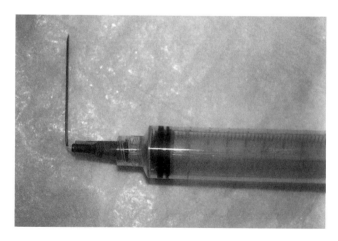

FIGURE 4.16. For the subcutaneous injection of anesthesia before stereotactic biopsy using a prone table, bending the needle at 90° can be helpful in directing the anesthetic into subcutaneous tissue.

be taped over the skin. Paper tape is often better tolerated. It can be helpful to keep sports bras available to apply additional pressure over the biopsied breast, particularly when there has been some difficulty with bleeding during the biopsy.

HISTOPATHOLOGIC ISSUES

The different methods by which gun–needle devices and vacuum-suction probes remove tissue can result in different qualities and quantities of the specimens obtained and different alterations in the breast at the biopsy site. It is important to understand how these differences may impact on the diagnostic efficacy of the procedure and the status of the breast.

Because they obtain larger cores and because these are contiguous, vacuum-suction probes have the ability to completely remove some lesions, particularly if they are small. In a summary of results of various studies, increasing likelihood of removal of lesions with increasing size of biopsy probes has been demonstrated.[31] Among three studies conducted with 14-gauge gun–needle devices, target lesions were totally removed in a mean of 7% of cases (range, 4–9%).[19,32,33] Using a 14-gauge vacuum-suction technique, target lesions were totally removed in a mean of 42% of women in six studies (range, 13–60%).[21,32–34,36,37] With the use of 11-gauge vacuum-suction probes in four studies, a mean of 65% (range, 46–71%) of lesions were completely excised.[33,35–37]

As has been noted above, the removal of larger amounts of tissue, particularly when the lesion is characterized mammographically as microcalcifications, may result in the greater likelihood of accurate diagnosis. However, caution on two issues is important. As has been discussed, it is inappropriate to totally remove a lesion unless the site of the biopsy can be identified for later localization. This might be required to obtain additional tissue for definitive diagnosis. It may also be necessary for therapy.

Second, the physician must be cognizant of the fact that the total removal of the lesion seen on imaging does not necessarily indicate that the entire lesion has been histopathologically excised. Because the true extent of the lesion is often greater than the volume of the lesion seen on mammography or sonography, complete excision of the lesion seen on imaging studies does not necessarily indicate complete removal of this lesion. In a study of 15 carcinomas in which the mammographic lesion was totally removed using 11-gauge vacuum-suction probes, residual carcinoma was found in 11 patients (73%) at surgery.[38] This reinforces the need for a localizing device to be placed at the biopsy site when the targeted lesion has been totally excised. These data also reinforce the need for surgical reexcision of carcinomas that appear to have been completely removed at the time of percutaneous biopsy. *These procedures should not be considered therapeutic.*

Although there is no therapeutic advantage to the total excision of benign lesions percutaneously, in some unusual instances it might be advantageous for the patient to have the targeted lesion totally removed. There is a small percentage of lesions that, although benign, will be observed to enlarge on follow-up examinations and will need to be excised. This event has been reported to occur in 7% to 9% of cases.[39,40] Complete removal of the imaged lesion might eliminate the need for excision due to interval enlargement in at least some of these cases.

Because of the different patterns of motion in the breast, the likelihood that these procedures displace epithelial cells within the breast may be different. Also, the vacuum used in the vacuum-suction probes may act to remove at least some dislodged cells from the breast. At least theoretically, this has the possibility of dislodging tumor cells within the breast or into the bloodstream and lymphatics. Because tumor cells might be displaced away from the site of an in situ carcinoma, this phenomenon also has the possibility of causing a misdiagnosis of invasive carcinoma. This could cause overtreatment with axillary surgery and/or chemotherapy of a noninvasive carcinoma.

The technique for biopsy with gun–needle devices requires repetitive thrusting of the cutting needle through the lesion. With vacuum-suction probes, only a single insertion of the biopsy probe into the site of the lesion is required; tissue is removed by repetitive suctioning of breast tissue into the tissue acquisition chamber. The motion of the vacuum-suction probes might be expected to be less likely to dislodge epithelial or tumor cells than the repetitive cutting motion of the gun–needle probes. In two studies from the same institution, 14-gauge gun–needle combinations were found to result in displacement of cells beyond the site of a carcinoma in 28% of 43 biopsies.[41] Using 11-gauge vacuum-suction probes, benign epithelium was displaced into surrounding stroma in only 7% of 28 cases.[42] In another study, epithelial cells were found to be displaced into the skin in two of eight women (25%) who underwent biopsy with 14-gauge gun–needle devices and none of those who underwent biopsy using vacuum-suction biopsy or with a coaxial sheath placed in the breast for sonographically guided gun-needle biopsy.[43] In a study that examined 352 surgical specimens for evidence of epithelial displacement, displaced tumor cells were found in 32% of carcinomas that had been preoperatively diagnosed with gun–needle combinations and 23% of those that had been preoperatively diagnosed with vacuum-suction probes.[44]

The clinical implication of this phenomenon is somewhat controversial, but there are data to suggest that although tumor cells are displaced by these procedures, they have minimal if any biological activity. A 15-year follow-up study has been reported on women matched stage for stage for their breast carcinomas, all of which were treated by mastectomy.[43] Women who were preoperatively diagnosed with needle aspiration of their tumors were compared with those without preoperative needling. No difference in long-term follow-up between the two groups was reported. Another study has looked at the difference in local recurrence of women who underwent preoperative needle localization versus those without this procedure.[45] Again, there was no difference in local tumor recurrence in the two groups. In still another study, it was found that displaced cells seemed to disappear with increasing time after core needle biopsy.[44] Among women in this study, tumor displacement was evident in 42% who underwent surgery within 15 days of biopsy; among those undergoing surgery 15–28 days after core biopsy, there was evidence of displaced tumor cells in 31%; and when surgery was performed more than 28 days after biopsy, epithelial displacement was only seen in 15%.

These studies suggest that there is very rarely, if ever, clinical significance to the displacement of tumor cells during percutaneous biopsy procedures. The higher incidence of this phenomenon during gun–needle procedures (especially if done without a coaxial guidance system) versus a directional vacuum-suction system does not need to influence the choice of biopsy probe.

It is important that pathologists interpreting core biopsy specimens be aware of the possibility of epithelial displacement by the biopsy probe and be able to differentiate artificially displaced tumor cells from those that are truly due to invasive carcinoma. Several characteristics have been described that are useful in making this distinction. These include the absence of surrounding tissue reaction, which would be expected with infiltrating carcinoma; the presence of epithelial cells in artificial spaces; and the association of questionable invasive tumor cells with histologic evidence of the needle tract, including hemorrhage, hemosiderin-laden macrophages, fat necrosis, granulation tissue, and inflammation.[41,42,46,47] Using these criteria, the overdiagnosis of DCIS as invasive carcinoma should be minimized.

COMPLICATIONS

Major complications of these procedures are rare. In a multiinstitutional study of more than 6,000 lesions, complications occurred in only 12 (0.2%).[48] These were defined as events that required additional medical or surgical intervention. They included three hematomas that needed surgical drainage and three infections that required drainage and/or antibiotics.

Although these complications are rare, they can compromise the ability to treat the disease diagnosed during the biopsy. One case has been reported in which a large hematoma developed after biopsy and made it impossi-

ble to resect a carcinoma found at biopsy for several months until the hematoma resolved.[49]

Sterile technique should be used during the biopsy, minimizing the likelihood of postbiopsy infection. If a coagulopathy exists, whether drug induced (e.g., aspirin, Coumadin) or due to an inherent clotting disorder in the patient, biopsy can be delayed until coagulation is normalized. Routine testing of coagulation before biopsy is usually not done.

Even in women with compromised coagulation, the performance of core biopsy has been described as being safely performed.[50] Icing the breast before the biopsy has been suggested to decrease the likelihood of hemorrhage in this setting. The application of ice to the breast in all women while pressure is applied to obtain hemostasis after the biopsy is useful to control bleeding at the biopsy site.

Minor complications are common after these procedures.[51] Although the physical impact of these biopsies is usually minimal, psychologically they can be extremely difficult. Anxiety surrounding the procedure commonly results in the inability of the patient to return to normal activities on the day of the biopsy.[52] It is worthwhile to advise women that they may not be able to return to work immediately after the biopsy because of this. It is also advantageous to have someone accompany the patient to the biopsy and on her return home after the procedure.

Other minor complications include bruising and pain at the biopsy site. Bruising occurs in about one half of women. Breast pain, requiring analgesics, occurs in about one third. Pain is usually readily controlled with over-the-counter analgesic agents. Women should be advised that aspirin and ibuprofin should be avoided for several days after the biopsy, as they can compromise coagulation.

REFERENCES

1. Nath ME, Robinson TM, Tobon H, Chough DF, Sumkin JH. Automated large-core needle biopsy of surgically removed breast lesions: comparison of samples obtained with 14-, 16- and 18-gauge needles. Radiology 1995;197:739–742.
2. Helbich TH, Rudas M, Haitel A, et al. Evaluation of needle size for breast biopsy: comparison of 14-, 16- and 18-gauge biopsy needles. AJR 1998;171:59–63.
3. Krebs TL, Berg WA, Severson MJ, et al. Large-core biopsy guns: comparison for yield of breast tissue. Radiology 1996; 200:365–368.
4. Liberman L, Dershaw DD, Rosen PP, Abramson AF, Deutch BM, Hann LE. Stereotaxic 14-breast biopsy: how many core biopsy specimens are needed? Radiology 1994;192:793–795.
5. Liberman L, Evans WP, Dershaw DD, et al. Specimen radiography of microcalcifications in stereotaxic mammary core biopsy specimens. Radiology 1994;190:223–225.
6. Berg WA, Krebs TL, Campassi C, Magder LS, Sun CCJ. Evaluation of 14- and 11-gauge directional, vacuum-assisted breast biopsy probes and 14-gauge biopsy guns in a breast parenchymal model. Radiology 1997;205:203–208.

7. Jackman RJ, Nowels KW, Shepard MJ, Finkelstein SI, Marzoni FA. Stereotaxic large-core needle biopsy of 450 nonpalpable breast lesions with surgical correlation in lesions with cancer or atypical hyperplasia. Radiology 1994;193:91–95.

8. Liberman L, Dershaw DD, Glassman J, et al. Analysis of cancers not diagnosed at stereotactic core breast biopsy. Radiology 1997;203:151–157.

9. Liberman L, Cohen MA, Dershaw DD, Abramson AF, Hann LE, Rosen PP. Atypical ductal hyperplasia diagnosed at stereotaxic core biopsy of breast lesions: an indication for surgical biopsy. AJR 1995;164:1111–1113.

10. Burbank F. Stereotactic breast biopsy of atypical ductal hyperplasia and ductal carcinoma in situ lesions: improved accuracy with a directional, vacuum-assisted biopsy instrument. Radiology 1997;202:843–847.

11. Jackman RJ, Burbank F, Parker SH, et al. Atypical ductal hyperplasia diagnosed at stereotactic breast biopsy: improved reliability with 14-gauge, directional, vacuum-assisted biopsy. Radiology 1997;204:485–488.

12. Jackman RJ, Burbank FH, Parker SH, et al. Atypical ductal hyperplasia diagnosed by 11-gauge, directional, vacuum-assisted breast biopsy: how often is carcinoma found at surgery (abstract)? Radiology 1997;205(P):325.

13. Philpotts LE, Shaheen NA, Carter D, Lange RC, Lee CH. Comparison of rebiopsy rates after stereotactic core needle biopsy of the breast with 11-gauge vacuum suction probe versus 14-gauge needle and automatic gun. AJR 1999;172:683–687.

14. Brem RF, Behrndt VS, Sanow L, Gatewood OMB. Atypical ductal hyperplasia: histologic underestimation of carcinoma in tissue harvested from impalpable breast lesions using 11-gauge stereotactically guided directional vacuum-assisted biopsy. AJR 1999;172:1405–1407.

15. Dershaw DD, Morris EA, Liberman L, Abramson AF. Nondiagnostic stereotaxic core breast biopsy: results of rebiopsy. Radiology 1996;198:323–325.

16. Liberman L, Dershaw DD, Rosen PP, et al. Stereotaxic core biopsy of breast carcinoma: accuracy at predicting invasion. Radiology 1995;194:379–381.

17. Jackman RJ, Burbank FH, Parker SH, et al. Accuracy of sampling ductal carcioma in situ by three stereotactic breast biopsy methods (abstract). Radiology 1998;209(P):197–198.

18. Won B, Reynolds HE, Lazaridis CL, Jackson VP. Stereotactic biopsy of ductal carcinoma in situ of the breast using an 11-gauge vacuum-assisted device: persistent underestimation of disease. AJR 1999;173:227–229.

19. Hann LE, Liberman L, Dershaw DD, Cohen MA, Abramson AF. Mammography immediately after stereotaxic core breast biopsy: is it necessary? AJR 1995;165:59–62.

20. Kaye MD, Vicinanza-Adami CA, Sullivan ML. Mammographic findings after stereotaxic core biopsy of the breast performed with large-core needles. Radiology 1994;192:149–151.

21. Liberman L, Hann LE, Dershaw DD, et al. Mammographic findings after stereotactic 14-gauge vacuum biopsy. Radiology 1997;203:343–347.

22. Canavese G, Catturich A, Vecchio C, et al. Pre-operative localization of nonpalpable lesions in breast cancer by charcoal suspension. Eur J Surg Oncol 1995;21:47–49.

23. Lamm RL, Jackman RJ. Mammographic abnormalities caused by percutaneous stereotactic biopsy of histologically benign lesions evident on follow-up mammograms. AJR 2000;174:753–756.

24. Lindfors KK, Rosenquist CJ. Needle core biopsy guided with mammography: a study of cost effectiveness. Radiology 1994;190:217–222.

25. Liberman L, Fahs MC, Dershaw DD, et al. Impact of stereotaxic core biopsy on cost of diagnosis. Radiology 1995;195:633–637.

26. Hillner BE, Bear HD, Fajardo LL. Estimating the cost-effectiveness of stereotaxic biopsy for nonpalpable breast abnormalities: a decision analysis model. Acad Radiol 1996;3:351–360.

27. Fajardo LL. Cost-effectiveness of stereotaxic breast core needle biopsy. Acad Radiol 1996;3:521–523.

28. Lee CH, Egglin TIK, Philpotts LE, Mainiero MB, Tocino I. Cost-effectiveness of stereotactic core needle biopsy: analysis by means of mammographic findings. Radiology 1997;202:849–854.

29. Liberman L, Feng TL, Dershaw DD, Morris EA, Abramson AF. Ultrasound-guided core breast biopsy: utility and cost-effectiveness. Radiology 1998;208:717–723.

30. Liberman L, Sama MP. Cost-effectiveness of stereotactic 11-gauge directional vacuum-assisted breast biopsy. AJR 2000;175:53–58.

31. Liberman L. Clinical management issues in percutaneous core breast biopsy. Radiol Clin North Am 2000;38:791–807.

32. Burbank F. Mammographic findings after 14-gauge automated needle and 14-gauge directional, vacuum-assisted stereotactic breast biopsies. Radiology 1997;204:153–156.

33. Jackman RJ, Marzoni FA, Nowels KW. Percutaneous removal of benign mamographic lesions: comparison of automated large-core and directional vacuum-assisted biopsy techniques. AJR 1998;171:1325–1330.

34. Burbank F, Parker SH, Fogarty TJ. Stereotactic breast biopsy: improved tissue harvesting with the Mammotome. Am Surg 1996;62:738–744.

35. Burbank F, Forcier N. Tissue marking clip for stereotactic breast biopsy: initial placement accuracy, long-term stability, and usefulness as a guide for wire localization. Radiology 1997;205:407–415.

36. Liberman L, Smolkin JH, Dershaw DD, et al. Calcification retrieval at stereotactic 11-gauge vacuum-assisted breast biopsy. Radiology 1998;208:251–260.

37. Liberman L, Dershaw DD, Morris EA, et al. Clip placement after stereotactic vacuum-assisted breast biopsy. Radiology 1997;205:417–422.

38. Liberman L, Dershaw DD, Rosen PP, et al. Percutaneous removal of malignant mammographic lesions at stereotactic vacuum-assisted biopsy. Radiology 1998;206:711–715.

39. Lee CH, Philpotts LE, Horwath LJ, et al. Follow-up of breast lesions diagnosed as benign with stereotactic core-needle biopsy: frequency of mammographic change and false-negative rate. Radiology 1999;212:189–184.

40. Jackman RJ, Nowels KW, Rodriguez-Soto J, et al. Stereotactic, automated, large-core needle biopsy of nonpalpable breast lesions: false-negative and histologic underestimation rates after long-term follow-up. Radiology 1999;210:799–805.

41. Youngston BJ, Liberman L, Rosen PP. Displacement of carcinomatous epithelium in surgical breast specimens following stereotaxic core biopsy. Am J Clin Pathol 1995;103:598–602.

42. Liberman L, Vuolo M, Dershaw DD, et al. Epithelial displacement after stereotactic 11-gauge directional vacuum-assisted breast biopsy. AJR 1999;172:677–681.

43. Stolier A. Seeding of the skin following core biopsy of the breast: a prospective study. *In* The Society of Surgical Oncology 52nd Annual Cancer Symposium Abstract Book. Arlington Heights, IL: Society of Surgical Oncology 1999; 27.

44. Diaz LK, Wiley EL, Venta LA. Are malignant cells displaced by large-gauge needle biopsy of the breast? AJR 1999;173: 1303–1313.

45. Berg JW, Robbins GF. A late look at the safety of aspiration biopsy. Cancer 1962;15:826–827.

46. Kopans DB, Gallagher WJ, Swann CA, et al. Does preoperative needle localization lead to an increase in local breast cancer recurrence? Radiology 1988;167:667–668.

47. Youngston BJ, Cranor M, Rosen PP. Epithelial displacement in surgical breast biopsies following needling procedures. Am J Surg Pathol 1994;18:896–903.

48. Parker SH, Burbank F, Jackman RJ, et al. Percutaneous large-core breast biopsy: a multi-institutional study. Radiology 1994;193:359–364.

49. Deutch BM, Schwartz MR, Fodera T, Ray DM. Stereotactic core breast biopsy of a minimal carcinoma complicated by a large hematoma: a management dilemma. Radiology 1997; 202:431–433.

50. Melotti MK, Berg WA. Core needle breast biopsy in patients undergoing anticoagulation therapy: preliminary results. AJR 2000;174:245–249.

51. Dershaw DD, Caravella BA, Liberman L. Limitations and complications in the utilization of stereotaxic core breast biopsy. Breast J 1996;2:13–17.

52. Maxwell JR, Bugbee ME, Wellisch D, et al. Imaging-guided core needle biopsy of the breast: study of psychological outcomes. Breast J 2000;6:53–61.

CHAPTER 5

Stereotactic Core Biopsy

Laura Liberman

Since its description in Sweden in the 1970s,[1] stereotactic biopsy has been increasingly used for breast diagnosis. Stereotactic biopsy provides an accurate, safe, and cost-effective alternative to surgical biopsy for mammographically evident lesions.[2] Although early studies of stereotactic biopsy used fine needles, fine needle aspiration has many limitations including benign nonspecific diagnoses, incomplete characterization of both benign and malignant lesions, and insufficient samples.[3] The limitations of the fine needles led to the development of techniques for stereotactic biopsy using larger tissue acquisition devices including automated core needles and directional vacuum-assisted biopsy probes. This chapter discusses the accuracy, safety, cost, indications and contraindications, equipment, and technique of stereotactic core biopsy and gives specific suggestions for biopsy of challenging cases.

ACCURACY OF STEREOTACTIC BIOPSY

Stereotactic core breast biopsy was pioneered in the United States by Parker and colleagues in a landmark article published in 1990.[4] Since that time, validation studies of stereotactic automated core biopsy with surgical correlation have shown 87–96% concordance between the results of stereotactic automated core biopsy and surgical biopsy with insufficient samples obtained in 0% to 17% of cases[5–9] (Table 5.1). The best results were obtained by those investigators who obtained multiple passes with a 14-gauge needle and long-excursion gun (Table 5.1).[5,6]

In clinical follow-up studies after stereotactic 14-gauge automated core biopsy, the frequency of missed carcinomas averaged 2.8% (range, 0.3% to 8.2%), with approximately 70% of missed cancers identified shortly after biopsy (immediate false-negatives) and 30% identified subsequently (delayed false-negatives).[2,10,11] This

frequency is comparable to the frequency of missed cancer at needle localization and surgical biopsy, which has an average cancer miss rate of 2.0% (range, 0% to 8%).[12] Steps that can minimize the likelihood and potential impact of a false-negative diagnosis include meticulous attention to technique (particularly with respect to lesion targeting), specimen radiography for calcifications, imaging–histologic correlation, and prompt recommendation for surgical excision when warranted by the stereotactic biopsy histology.

ADVANTAGES OF STEREOTACTIC BIOPSY: COST

Stereotactic biopsy has many advantages compared to surgical biopsy. It is faster, less invasive, causes minimal to no scarring, and is less expensive than surgical biopsy.[2] In previous studies, stereotactic 14-gauge automated core biopsy spared the patient a surgical procedure in 76–81% of cases, decreasing the cost of diagnosis by 40% to 58%.[13–15] Liberman et al.[13] calculated that if stereotactic 14-gauge automated core biopsy were used instead of surgical biopsy for histologic diagnosis of nonpalpable breast lesions, annual national savings would approach $200 million.

The 11-gauge vacuum-assisted devices are more expensive than the 14-gauge automated needles, but expand the population of women who are candidates for stereotactic biopsy. In one study, stereotactic 11-gauge vacuum-assisted biopsy spared a surgical procedure in 76% of lesions, yielding a 20% decrease in cost of diagnosis.[13] Liberman and Sama[16] calculated that selective use of 11-gauge vacuum-assisted biopsy for calcifications and lesions not amenable to stereotactic 14-gauge automated core biopsy would increase annual national savings by over $50 million.

TABLE 5.1. *Stereotactic automated core breast biopsy studies with surgical correlation*

Investigator	Year	No. of cases	No. of passes	Needle	Gun	Concordance (%)	Insufficient (%)
Parker[5]	1991	102[a]	3–4	14G	Long	96	0
Elvecrog[6]	1993	100[a]	≥5	14G	Long	94	0
Gisvold[8]	1994	104[a]	≥5	14G	Long	90	0
Dronkers[7]	1992	53[b]	2	18G	Short	91	6
Parker[4]	1990	10[c]	3–4	18G (n = 65), 16G (n = 9), 14G (n = 29)	Long (n = 101), short (n = 2)	87	1
Gisvold[8]	1994	56[a]	<5	14G	Long	80	2
Dowlatshahi[a]	1991	250[a]	2–3	20G	Long (n = 130), short (n = 120)	67–69	

G, gauge.
[a]Prone.
[b]Upright.
[c]Upright in 30, prone in 73.

INDICATIONS AND CONTRAINDICATIONS

Breast Imaging Reporting and Data System (BI-RADS) Category

Stereotactic biopsy is used to obtain histologic diagnoses on mammographically evident lesions that would otherwise warrant surgical biopsy.[17] Stereotactic biopsy is most often used for biopsy of lesions that are suspicious (Breast Imaging Reporting and Data System, or BI-RADS, category 4). Category 4 lesions account for approximately 70% of lesions referred for biopsy; of these, 30% to 40% are malignant.[19,20] Stereotactic biopsy also decreases the number of operations performed in women who have lesions that are highly suggestive of malignancy (BI-RADS Category 5).[21,22] Category 5 lesions account for approximately 20% of lesions that undergo biopsy; of these, approximately 80–90% are malignant.[19,20] "Probably benign" (BI-RADS Category 3) lesions have an extremely low (0.5–2%) frequency of cancer,[23,24] and are best managed with short-term follow-up mammography rather than biopsy except under special circumstances (e.g., if the patient is unable to comply with follow-up, is extremely anxious, or has a synchronous breast cancer).

Stereotactic Versus Ultrasound Guidance

Core biopsy can be performed under stereotactic or ultrasound guidance[25]; considerations impacting on the choice of guidance modality include lesion visibility, equipment availability, physician and patient preferences, and cost. Stereotaxis is the guidance modality of choice for lesions evident as calcifications without an associated soft tissue mass. Stereotactic guidance is also preferable for mass lesions that are sonographically inapparent or too subtle to target sonographically, if breast immobilization is considered necessary, or if the patient is unable to cooperate with the ultrasound-guided biopsy procedure. For masses visible mammographically and sonographically, ultrasound-guided biopsy is faster, does not require ionizing radiation, and allows real-time visualization of the needle.[26] Furthermore, although both stereotactic and ultrasound-guided core biopsy are less expensive than surgery, cost savings are greater for biopsies performed under ultrasound guidance.[27]

Contraindications

Stereotactic biopsy is contraindicated for lesions that cannot be targeted (i.e., cannot be definitively identified on stereotactic images) or cannot be included on the images (e.g., due to extreme posterior position). Stereotactic biopsy is also contraindicated for patients who cannot cooperate with the procedure or who have bleeding diatheses. Inability to tolerate local anesthesia is a contraindication but is rare, particularly to local anesthetics of the amide type (e.g., lidocaine); allergy most often occurs with ester-type agents (e.g., procaine) and is generally limited to structurally similar compounds.[28]

Some investigators considered small lesion size (e.g., <5 mm) to be a contraindication to stereotactic 14-gauge automated core biopsy,[13] but with the advent of vacuum-assisted devices that allow insertion of a localizing clip,[29,30] small lesion size has ceased to be a contraindication to stereotactic biopsy. Insufficient breast thickness to accommodate the excursion of the gun had also previously been considered a contraindication to stereotactic biopsy,[13,31] but with the use of vacuum-assisted devices that do not require firing in the breast stereotactic biopsy may be feasible in such cases.[16]

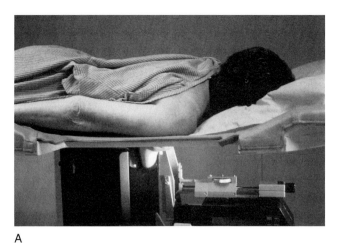

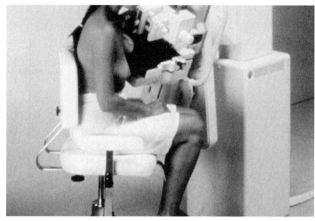

A

B

FIGURE 5.1. Patients positioned for stereotactic biopsy on different equipment. (**A**) Patient prone on dedicated table. (**B**) Patient upright in add-on stereotactic unit.

PRINCIPLES OF STEREOTAXIS

The primary principle of stereotaxis is that the three-dimensional location of a lesion can be determined by analyzing its change in position on angled views.[32] This three-dimensional information is calculated as the x (horizontal), y (vertical), and z (depth) coordinates of the lesion. The angled stereotactic images are obtained by moving the X-ray tube an equal distance to the right and left of midline; by convention, manufacturers have established this to be $+15°$ and $-15°$ along the x (horizontal) axis.

The x position of the lesion is the mean of the x positions of the lesion on the two stereotactic images. The y position is constant on the two images, because the change in direction of the X-ray beam only occurs along the horizontal axis. The depth of the lesion is a function of the apparent displacement of the lesion relative to two reference points (at the level of the back breast support) and can be calculated mathematically[32] as:

$$\Delta a\, z = \Delta x\, /\, 2 \tan (15°) = 1.866\ \Delta x$$

EQUIPMENT

Upright Versus Prone

Stereotactic biopsy can be performed with the patient in the prone or upright position (Figure 5.1). The upright units are less expensive, take up less space, and may allow better access to the posterior breast and axillary region. However, they have several disadvantages, such as higher likelihood of patient motion, higher frequency of vasovagal reactions, and more limited work space. The use of decubitus positioning with the upright unit has been described and may improve results with upright equipment.[33] The prone dedicated tables have more work space, are compatible with a variety of tissue acquisition devices, and are probably easier for the patient, but they take up more room and are more expensive.

Digital Imaging

The ability to acquire and display mammographic images digitally has dramatically improved the capabilities of stereotactic equipment (Figure 5.2). Just as digital imaging decreases the length of time needed to perform needle localization by approximately 50%,[34] it substantially decreases the time necessary to perform stereotactic biopsy. The ability to perform the procedure more quickly minimizes motion and thereby increases the accuracy of needle placement. In a series of 305 patients who had digital stereotactic core biopsy, Parker et al.[35] reported that the average time required for biopsy was 17 minutes. Dig-

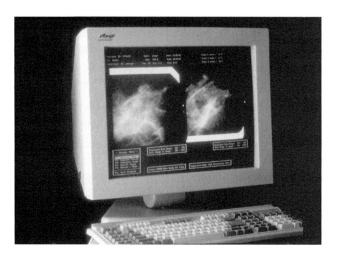

FIGURE 5.2. Digital display for stereotactic biopsy.

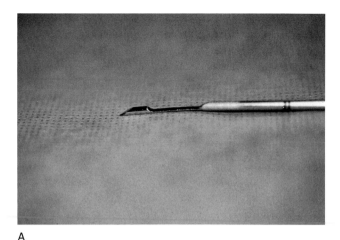
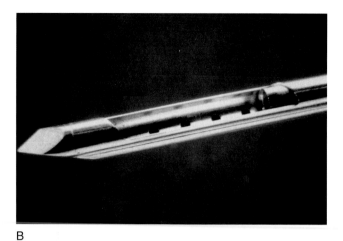

A   B

FIGURE 5.3. Tissue acquisition devices for stereotactic biopsy. (**A**) Automated needle, 14 gauge. (**B**) Vacuum-assisted biopsy probe, 11 gauge.

ital stereotactic biopsy systems also have a lower radiation dose than film-screen systems. The main disadvantages of digital imaging are small field of view (5 × 5 cm in current systems), occasional difficulty with subtle lesions or faint calcifications, and expense.

Tissue Acquisition Device

Tissue acquisition for stereotactic biopsy is generally accomplished with automated needles or directional vacuum-assisted biopsy probes (Figure 5.3). Automated core needles are excellent for masses, but have substantial limitations in the assessment of calcifications, including occasional failure to retrieve calcifications and histologic underestimation of lesions containing atypical ductal hyperplasia (ADH) or ductal carcinoma in situ (DCIS). Another limitation of the automated needles is the lack of a reliable method for placing a localizing marker.

Directional vacuum-assisted biopsy devices (Mammotome, Biopsys, Ethicon Endo-Surgery, Cincinnati, OH, and Minimally Invasive Breast Biopsy [MIBB], US Surgical, Norwalk, CT) are advantageous for calcific lesions, because of the higher frequency of calcification retrieval[36–38] and more accurate characterization of calcific lesions, particularly those that contain ADH[39–41] and/or DCIS.[39,42,43] For small lesions, the vacuum-assisted biopsy devices (e.g., 11-gauge Mammotome or MIBB) are preferable because they allow placement of a localizing marker.[29,30] The vacuum-assisted devices may also be useful if removal of a larger volume of tissue is desired.[16]

PREBIOPSY PREPARATION

Philpotts et al.[31] reported that of 572 scheduled stereotactic core-needle biopsies, 89 (16%) were canceled. Reasons for cancelation included lesion not recognized in

29%, lesion reassessed as benign in 19%, cysts diagnosed with sonography or aspiration in 25%, suboptimal lesion location in 13%, patient intolerant of the procedure in 8%, and other in 4%. Fifty (57%) of the canceled cases were referred from outside facilities. These data underscore the importance of completing a thorough imaging evaluation prior to scheduling stereotactic breast biopsy.

Stereotactic biopsy should not be used to circumvent appropriate imaging workup. Additional views or ultrasound should be performed, if indicated, prior to undertaking the procedure. Every attempt should be made to identify the location of the lesion in three dimensions prior to biopsy, rather than to rely on the use of stereotactic techniques to localize a lesion seen on one view only. It is rare that a real lesion cannot be found on two conventional mammographic images if a thorough workup is performed. If the stereotactic biopsy is scheduled on the basis of mammograms performed at another facility, those films should be submitted and reviewed prior to the procedure.

Percutaneous biopsy is usually not performed in patients on anticoagulants such as Coumadin (warfarin), although a few such cases have been reported without significant complications.[44] It is important to carefully consult with the referring clinician prior to scheduling the biopsy in these women. If percutaneous biopsy is considered the best diagnostic approach and if it is clinically acceptable to temporarily discontinue anticoagulation, Coumadin may be stopped approximately 4 days before the procedure and the international normalization ratio (INR) checked the day before the biopsy; Coumadin can be restarted after the biopsy is complete. If it is desirable to continue anticoagulation as long as possible, then upon discontinuing the Coumadin, the patient may start Fragmin (dalteparin sodium), a low-molecular weight heparin, at a dose of 100 units per kilogram injected subcutaneously twice a day, with the last dose given 24 hours prior to biopsy. After the biopsy, the patient restarts both Fragmin and Coumadin, and then discontinues the Fragmin when the INR approaches the therapeutic level (approximately 2).

Routine prophylactic antibiotics are not indicated for stereotactic biopsy. It is desirable that patients avoid aspirin for 1 week and nonsteroidal antiinflammatory agents for 48 hours prior to the procedure, but they may take acetaminophen.

INFORMED CONSENT AND POTENTIAL COMPLICATIONS

Informed consent should be obtained for all stereotactic biopsy procedures. Potential risks include bleeding and infection. In a multiinstitutional study of 6152 stereotactic 14-gauge automated core biopsy procedures, clinically significant complications occurred in 12 cases (0.2%): There were three hematomas requiring surgical drainage and three infections.[45] In a multiinstitutional study of 14-gauge directional vacuum-assisted biopsy, the frequency of complications was 0.1% (3/2093).[40]

The patient should be told that minor discomfort and bruising are common.[46] She should also be informed of the possibility of a nondiagnostic result or that the findings may indicate the need for surgical biopsy. In previous studies, repeat biopsy was recommended after percutaneous biopsy in 9% to 18% of cases,[47–49] most often for specific histologic entities such as atypical ductal hyperplasia [40,41,50,51] or possible phyllodes tumors,[47] or because of discordance between histologic findings and imaging characteristics.[52]

Patients sometimes ask whether stereotactic biopsy will result in long-term changes on their mammograms. In a study of 24 patients who had 6-month follow-up mammograms after stereotactic biopsy, the only changes were the results of tissue sampling (defects in lesions from which tissue was extracted or a decrease in the number of calcifications).[53] No parenchymal scarring, fat necrosis, architectural distortion, or other sequelae of surgical biopsy were observed. Burbank [54] reviewed follow-up mammograms after 14-gauge directional vacuum-assisted biopsy and also found no evidence of postbiopsy scarring. Lamm and Jackman[55] reported a mammographic density seen well only in the projection parallel to the biopsy needle tract in 2% (5/226) of lesions that had undergone stereotactic 11-gauge vacuum-assisted biopsy. These densities were small (mean diameter, 8 mm; range, 5–10 mm), dense, and round or oval with irregular or spiculated margins; all were seen in the craniocaudal projection only, the approach used for the stereotactic biopsy. Lamm and Jackman [55] found no such densities among 96 lesions that had undergone 14-gauge vacuum-assisted biopsy or 422 lesions that had had a 14-gauge automated core biopsy.

STEREOTACTIC BIOPSY TECHNIQUE

Preliminary Steps

Techniques for the two most commonly used methods of stereotactic biopsy (14-gauge automated core biopsy and directional vacuum-assisted biopsy) are discussed below. The equipment necessary to perform stereotactic biopsy is shown in Table 5.2. The preliminary steps (selecting the approach, patient positioning, and lesion targeting) and some of the later steps (specimen radiography, specimen processing) are common to both automated core and directional vacuum-assisted biopsy procedures. The methods diverge in several important areas, including needle positioning, tissue acquisition, imaging during and after the biopsy, and localizing marker placement. A summary of the steps needed to perform stereotactic automated core biopsy is given in Table 5.3, and a summary of the steps needed to perform stereotactic 11-gauge vacuum-assisted biopsy is shown in Table 5.4.

Selecting the Approach

The approach should allow clear visualization of the lesion. It is usually preferable to choose the approach that requires traversing the shortest distance from skin to lesion for two reasons. First, the shortest distance allows the greatest accuracy in needle placement: a small error in the angle of placement will result in a smaller error in position if the distance traversed is shorter. Second, the shortest approach provides more tissue on the far side of the lesion to accommodate the excursion of the needle.

TABLE 5.2. *Equipment for stereotactic core biopsy*

For all core biopsy procedures
  Stereotactic unit
  Sterile gloves
  Sterile gauze
  Alcohol and/or hydrogen peroxide
  Betadine
  Lidocaine (1%)
  Syringes (3 and 10 cc)
  Needles (25 gauge, 0.75 inch, and 22 gauge)
  Scalpel (no. 11 straight edge)
  X-ray film (for specimen radiography)
  Sterile tweezers
  Cassette (for specimens containing calcium)
  Jar of formalin (10% neutral buffered)
  Steri-Strips (0.25 inch)
Additional equipment for automated core biopsy
  Automated gun
  Biopsy needle (14 gauge)
  Sterile needle holder
Additional equipment for vacuum-assisted biopsy
  Vacuum-assisted pump, driver, connecting tubing
  Biopsy probe (11 gauge)
  Localizing clip

TABLE 5.3. *Stereotactic automated core biopsy: summary of steps*

1. Obtain preliminary grid-localizing film; mark skin.
2. Position patient in stereotactic unit; obtain scout film.
3. Obtain two angled stereotactic (targeting) images; determine coordinates and transmit to stereotactic unit.
4. Calculate if thickness is adequate to fire in breast ($z - 5 + 22$ = less than compressed breast thickness).
5. Cleanse breast with Betadine.
6. Place needle in gun, position needle-holder, and mount gun on stereotactic unit; zero needle.
7. Position needle at skin entry site.
8. Inject local anesthesia (1% lidocaine without epinephrine).
9. Place needle to prefire position ($z - 5$).
10. Obtain prefire stereotactic images. Needle tip should be at leading edge of lesion on both views.
11. Fire needle and obtain postfire images. Needle should traverse lesion on both views.
12. For masses: If initial specimen is through the center of the lesion, obtain subsequent cores at 12, 6, 3, and 9 o'clock. Five cores are usually sufficient.
13. For calcifications: If initial specimen is through the center, obtain subsequent cores at 12, 6, 3, and 9 o'clock or according to the geometry of distribution of calcifications in breast parenchyma.
14. Do specimen radiography for calcifications. Continue obtaining specimens until calcifications are retrieved or specimens are composed predominantly of blood and not breast tissue. It may be preferable to obtain at least 10 specimens.
15. Remove the needle, clean the biopsy site with alcohol, and compress for 5 minutes. Apply Steri-Strips and sterile gauze. Give the patient postbiopsy instructions verbally and in writing.

TABLE 5.4. *Stereotactic 11-gauge vacuum-assisted biopsy: summary of steps*

1. Obtain preliminary grid-localizing film; mark skin.
2. Position patient in stereotactic unit; obtain scout film.
3. Obtain two angled stereotactic (targeting) images.
4. Determine coordinates and transmit to stereotactic unit.
5. Calculate if there is adequate thickness to fire in breast ($z - 2 + 19.3$ = less than compressed breast thickness).
6. Position patient in stereotactic unit; obtain scout film.
7. Obtain two angled stereotactic (targeting) images.
8. Cleanse breast with Betadine.
9. Position the needle-holder, place probe in driver, mount driver, connect to vacuum pump, turn on pump.
10. Zero and flush probe; position probe at skin entry site.
11. Inject local anesthesia: 1% lidocaine without epinephrine (superficial), 1% lidocaine with epinephrine (deep).
12. If firing in breast: Place needle to prefire position ($z - 2$) and obtain prefire stereotactic images; tip of probe should be at leading edge of lesion on both views. Fire probe in breast, collect first specimen, and obtain postfire images; probe should traverse lesion or be immediately adjacent to lesion on both views.
13. If firing outside breast: Fire probe and place at the postfire position ($z - 2$). Obtain postfire stereotactic images; needle tip should traverse lesion or be immediately adjacent to lesion on both views. Collect first specimen.
14. Obtain subsequent specimens; choose direction of tissue acquisition based on location of probe with respect to lesion. For masses: At least eight specimens (e.g., 1.5-hour increments at 12:00, 1:30, 3:00, 4:30, 6:00, 7:30, 9:00, 10:30). For calcifications: Usually at least 10–20 specimens with calcification retrieval documented by specimen radiography.
15. Specimen radiography for calcifications: After approximately eight specimens are obtained. They are handed to the technologist for radiography on the Faxitron unit in another room. More specimens can be collected while the first specimens are being radiographed. Specimens containing calcium are placed in a cassette in the container of formalin; specimens without calcium float freely in the formalin.
16. Postexamination stereotactic images are obtained after tissue acquisition is complete to determine if the mammographic lesion has been removed. If so, a clip should be placed; if not, the bowl of the probe is closed and the probe removed from the breast.
17. For clip placement: Suction the biopsy cavity, perform the "tap" maneuver, close the bowl, withdraw the probe to a depth of $z - 7$, and pull the cutter all the way back. While the technologist presses the "VAC" button and pinches off the back tubing, introduce and deploy the clip.
18. Obtain postclip stereotactic images to confirm clip deployment; target the clip to obtain coordinates and compare them to coordinates of the original lesion.
19. With vacuum off, close bowl, turn probe 180°, and remove probe from breast.
20. Apply compression with ice for approximately 20 minutes; apply Steri-Strips.
21. Obtain a postbiopsy two-view mammogram. Mark the biopsy site on films with wax pencil.
22. Apply sterile gauze. Give postbiopsy instructions to patient verbally and in writing.

Preliminary Grid-Localizing Film

After the approach is selected, it is helpful to obtain a preliminary image on the conventional mammography unit with the alphanumeric grid used for needle localizations. The skin over the lesion is marked with a felt-tip pen, and this mark is used to position the patient for the biopsy procedure (Figure 5.4). If stereotactic biopsy is performed with the patient in the prone position, it should be remembered that gravity may result in the lesion dropping closer to the floor than the mark on the skin (which was made with the patient sitting). The preliminary grid-localizing film minimizes the number of scout films necessary on the stereotactic unit.

Positioning the Patient

Excellent patient positioning for stereotactic biopsy is essential and requires close cooperation of radiologist, technologist, and patient. If stereotactic biopsy is performed with the patient prone, the patient is usually positioned with her head turned away from the radiologist's working area and with both arms at her sides. A thin pillow can be placed between the table and the patient's abdomen. The breast must be immobilized during stereotactic biopsy. Compression is applied at the time of the scout film and maintained throughout the biopsy proce-

dure. The amount of compression should be adequate to prevent motion and obtain high quality images, but must be tolerable.

Scout Film and Stereotactic Images

Ideally the lesion should be centered on the horizontal, or x, axis on the scout image, so that the lesion remains within the field of view for the angled stereotactic images. After the scout image is obtained, it is helpful to mark the location of the corners of the aperture of the compression paddle with a felt-tip pen, so that any patient motion will be readily identified. The two 15° oblique stereotactic images are then obtained. The Fischer table (Mammotest, Fischer Imaging, Denver, CO) has "target on scout" software that allows the operator to substitute the scout image for one of the two stereotactic images if desired.

Targeting the Lesion and Preparing the Breast

Successful targeting requires that the same point be identified on both angled stereotactic views. For masses, the initial target is usually the center of the lesion. For calcifications, the same calcification must be selected on both images—either a calcification centrally located within the cluster or one particularly distinctive in its mor-

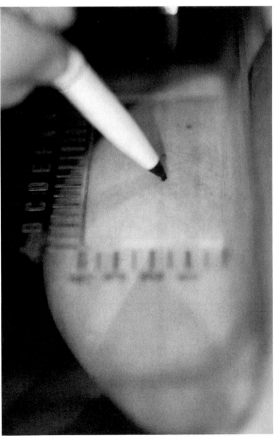

A

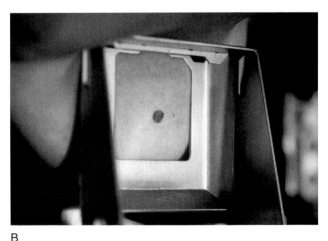

B

FIGURE 5.4. Marking the skin and positioning for stereotactic biopsy. (**A**) Preliminary film is obtained with the breast under compression in an alphanumeric grid. The lesion is identified, and a mark is made on the skin overlying the lesion. (**B**) Patient is positioned on a prone dedicated table with the aperture of the compression paddle centered over the lesion. If the biopsy is being performed with the patient prone, the lesion may be closer to the floor than the mark on the skin owing to the effect of gravity in the prone position.

phology so that it can be reliably identified on the two stereotactic images.

For digital systems, the location of the first target is communicated to the stereotactic equipment via a mouse. The computer then calculates the x, y, and z coordinates of the lesion. These coordinates can be transmitted from the viewing monitor to the biopsy unit by pressing a button.

Stereotactic Automated Core Biopsy: Tissue Acquisition

A summary of the steps needed to perform stereotactic automated core biopsy is shown in Table 5.3.

Determination of Adequate Thickness for Firing

After lesion coordinates are obtained, a calculation is performed to determine whether the compressed breast thickness is adequate to accommodate the excursion of the gun. The compressed breast thickness is indicated on the equipment in a digital readout that is displayed on the stereotactic unit. The desired prefire position of the needle is at the leading edge of the lesion; for the 14-gauge automated core biopsy, this is usually at a depth 5 mm proximal to the depth of the center of the lesion (i.e., $z - 5$ mm). It is safe to fire the needle in the breast if the sum of the depth of the pre-fire needle position ($z - 5$ mm) plus the excursion of the gun (22 mm for a Pro-Mag 2.2, Manan Medical Products, Northbrook, IL) is less than the thickness during compression. If this sum is equal to or greater than the thickness during compression, repositioning is necessary.

Preparing the Automated Needle

A sterile needle holder is positioned between the gun holder and the skin. The biopsy needle is placed in the spring-loaded automated gun. It is helpful to explain to the patient that when the biopsy is performed she will hear a loud clicking noise and then to fire the gun in the air so she will be familiar with the sound. The gun is mounted into position and tightened with a side screw. For some equipment, the data regarding needle length must be entered. For other equipment, the needle must be "zeroed" by lining up the tip of the needle with the upper, outer edge of the aperture of the compression paddle. The needle is then set to the appropriate x and y coordinates and brought to the skin surface.

Local Anesthesia

The skin in the aperture of the compression plate is cleansed with iodine soap, such as Betadine. Local anesthesia is given with a 25-gauge hypodermic needle. A subcutaneous wheal is raised, and deep anesthesia is given. Patients may experience less discomfort if the deep anesthesia is given first. For 14-gauge automated core

biopsies, approximately 5–10 cc of 1% lidocaine without epinephrine is commonly administered.

Placing the Needle and Obtaining Prefire Images

A small linear scalpel incision is made to break up subcutaneous tissue; in general, a vertical incision is preferable because it parallels the direction in which patients tend to move. The needle is then placed to the desired depth, which is proximal to the center of the lesion (Figure 5.5). If the lesion is centered at a depth of z, the 14-gauge automated core needle tip is placed proximal to that, at a depth of $z - 5$ (i.e., 5 mm less than the calculated distance to the center of the lesion). Pre-fire stereotactic images are then obtained and should ideally demonstrate the needle tip at the leading edge of the lesion on both stereotactic images.

First Pass and Post-fire Images

The "stroke margin," which is indicated in a digital readout on the stereotactic unit, is a measure of the distance that will remain between the needle and the Bucky if the needle is fired from its current position. The needle should only be fired if the stroke margin is a positive number.

If the needle position is appropriate and the stroke margin is positive, the needle is fired, and two postfire stereotactic images are obtained. The needle should have traversed the lesion on both postfire images. For a stereotactic 14-gauge automated core biopsy, if pre- and postfire images reflect good needle position on the first pass, and if specimen radiography (discussed below) confirms lesion sampling for calcifications, no further stereotactic images are required.

Specimen Radiography

For lesions evident as calcifications, specimen radiography is performed to document that calcifications have been retrieved.[56,57] The likelihood of obtaining diagnostic material is significantly higher if calcifications are present on specimen radiographs than if they are not present. Liberman et al.[57] found that the likelihood of obtaining a specific histologic diagnosis was 81% if calcium was seen at specimen radiography versus 38% if calcium was not seen.

To perform specimen radiography, the specimens can be placed on a piece of film and irrigated with sterile saline. They can be radiographed on standard mammography equipment using magnification (×1.8) without compression at kVp = 22 and mAs = 4. Alternatively, specimen radiography can be performed on a Faxitron unit, or a digital specimen radiograph may be obtained. If the biopsy is performed for calcifications, a benign result is not considered definitive unless calcifications are identified on the radiographs of the core biopsy specimens. At our institution, we do not perform specimen ra-

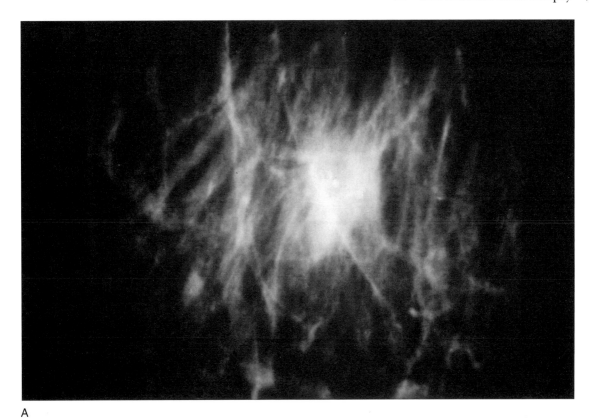

A

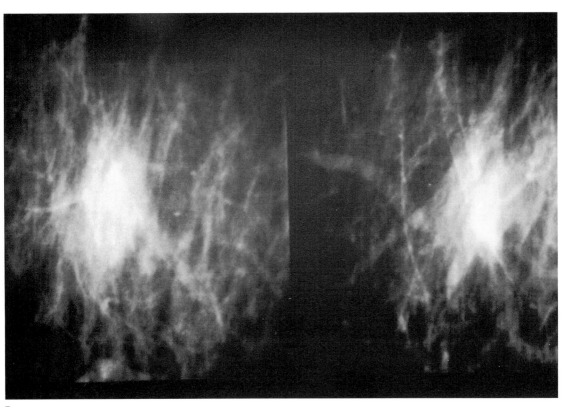

B

FIGURE 5.5. Automated core biopsy (14 gauge) in a 66-year-old woman with a spiculated right breast mass. **(A)** Scout digital image shows the spiculated mass centered in the aperture of the compression paddle. **(B)** Targeting stereotactic images show the spiculated mass on both 15° angled views.

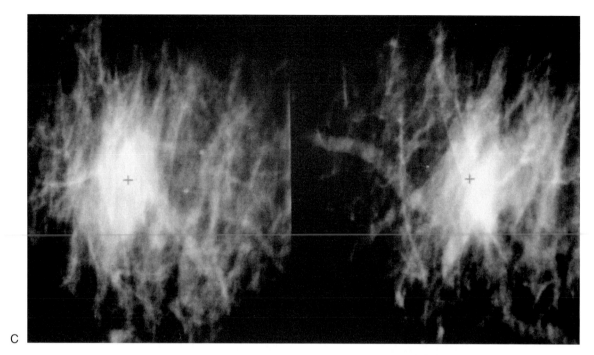

C

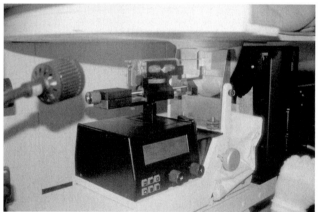

D

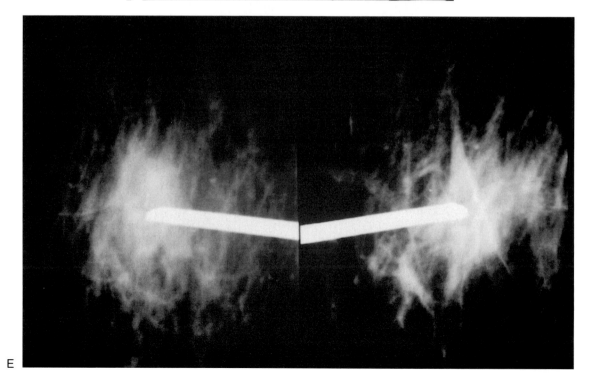

E

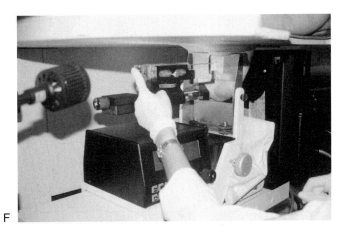

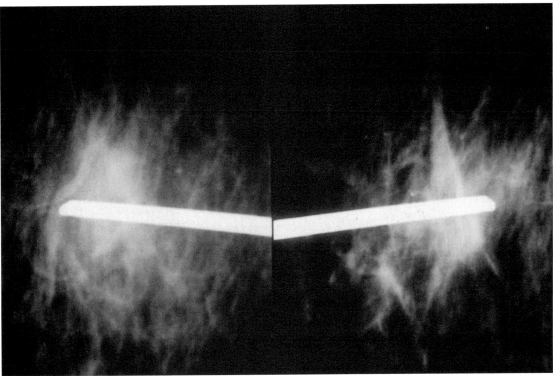

FIGURE 5.5. (C) Using the handheld mouse, a cursor is placed over the center of the lesion to obtain the three-dimensional (x, y, z) coordinates of the lesion. (D) After cleansing the skin and giving local anesthesia, the 14-gauge needle is inserted to the appropriate depth. (E) Prefire stereotactic images confirm that the needle tip projects over the proximal aspect of the lesion on both projections. (F) The needle is fired in the breast. (G) Postfire stereotactic images confirm that the needle has traversed the lesion in both projections.

diography for stereotactic biopsy of uncalcified masses, although there is one such report in the literature.[58]

Subsequent Cores

Previous studies have demonstrated the importance of obtaining an adequate volume of tissue. In a study of stereotactic 14-gauge automated core biopsy, Liberman et al.[59] found that five cores were sufficient to make a histologic diagnosis in 97% of masses, but allowed a diagnosis in only 87% of calcification lesions. Based on these data,

our protocol for the 14-gauge automated stereotactic core biopsy has been to obtain five samples for masses and at least five for calcifications with specimen radiography (discussed below) for the calcification lesions. Parker[60] has suggested taking a minimum of 10 samples for 14-gauge automated core biopsy of calcifications.

For 14-gauge automated core biopsy of a mass, the initial biopsy point is generally the center of the mass with additional specimens obtained from the 12, 6, 3, and 9 o'clock position of the lesion through the same scalpel incision. The literature strongly supports use of directional vacuum-assisted biopsy rather than automated core biopsy for calcifications[36,38,61]; however, if 14-gauge automated core biopsy of calcifications is performed, the subsequent specimens can be taken from the 12, 6, 3, and 9 o'clock positions, or according to the geometric distribution of calcification in the breast parenchyma.

Subsequent cores are generally obtained without additional stereotactic imaging, unless the first pre- and postfire images indicated suboptimal positioning, or specimen radiography fails to confirm sampling of calcifications. Data from Hann et al.[62] suggest that a postbiopsy mammogram immediately after stereotactic 14-gauge automated core biopsy is not necessary.

Stereotactic Directional Vacuum-Assisted Biopsy: Tissue Acquisition and Afterward

A summary of the steps needed to perform stereotactic directional vacuum-assisted biopsy is given in Table 5.4. The equipment needed to perform stereotactic directional vacuum-assisted biopsy is shown in Figure 5.6.

Determination of Adequate Thickness for Firing

After lesion coordinates are obtained, a calculation can be performed to determine whether the compressed breast thickness, as indicated in a digital readout in the stereotactic equipment, is adequate to allow firing the probe inside the breast. For 11-gauge vacuum-assisted biopsy, the desired prefire position of the probe is 2 mm proximal to the center of the lesion (i.e., $z - 2$). If the sum of the prefire position ($z - 2$ mm) and the excursion of the probe (19.3 mm) is less than the compressed breast thickness (in millimeters), the probe can be fired inside the breast without striking the back breast support. If the sum of the prefire position ($z - 2$ mm) and the excursion of the probe (19.3 mm) is equal to or more than the compressed breast thickness (in millimeters), the breast can be repositioned in an attempt to achieve adequate thickness to

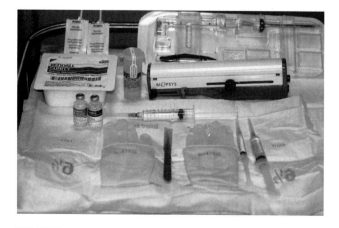

FIGURE 5.6. Equipment tray for stereotactic 11-gauge directional vacuum-assisted breast biopsy.

allow firing in the breast. Alternatively, the biopsy can be performed by firing the probe outside the breast and placing it at the postfire position (described below).

Preparing the Probe and the Breast

After targeting images are obtained and the coordinates are transmitted to the stereotactic unit, the skin in the aperture of the compression paddle is cleansed with iodine soap such as Betadine (Figure 5.7). A sterile needle holder is positioned between the driver and the skin. The biopsy probe is placed in the driver, and the driver is then mounted into position (Figure 5.7). For some equipment, the data regarding needle length must be entered. For other equipment, the needle must be "zeroed" prior to firing by lining up the tip of the needle with the upper edge of the aperture of the compression paddle (Figure 5.7). The needle is then set to the appropriate x and y coordinates and brought to the skin surface. It is important to flush the vacuum-assisted biopsy probe with 5–10 cc sterile saline before obtaining tissue to minimize the chance of clogging during the procedure (Figure 5.7), and to observe flushing in both the front and back tubing.

Local Anesthesia

Local anesthesia is given with a 25-gauge hypodermic needle in the subcutaneous tissues at the skin entry site (Figure 5.8), and with a 22-gauge needle in the deeper tissues. For vacuum-assisted biopsy, we administer lidocaine (1%) without epinephrine in the skin, but use lidocaine (1%) with epinephrine (1:100,000, 10 μg/ml) for deep anesthesia unless the patient has cardiac disease or other contraindications to adrenergic stimulation. Epinephrine approximately doubles the duration of anesthesia and assists with hemostasis but should not be used in the skin or subcutaneous tissue because of its potential to cause tissue necrosis. We routinely administer 10–15 cc of lidocaine for vacuum-assisted biopsy, a higher volume than that used for 14-gauge automated core biopsy. The maximal dose of epinephrine for local infiltration in adults is 200–250 μg or 20–25 ml of solution that contains 10 μg/ml of epinephrine.[63]

A small linear scalpel incision is made to break up subcutaneous tissue, and it should be sufficiently large to accommodate the directional vacuum-assisted biopsy probe (Figure 5.8).

Placing the Probe and Obtaining Prefire Images

For directional vacuum-assisted breast biopsy, firing is not essential for tissue acquisition. One may place the probe to the prefire position and fire in the breast or one may fire the probe outside the breast and place the probe at the postfire position (Figure 5.9). Firing outside the breast decreases the radiation exposure and saves time (by sparing prefire images) and is particularly helpful for breasts too thin to

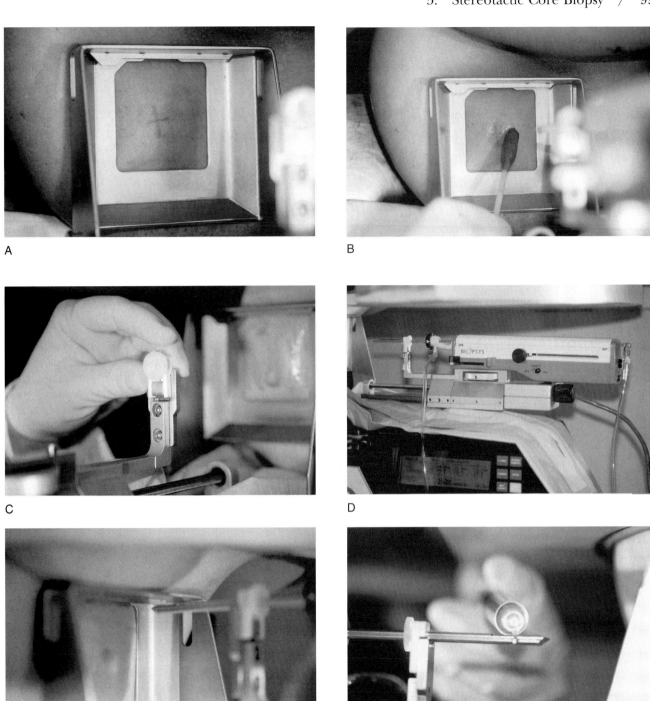

FIGURE 5.7. Preparing the breast and probe for stereotactic 11-gauge directional vacuum-assisted breast biopsy. **(A)** After obtaining a grid-localizing film, the breast is positioned with the lesion in the aperture of the compression paddle. **(B)** After obtaining a scout digital image, targeting stereotactic images, and obtaining lesion coordinates, the breast within the aperture of the compression paddle is cleansed with iodine soap such as Betadine. **(C)** The needle guide is positioned. **(D)** The 11-gauge probe is placed in the driver, and the driver is mounted on the holder. **(E)** The tip of the 11-gauge probe is lined up with the overhanging part of the compression paddle. **(F)** The 11-gauge probe is flushed with 5–10 cc sterile saline. Flushing minimizes the likelihood of clogging during the procedure, which could potentially interfere with tissue acquisition.

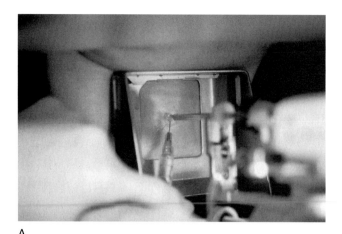
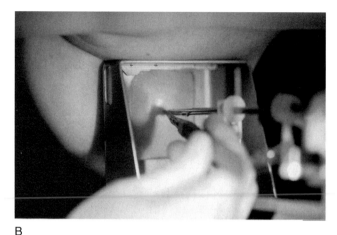

A   B

FIGURE 5.8. Anesthesia and incision for stereotactic biopsy. (**A**) The probe is brought to the skin surface overlying the lesion, and local anesthesia is injected. (**B**) An incision is made with a scalpel over the lesion site.

accommodate the excursion of the biopsy probe or for lesions so superficial that the prefire position of the probe would be partly outside the breast. However, it has been suggested that if the probe is not fired within the breast, the lesion may be displaced rather than pierced by the needle, increasing the likelihood of failure; therefore, some have recommended firing inside the breast when possible.[61]

The ideal prefire position is $z - 5$ (i.e., 5 mm proximal to the center of the lesion) for 14-gauge vacuum-assisted biopsy and $z - 2$ (i.e., 2 mm proximal to the center of the lesion) for the 11-gauge vacuum-assisted biopsy. The probe should project over the leading edge of the lesion on both prefire stereotactic images (Figure 5.10).

Biopsy (First Pass) and Postfire Images

If the vacuum-assisted biopsy probe has been set to the prefire position and prefire images are obtained, the probe is then fired inside the breast. The first sample is acquired by manually bringing the cutter forward and turning it to close the bowl. Postfire stereotactic images are then obtained, which ideally show that the probe has traversed

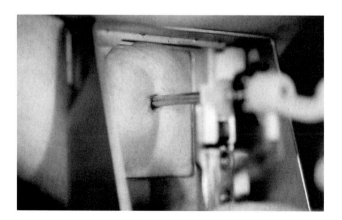

FIGURE 5.9. The 11-gauge probe is placed in the breast.

the lesion (Figure 5.10). The cutter is then retracted to acquire the first specimen.

For directional vacuum-assisted biopsies where the probe has been fired outside the breast and placed to the postfire position, the postfire images are obtained prior to tissue acquisition. Note that if the probe is "zeroed" prior to firing, the fired probe is set to a position 2 mm proximal to the depth of the center of the lesion (i.e., $z - 2$ mm). The cutter is then retracted, the vacuum engaged, and the first specimen obtained and retrieved.

Subsequent Cores

Few data address the number of specimens to be obtained in stereotactic directional vacuum-assisted biopsy, particularly for mass lesions. Jackman et al.[40] found more accurate characterization of lesions containing atypical ductal hyperplasia, with fewer histologic underestimates, if a minimum of 10 specimens were obtained at 14-gauge directional vacuum-assisted biopsy. Parker and Klaus [64] suggest removal of at least 15 specimens during directional vacuum-assisted breast biopsy. At our institution, we generally obtain 10–20 specimens for stereotactic vacuum-assisted breast biopsy; since each specimen is approximately 100 mg,[65] this usually translates into at least 1 gram of tissue.

For directional vacuum-assisted biopsy, if the first specimen is obtained from the center of the lesion, subsequent specimens can be from different sites by turning the thumbwheel (Figure 5.11), which rotates the bowl around according to the clock face. Eight specimens obtained at 1.5-hour (positional) increments (i.e., 12, 1:30, 3, 4:30, 6, 7:30, 9, 10:30 o'clock) results in contiguous sampling. If the probe is placed "low" with respect to the lesion, the specimens can be acquired from the upward hemisphere (i.e., 9 to 3 o'clock, in the upward direction); if the probe is placed "high" with respect to the lesion, the specimens can be acquired from the downward hemisphere (i.e., 3 to 9 o'clock, in the downward direction).

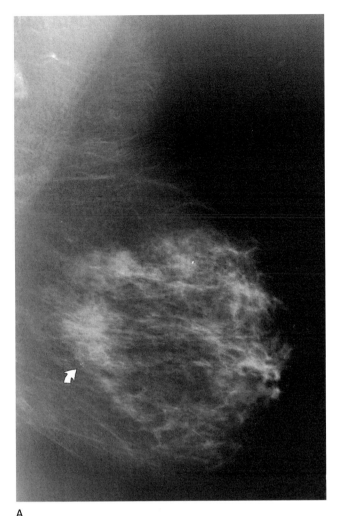

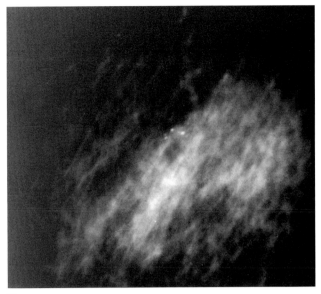

B

A

FIGURE 5.10. Stereotactic 11-gauge vacuum-assisted biopsy in a 77-year old woman with a 1.2 cm cluster of pleomorphic calcifications in the right breast, lower outer quadrant. (**A**) Mediolateral oblique view of right breast shows calcifications in the right lower outer quadrant (arrow). (**B**) Digital scout stereotactic image shows calcifications. (**C**) Targeting stereotactic images demonstrate calcifications on both projections (arrows).

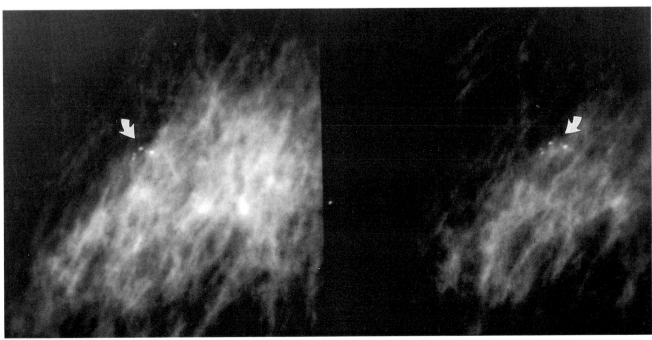

C

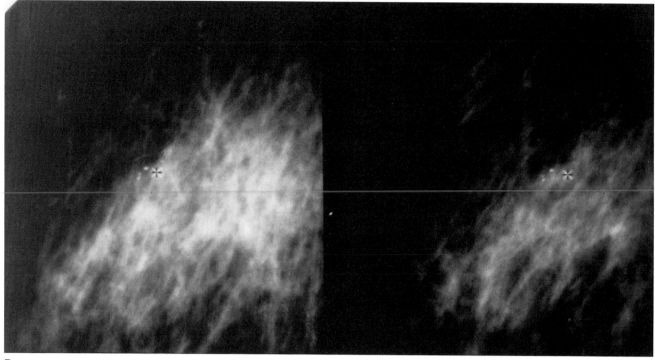

D

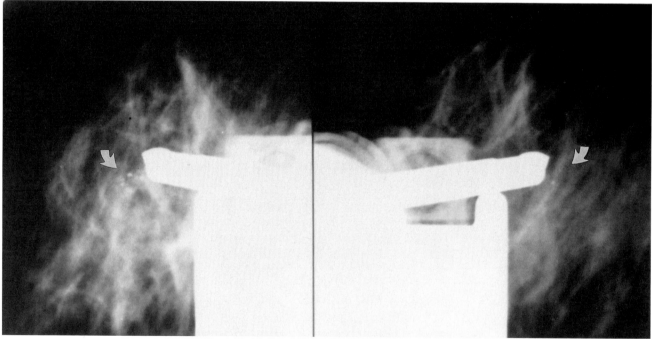

E

FIGURE 5.10. (**D**) Cursor is placed over a single calcification identified in both projections to obtain coordinates. (**E**) After positioning the probe proximal to the lesion (to a depth of $z - 2$, i.e., 2 mm superficial to the calculated depth coordinate), stereotactic images are obtained. The calcifications (arrows) are just deep to the biopsy probe and "below" it (i.e., toward the 6 o'-clock axis).

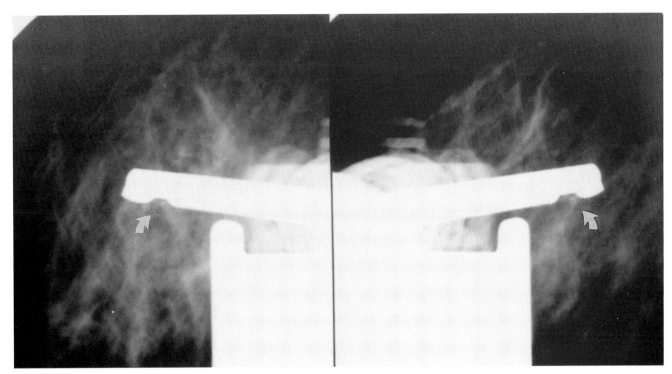

F

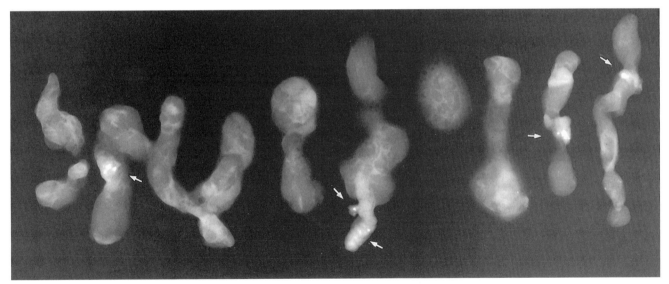

G

FIGURE 5.10. (F) The probe is turned so that the bowl faces "downward" (i.e., toward 6 o'clock, the location of the calcifications), and the probe is fired in the breast. Postfire images demonstrate calcifications (arrows) in the bowl of the probe. **(G)** Specimen radiographs demonstrate calcifications (arrows) in multiple cores.

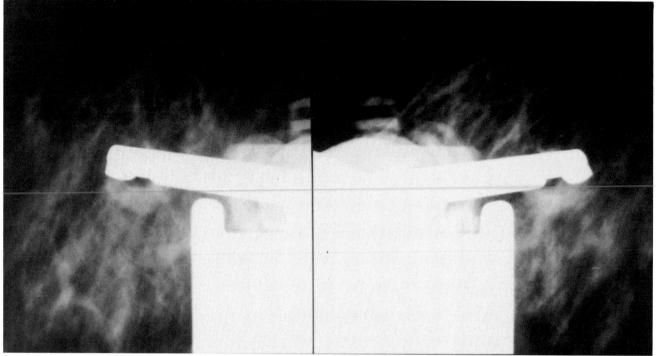

H

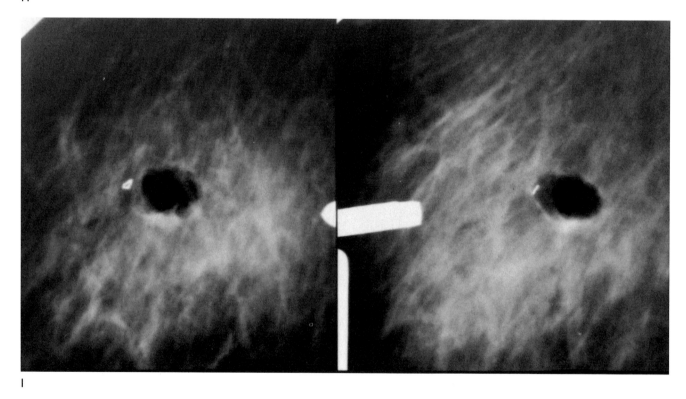

I

FIGURE 5.10. (H) Stereotactic images after tissue acquisition is complete show no residual calcifications, so a localizing clip was placed at the biopsy site. (I) Stereotactic images after clip placement show the clip in the biopsy cavity. (J) Cursor can be placed over the clip and coordinates obtained. These coordinates can be compared to the coordinates of the original lesion.

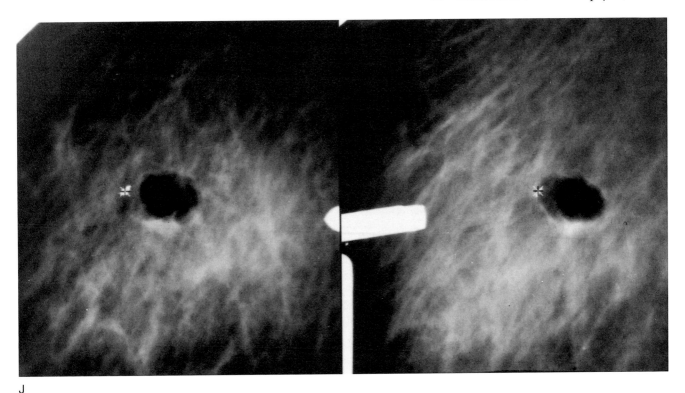

J

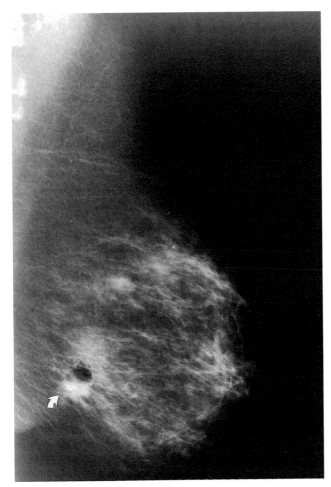

K

FIGURE 5.10. (J) Cursor can be placed over the clip and coordinates obtained. These coordinates can be compared to the coordinates of the original lesion. **(K)** Mediolateral oblique view of the right breast obtained as part of a two-view mammogram immediately after stereotactic biopsy and clip placement. It shows the clip in good position in the biopsy cavity (arrow). Histologic analysis yielded benign fibroadenoma with calcification.

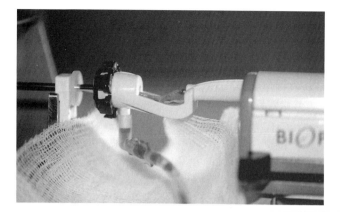

FIGURE 5.11. The specimen is evident in the collecting area of the probe. The direction of tissue acquisition can be controlled by turning the thumbwheel.

If the patient experiences discomfort during the procedure, additional anesthetic can be administered through the back of the probe (Figure 5.12).

The "Tap" Maneuver for Vacuum-Assisted Breast Biopsy

If attempt at tissue acquisition yields no material at directional vacuum-assisted breast biopsy (Mammotome), the "tap" maneuver, originally described by Parker and Burbank, is performed.[63] To perform this, the cutter is pulled back, the vacuum on the driver is shut off, and the front vacuum tube is pinched off. The cutter is then brought forward to the precut stop position so that the tip of the cutter is at the proximal end of the bowl. The operator then toggles the vacuum and manipulates the cutter manually from the proximal to distal end of the bowl and back many times by turning the dial on the probe driver. Additional short bursts of vacuum are applied while the cutter is pulled back. This maneuver allows tissue fragments in the bowl or shaft of the probe to be pulled into the cutter lumen, collected, and cleared from the system.

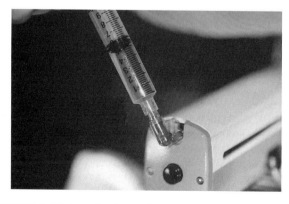

FIGURE 5.12. Anesthesia can be administered directly to the biopsy site through the back of the probe if there is discomfort during the stereotactic biopsy procedure.

Specimen Radiography

Specimen radiography is performed during stereotactic biopsy for all lesions evident as calcifications, using the technique discussed above (Figure 5.10). In general, at our institution, after we obtain the first 8–10 samples at 11-gauge vacuum-assisted biopsy, we give the specimens to our technologist for specimen radiography. While the first set of specimens is being radiographed, an additional 8–10 specimens are often acquired. If calcification retrieval is not confirmed, it can be useful to "retarget" with a new set of stereotactic images, make appropriate adjustments in needle position, and acquire more specimens.

Postexamination Stereotactic Images

When tissue acquisition is complete at stereotactic directional vacuum-assisted breast biopsy (i.e., calcification retrieval documented at specimen radiography for calcifications or appropriate volume of tissue removed for masses), it is helpful to obtain a pair of postexamination stereotactic images (Figure 5.10). These images help determine if the mammographic lesion has been removed, and if placement of a localizing clip is necessary. Prior to obtaining the images, the biopsy cavity should be suctioned to remove blood and debris. This will allow the best evaluation of the air-filled biopsy cavity.

Clip Placement

A stainless steel clip can be placed after 11-gauge directional vacuum-assisted breast biopsy.[29,30] For clip placement, the 11-gauge directional vacuum-assisted biopsy probe is withdrawn an additional 5 mm from the biopsy position (i.e., to $z = -7$ from $z = -2$) for clip placement. The probe should be cleaned with the "tap" maneuver to remove adherent tissue fragments. The clip introducer is placed into the probe (Figure 5.13). The technologist engages vacuum by pressing the "VAC" button with the rear tubing pinched off, and the radiologist deploys the clip by pressing the squeeze handles on the clip applier. When the clip deploys, the color indicator turns from gray to blue. After clip deployment, the vacuum is released and the probe is turned 180°, closed, and withdrawn.

Two stereotactic images should be obtained to confirm the location of the clip. It is helpful to remove the probe after clip placement but before obtaining these stereotactic images for three reasons. First, if the probe is left in place, it can obscure the clip. Second, the clip can be inadvertently removed when the probe is removed; if the images are obtained after probe removal, this can be appreciated and a new clip placed prior to releasing compression. Third, the most common reason for failure of clip deployment is clipping a tissue fragment in the holes of the bowl; if this occurs, the probe should be removed, "flushed" as at the beginning of the procedure, and repositioned to the appropriate depth ($z - 7$) so that a new

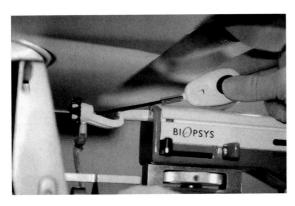

FIGURE 5.13. Placement of a localizing clip after stereotactic 11-gauge vacuum-assisted breast biopsy. The clip introducer is placed directly into the probe as shown.

clip can be placed. On the stereotactic images confirming clip deployment, the clip can be "targeted" and the coordinates compared to those of the original lesion to assess clip location (Figure 5.10).

A two-view mammogram is of some value after all stereotactic 11-gauge vacuum-assisted biopsy procedures, but it should be routinely obtained after clip placement. Close proximity of the clip to the lesion site on stereotactic images does not ensure close proximity on conventional images. The compressed breast is like an accordion: Areas of the breast that are far apart are brought close together; when compression is released, those areas move farther apart.[29] If the clip is slightly removed from the lesion site in the depth (z) direction on the stereotactic images obtained with the breast compressed along the depth (z) axis, the clip may be far distant from the lesion when compression is released. The two-view mammogram obtained after clip placement allows the best assessment of the location of the clip relative to the biopsy site and can serve as a guide for subsequent localization if necessary.

Final Steps

Specimen Processing

For mass lesions, all specimens are sent to the laboratory in one container of neutral buffered formalin. For calcification lesions, specimens can be sent in one container, but it is helpful to identify for the pathologist the specimens that contain radiographically evident calcification. This can be accomplished by placing the specimens with calcifications identified on specimen radiography in a cassette inside the container whereas the specimens without radiographic evidence of calcification are floating freely in the formalin[66] (Figure 5.14); the pathologist is then asked specifically to address whether calcification

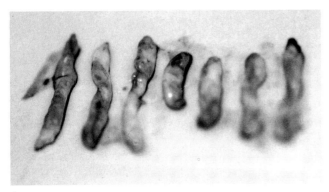

A

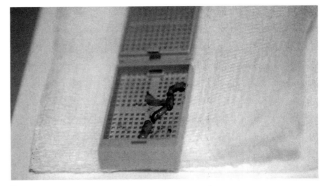

B

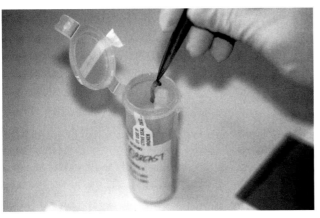

C

FIGURE 5.14. Specimen processing during stereotactic 11-gauge vacuum-assisted biopsy of microcalcifications. (**A**) Specimens are initially placed on film and irrigated with saline. Specimen radiography is performed to identify the specimens containing calcification. (**B**) Specimens containing radiographically evident calcification are placed in a cassette. (**C**) Specimens without radiographically evident calcification are placed so they are floating freely in formalin. The pathologist is asked to comment specifically on the presence and location of calcifications within the specimens.

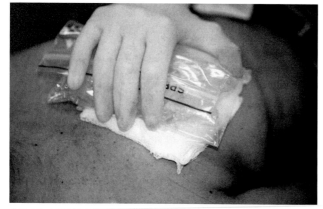

A

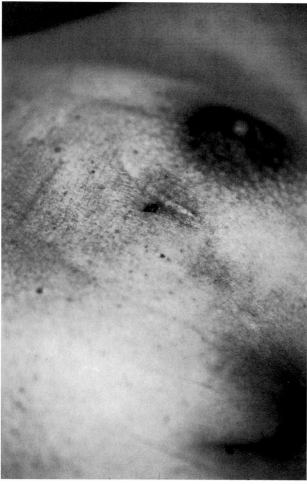

B

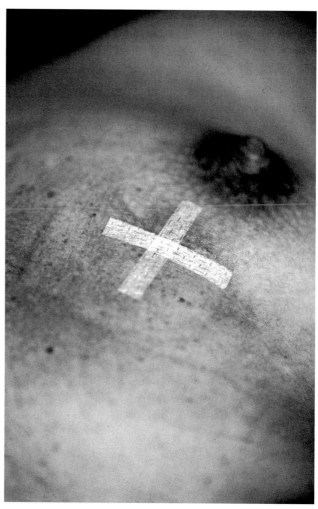

C

FIGURE 5.15. Care of the biopsy site after stereotactic 11-gauge vacuum-assisted biopsy. (**A**) Sterile gauze is placed over the biopsy site, and compression with ice is held for approximately 20 minutes. (**B**) Only a small skin nick is evident after stereotactic biopsy. (**C**) The skin nick is covered with sterile strips (shown) and sterile gauze.

is present in the specimens, and (if so) whether it is identified in tumor, benign tissue, or both.

If calcifications are seen at specimen radiography but the pathologist does not identify calcifications histologically, there are several steps that can be helpful. First, the tissue blocks can be radiographed to identify the cores that contain calcifications for the pathologist. Second, the pathologist can look with polarized light, which can help identify calcium oxalate (weddellite) crystals.[67] Third, the pathologist can take deeper sections (levels) of the specimens in order to identify calcifications.

Postbiopsy

After the procedure, compression is held to achieve hemostasis. We generally hold compression for approximately 5 minutes for 14-gauge automated core biopsy and 10–20 minutes (with ice) for directional vacuum-assisted biopsy. The wound is cleansed with alcohol, and a sterile bandage is applied (Figure 5.15). The patient is told she can shower in the morning but is asked not to completely immerse the breast in water for 2 days and to avoid strenuous activity for a few days. Postbiopsy instructions are given to her verbally and in writing. She is also given the phone number of the radiologist who performed the biopsy and is told when she will be contacted with the results.

At our institution, the radiologist performing the biopsy reviews the pathology report and communicates all biopsy results to the patient and to the referring physician. The biopsy report is not finalized until the pathology results are available. The radiologist then dictates an addendum with the pathologic findings and specific recommendations for future management. The final written biopsy report should include the pathology results and management recommendations and should document to whom the results were communicated.

TROUBLESHOOTING

Needle Placement Errors

Obtaining diagnostic results at stereotactic biopsy requires that the needle be appropriately placed in the breast, but needle position is only accurate if it is accurate on both stereotactic images. This section addresses analysis of needle placement on stereotactic images and how to recognize and correct errors in needle placement.

14-Gauge Automated Core Biopsy

The 14-gauge automated core needles require pinpoint precision in needle placement, because tissue is only acquired along the line of fire. For 14-gauge automated core biopsy, the prefire stereotactic images are the last images obtained prior to tissue acquisition, and these are analyzed to determine the accuracy of needle placement. Needle position is only accurate if it is accurate on both prefire stereotactic images. For prefire images there are two options for placement of the 14-gauge automated needle. It can be placed to the position of the center of the lesion (z), imaged, and then pulled back the 5 mm pull-back distance before firing; alternatively, it can be placed at the leading edge of the lesion, a depth of "z minus the pull-back" (i.e., $z - 5$ mm) (Figure 5.16). On postfire images, the needle should traverse the lesion (Figure 5.17).

Errors in needle placement may occur on one or more of the x, y, or z axes (Figure 5.18). X-axis error results in the needle being displaced to the right or left of the desired location (as determined when one is looking directly

Appropriate Pre-fire Placement of Automated Needle

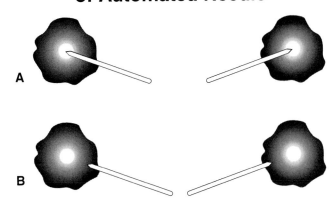

FIGURE 5.16. Appropriate prefire needle position for a 14-gauge automated core biopsy: two alternatives. (**A**) Prefire images, obtained after placing the needle at a depth of z, show the needle tip projected over the center of the lesion on both projections. If prefire images are obtained at this position, the needle tip should be pulled back 5 mm before firing. (**B**) Prefire images, obtained after placing the needle to a depth of "z minus 5 mm pull-back," show the needle tip at the leading edge of the lesion on both views.

at the aperture of the compression plate) on both prefire stereotactic images. A y-axis error results in the needle tip being displaced either too close or too far from the desired distance from the chest wall on the two prefire stereotactic images. A z-axis error results in the needle tip being either too deep or too superficial to the desired location on both prefire stereotactic images. Analysis of needle position requires review of both angled stereotactic images (Figure 5.19); positioning cannot be determined to be accurate unless it is accurate on both projections. In a study of cancers not diagnosed at stereotactic 14-gauge automated core biopsy, Liberman et al.[68] found that incorrect needle placement was the most common reason for failure to diagnose cancer, with horizontal (x-axis) errors most frequently observed.

Appropriate Post-fire Placement of Automated Needle

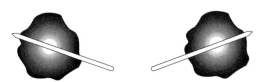

FIGURE 5.17. Appropriate postfire position for the 14-gauge automated needle. The needle has traversed the lesion on both projections.

Errors in Pre-fire Position of Automated Needle

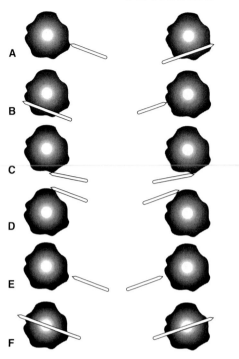

FIGURE 5.18. Errors in 14-gauge automated needle positions as determined on prefire stereotactic images. (**A**) An *x* (horizontal) axis error. The needle tip is to the right of the lesion. (**B**) An *x* (horizontal) axis error. The needle tip is to the left of the lesion. (**C**) A *y* (vertical) axis error. The needle tip is below the lesion. (**D**) A *y* (vertical) axis error. The needle tip is above the lesion. (**E**) A *z* (depth) axis error. The needle tip is superficial to the lesion. (**F**) A *z* (depth) axis error. The needle tip is deep to the lesion.

If the needle placement is incorrect, the radiologist has two options. One is to use the location of the needle tip with respect to the target on the prefire images to estimate the necessary correction; the needle is then repositioned as needed. This approach requires some experience. The second option is to "retarget" (i.e., obtain another set of stereotactic coordinates). This approach usually can be achieved using the prefire stereotactic images with the needle in place. If the needle tip obscures the desired target, however, the needle should be removed and a new set of "targeting" stereotactic images obtained. The needle is then placed in the breast in accordance with the new coordinates. Accurate positioning should then be confirmed with a new set of prefire stereotactic images.

If the error in needle placement is in the depth (*z*) axis, the needle can be advanced or pulled back without completely removing it from the breast. If the error in needle placement is in the horizontal (*x*) or vertical (*y*) axis, it is advantageous to remove the needle tip from the area of the lesion, usually to outside or just under the skin,

and then reintroduce it to the new position. If needle positioning is adjusted in the horizontal or vertical axis without removing the needle from the area of the lesion, the lesion may move its position when the needle is moved to its new coordinates.

Vacuum-Assisted Biopsy

Targeting requirements are slightly more relaxed for vacuum-assisted biopsy than for 14-gauge automated core biopsy because vacuum suction allows tissue acquisition from outside the line of fire; however, it is equally important to be able to determine the location of the lesion with respect to the biopsy device. For vacuum-assisted biopsy, the probe may be positioned immediately

Importance of 2 Views in Evaluating Pre-fire Needle Position

Case 1

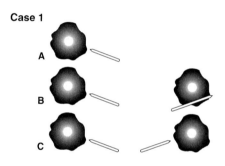

Case 2

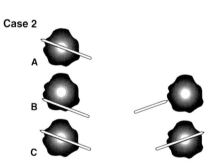

FIGURE 5.19. Importance of both stereotactic images in assessing the prefire position of the 14-gauge automated needle. (**Case 1**) A, A single prefire stereotactic image shows that the needle is not in optimal position, but cannot distinguish between error in the *x* (horizontal) or *z* (depth) axis. B, If the stereotactic pair is as shown, the error is in the *x* (horizontal) axis: the needle tip is to the right of the lesion. C, If the stereotactic pair is as shown, the error is in the depth (*z*) axis: the needle tip is superficial to the lesion. (**Case 2**) A, The single prefire stereotactic image shows that the needle is not in optimal position but cannot distinguish between an error in the *x* (horizontal) or *z* (depth) axis. B, If the stereotactic pair is as shown, the error is in the *x* (horizontal) axis: needle tip is to the left of the lesion. C, If the stereotactic pair is as shown, the error is in the depth (*z*) axis: needle tip is deep to the lesion.

adjacent to, rather than within, the lesion and still succeed in acquiring lesional tissue. Note that for vacuum-assisted biopsy the images obtained immediately before tissue acquisition are the post-fire images.

If the probe is adjacent to, rather than within, the lesion, tissue should be acquired from the appropriate direction (Figure 5.20). If the lesion is to the right of the biopsy probe, for example, tissue can be acquired in the rightward direction (i.e., from 12 to 6 o'clock in the right hemisphere). If the lesion is to the left of the biopsy probe, tissue can be acquired in the leftward direction (i.e., from 6 to 12 o'clock in the left hemisphere). If the lesion is cephalad to the probe, tissue can be acquired from 9 to 3 o'clock in the upward hemisphere; and if the lesion is caudal to the probe, tissue can be acquired from 3 to 9 o'clock in the downward hemisphere.

Challenging Cases

Challenging cases at stereotactic biopsy include lesions that are posterior in location or in the axillary region, thin breasts, superficial lesions, small lesions, amorphous (faint) calcifications or other subtle lesions, and multiple lesions.[69]

Posterior/Axillary Tail Lesions

Posterior lesions pose a challenge for stereotactic biopsy, because of the difficulty of including the lesion on the mammographic images. In the study by Philpotts et al.[31]

of 89 canceled cases at stereotactic 14-gauge automated core biopsy, a posterior or superficial lesion location was the cause of cancelation in 8 cases (9%).

The technologist plays a critical role in positioning the patient for stereotactic biopsy and can be most helpful in

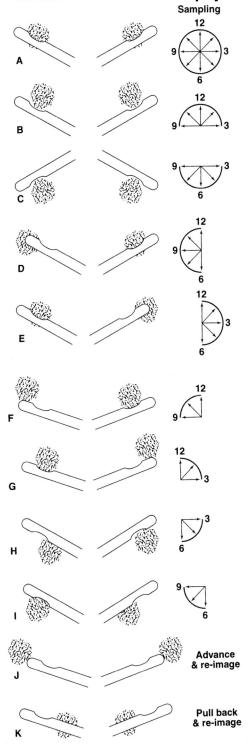

Post-fire Probe Position in Vacuum-Assisted Biopsy

FIGURE 5.20. Analysis of the position of the vacuum-assisted biopsy probe with respect to the lesion on postfire stereotactic images and determining the direction of sampling. A, The probe is through the center of the lesion. Sampling can proceed "around the clock." B, The probe is below the lesion. Sampling should occur from 9 to 3 o'clock in the upward hemisphere. C, The probe is above the lesion. Sampling should occur from 3 to 9 o'clock in the downward hemisphere. D, The probe is to the right of the lesion. Sampling should occur from 12 to 6 o'clock in the leftward hemisphere. E, The probe is to the left of the lesion. Sampling should occur from 12 to 6 o'clock in the rightward hemisphere. F, The probe is below and to the right of the lesion. Sampling should occur from 9 to 12 o'clock (i.e., up and to the left). G, The probe is below and to the left of the lesion. Sampling should occur from 12 to 3 o'clock (i.e., up and to the right). H, The probe is above and to the left of the lesion. Sampling should occur from 3 to 6 o'clock (i.e., down and to the right). I, The probe is above and to the right of the lesion. Sampling should occur from 6 to 9 o'clock (i.e., down and to the left). J, The probe is superficial to the lesion. The probe should be advanced and the postfire images repeated before sampling. K, The probe is deep to the lesion. The probe should be withdrawn and the postfire images repeated before sampling.

difficult cases. The posterior breast and axillary region may be more accessible on upright than on prone equipment. Posterior lesions may also be more accessible on the Fischer (Denver, CO) table, which allows slight upward angulation of the needle, rather than the LoRad (Danbury, CT) table, with which the needle entrance is horizontal.

For posterior lesions undergoing biopsy with the patient prone on a dedicated table, placement of the patient's arm through the hole is useful.[70] If this is done, it is helpful to have something for the dependent hand to grasp. This increases patient comfort and tolerance and may improve visualization of the posterior tissues.

Thin Breasts

Thin breasts or lesions in a thin portion of the breast (e.g., the retroareolar region) may pose a problem for stereotactic biopsy. For stereotactic 14-gauge automated core biopsy, firing the needle is essential for tissue acquisition. If the breast is too thin to accommodate the 2.2 to 2.3-cm excursion of the long-throw gun, stereotactic 14-gauge automated core biopsy may not be feasible. In the study by Philpotts et al.[31] of 89 canceled cases at stereotactic 14-gauge automated core biopsy, inadequate thickness of compressed breast parenchyma was the cause of cancelation in 4 (4%) cases.

The thickness of compressed breast parenchyma can be anticipated prior to scheduling stereotactic biopsy. Sometimes the compressed breast thickness is indicated on the identification flasher on the mammography films; if not, the compressed breast thickness can be measured during the diagnostic evaluation.[31] Because firing inside the breast is not essential for tissue acquisition during directional vacuum-assisted biopsy, vacuum-assisted biopsy may be performed even in breasts too thin to undergo stereotactic 14-gauge automated core biopsy: The probe can be fired outside the breast and placed at the postfire position. During 11-gauge vacuum-assisted biopsy, the compressed breast thickness must at least be adequate to accommodate the collecting area (bowl) and tip of the biopsy probe (19 + 8 = 27 mm).

When performing stereotactic biopsy of thin breasts, it can be helpful to use the approach that allows maximum breast thickness. The thickness of compressed breast parenchyma is generally greater when the breast is compressed in a mediolateral direction rather than a craniocaudal direction.[71] Sometimes rolling the breast can be of use. Raising a generous wheal of anesthetic is also helpful for increasing breast thickness.[61]

The "reverse compression paddle" technique is particularly helpful in thin breasts.[72] This involves use of two parallel compression paddles with the apertures lined up, one on the near surface of the breast and the other on the far surface (taped to the Bucky). The scout and targeting images are then obtained, and the directional vacuum-assisted biopsy probe is fired outside the breast and placed to the postfire position. The second paddle will allow the tissue to be pushed through the aperture on the far side, often allowing enough room to successfully perform the biopsy. Alternatively, Bober and Russell[73] have described the use of a breast bolster consisting of an elongated plastic sponge at the periphery of the breast pushing inward; this method decreases the breast radius and thereby increases the depth of the compressed breast.

Superficial Lesions

Superficial lesions pose a problem similar to that posed by thin breasts: They may not allow firing the needle inside the breast because the prefire position of the collecting area of the needle would be in part outside the breast. Since firing the needle inside the breast is not essential for vacuum-assisted biopsy, superficial lesions may undergo biopsy with the vacuum-assisted probes.

To perform 11-gauge vacuum-assisted biopsy of a superficial lesion, the probe is fired outside the breast and then placed at the postfire position. It is of note that the bowl (collecting area) of the probe must be fully inside the breast during tissue acquisition in order to get an adequate seal to obtain vacuum. If the postfire position of the probe is such that some of the bowl is still outside the breast, the probe is then advanced until the bowl is just buried in the breast (Figure 5.21). The lesion will not be in the center of the bowl, but it will still be within the bowl, and therefore should be sampled during the biopsy procedure. Other techniques useful for biopsy of superficial lesions include raising a generous wheal of local anesthetic in the skin to increase the depth of the lesion and use of a skin hook to pull tissue over the probe entry site.

Small Lesions

At our institution, we have avoided performing stereotactic 14-gauge automated core biopsy of lesions measuring less than 5 mm. The reason for excluding these lesions is the theoretical possibility of removing the entire mammographic lesion with the automated needle without a reliable method of placing a localizing marker, rendering subsequent surgical excision more difficult. The 11-gauge vacuum-assisted biopsy probe can be used for stereotactic biopsy of small lesions, because it allows ready placement of a localizing marker.

When performing directional vacuum-assisted biopsy of small lesions, it is often helpful to position the probe slightly underneath the lesion (closer to the floor) to allow visualization of both the probe and the lesion[61] (Figure 5.22). Tissue is then acquired in the upward direction (from 9 to 3 o'clock in the upward hemisphere). It is par-

Post-fire Probe Placement For Vacuum-Assisted Biopsy of a Superficial Lesion

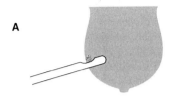

A

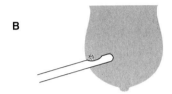

B

FIGURE 5.21. Postfire probe placement for vacuum-assisted biopsy of a superficial lesion. (A) Unacceptable probe position. If the probe is placed to the usual depth ($z - 2$ mm) for this superficial lesion, part of the collecting area (bowl) of the probe will be outside the breast, and vacuum will not be achieved. (B) Acceptable probe position. To biopsy this superficial lesion, the bowl of the probe is advanced until it is just inside the breast. The lesion will not be in the center of the bowl but should still be within the bowl, enabling tissue sampling.

ticularly important in these cases to obtain images after tissue acquisition is complete to determine if the mammographic lesion has been removed; if it has, placement of a localizing clip is prudent.[29,30]

Amorphous Calcifications

Amorphous (faint) calcifications may be particularly challenging. In a study of stereotactic 11-gauge directional vacuum-assisted biopsy, Liberman et al.[61] reported that calcification retrieval was successful in 95% (106/112) of cases. Failure to retrieve calcifications was significantly more likely in lesions measuring 5 mm or smaller (5/43 = 12% vs. 1/69 = 1%, $p = 0.03$), in calcifications with amorphous morphology (3/14 = 21% vs. 3/98 = 3%, $p < 0.03$), or if the probe was fired outside the breast (5/40 = 12% vs. 1/72 = 1%, $p = 0.02$).

As in all cases of calcifications that undergo stereotactic biopsy, it is essential to identify the same calcification on both stereotactic images to achieve proper needle placement. Ideally, the targeted calcification should be suspicious and should be located in the center of the group. However, if the calcifications are amorphous and/or loosely arranged, it may be helpful to target a calcifi-

cation that is distinctive enough that it can be confidently identified on both stereotactic images ("Mr. Bright"), even if it is neither the most suspicious nor the most centrally located. If this calcification is immediately adjacent to the other calcifications in the group, its retrieval should be accompanied by retrieval of its neighbors.[69]

For example, suppose that there is a single dense, easily visible calcification accompanied by numerous amorphous forms posterior to it that are difficult or impossible to see on the stereotactic images. The radiologist can target the dense calcification and specifically sample the tissue posterior to it in order to retrieve the amorphous forms. In cases where the amorphous forms are superficial to the dense and easily visible calcification, if the directional vacuum-assisted biopsy instrument is used, one can target the dense calcification and withdraw the probe

Post-fire Probe Placement For Vacuum-Assisted Biopsy of a Small Lesion

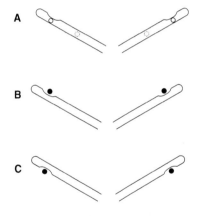

A

B

C

FIGURE 5.22. Post-fire position of vacuum-assisted biopsy probe when performing biopsy of small lesions. (A) Suboptimal postfire position of vacuum-assisted biopsy probe for small (i.e., subcentimeter) lesions. Positioning the probe directly over the lesion may obscure the lesion. If the lesion is obscured, it cannot be determined if the lesion is under the bowl of the probe (which would be a good position for sampling) (solid line circle) or under the shaft of the probe (which would not be appropriate for sampling) (dotted circle). (B) Acceptable postfire position of vacuum-assisted biopsy probe for small lesions. The bowl of the probe is immediately beneath the lesion, enabling visualization of the probe and the lesion. Tissue sampling should proceed from 9 to 3 o'clock in the upward hemisphere. (C) Acceptable postfire position of vacuum-assisted biopsy probe for small lesions. The bowl of the probe is immediately above the lesion, enabling visualization of the probe and the lesion. Tissue sampling should proceed from 3 to 9 o'clock in the downward hemisphere.

an appropriate distance in the z (depth) direction prior to tissue retrieval.

The prefire location of the needle or probe should be carefully assessed. The bowl of the directional vacuum-assisted biopsy instrument should be turned in the direction of the lesion prior to obtaining the first specimen. It may be helpful to refrain from giving some of the deep anesthetic until needle placement is confirmed because the anesthesia may obscure the already faint calcium. It is essential to work as quickly as possible, particularly for subtle lesions such as amorphous calcifications. The longer it takes to do the procedure, the higher the likelihood that the patient will move or that the lesion will be obscured by hematoma.

Subtle Lesions

Subtle lesions, such as isodense masses in nodular breasts or subtle areas of architectural distortion, can be difficult to identify on stereotactic images. For such lesions one can sometimes predict whether the lesion can be successfully targeted prior to scheduling the stereotactic biopsy procedure. If stereotactic biopsy is being considered for a subtle area, it may be helpful to perform two 15° angled views from the projection that allow the best visualization of the lesion, simulating the two projections that would be used for stereotactic biopsy. If the lesion cannot be reliably identified on those two views, it likely will not be well visualized on the targeting views obtained during the stereotactic biopsy procedure.

For subtle lesions scheduled for stereotactic biopsy, several steps are helpful in targeting. First, select the approach that allows optimal lesion visualization. Second, obtain a preliminary scout film with the alphanumeric grid that is used for needle localizations and mark the skin overlying the lesion prior to positioning the patient in the stereotactic unit. Third, use adjacent landmarks, including benign calcifications (if present), fat lobules, or stromal architecture. Fourth, if there is one particular portion of the lesion that is more distinctive or more reliably targeted, target that. Fifth, if available, it can be helpful to use a technique such as "Target on Scout" (Fischer Imaging Corporation, Denver, CO), which allows the radiologist to use the scout view and one 15° oblique projection in lieu of the two 15° oblique stereotactic images for targeting. Finally, it may be helpful to refrain from giving too much deep anesthesia until after stereotactic images confirm accurate needle placement.

Ultrasound is an excellent guidance modality for percutaneous biopsy of breast masses, particularly for masses that are subtle on the mammogram but well seen on sonography. For subtle masses that undergo percutaneous biopsy under stereotactic or ultrasound guidance, a two-view mammogram obtained immediately after percutaneous biopsy may show air and hematoma at the bi-opsy site and can help confirm that the area identified on the mammogram was sampled.

Multiple Lesions

Stereotactic biopsy is useful for women with multiple lesions.[74,75] Stereotactic biopsy diagnosis of two benign lesions spares a woman the expense and deformity of two benign surgical excisions. Stereotactic biopsy diagnosis of two carcinomas in different quadrants (multicentric disease) may enable the woman to proceed with mastectomy as a one-stage definitive treatment. Stereotactic biopsy diagnosis of one carcinoma and one benign lesion may indicate that the woman is a candidate for breast conservation and spare her a benign surgical biopsy that would compromise her cosmetic result.

When performing stereotactic biopsy of multiple lesions, each lesion should undergo biopsy with a new set of instrumentation, including a new anesthetic syringe and needle and a new probe. It is important to pay meticulous attention to labeling the specimen containers as well as the postbiopsy mammogram.[69] It is preferable to perform biopsy of the most suspicious lesion first: All interventional procedures should be approached as if the first thing done may be the last thing accomplished, and it is essential to prioritize.

Clip Problems

Why Clip?

The entirety of a small mammographic lesion can be removed at stereotactic biopsy, but complete removal of the mammographic lesion does not ensure complete excision of the histologic process. Of 15 carcinomas in which the entire mammographic lesion was removed at stereotactic 11-gauge vacuum-assisted biopsy in a study by Liberman et al.,[76] surgery revealed residual carcinoma in 11 (73%). Therefore, if the entire mammographic lesion is removed, it is prudent to place a localizing marker at the lesion site to facilitate subsequent needle localization if warranted.

Accuracy of Clip Placement

The clip is usually placed in close proximity to the biopsy site after stereotactic 11-gauge vacuum-assisted biopsy. A study that evaluated clip location on postbiopsy stereotactic images found that the clip was placed within 1 cm of the lesion site in 40 (95%) of 42 lesions that had stereotactic 11-gauge vacuum assisted biopsy.[29] In two studies that assessed clip location on two-view mammograms obtained after stereotactic 11-gauge vacuum-assisted biopsy, Burbank and Forcier[30] found that the initial marker clip deployment averaged 5 mm above baseline from the center of the target lesion with deployment >2.4 cm from the lesion center in 7% of cases. Rosen and Vo [77] found that the clip was placed within 5 mm of the target in 62 (56%) of 111 cases, within 6–10 mm in 18 (16%), and <1 cm removed from the target in 31 (28%).

Few studies address the long-term stability of clip position. However, Burbank and Forcier [30] found that compared with baseline variability, marker clips remained stable in position from initial deployment to first imaging follow-up (mean, 8.6 months).

Failure of Clip Deployment

Occasionally, the clip fails to deploy after stereotactic biopsy, usually because the clip adheres to retained tissue fragments in the bowl of the probe rather than deploying in the breast.[29] Suctioning out the biopsy cavity and performing the "tap" maneuver after tissue acquisition and before clip placement can remove retained fragments and increase the likelihood of successful clip deployment. If the clip is not evident on the stereotactic images obtained after clip placement and probe removal, the bowl of the probe should be inspected to identify tissue fragments (and, if fragments are identified, these should be radiographed); then the probe should be flushed as at the beginning of the procedure, placed back to the appropriate depth ($z - 7$), and a new clip placed with its appropriate location confirmed on stereotactic images after probe removal.[29]

It is possible that even after successful deployment the clip may be dislodged while withdrawing the probe from the breast. It is desirable to obtain stereotactic images after (rather than before) removal of the probe; if the clip was inadvertently removed it will be recognized on these images, and a new clip can be deployed while the breast is in position.

Errors in Clip Placement

When clip placement is imperfect, the most common error is in the depth (z) direction because of the accordion effect of breast compression (described above). The two-view mammogram after clip deployment is essential to identify the location of the clip with respect to the biopsy site.

If the clip is slightly deep or superficial to the lesion and the histologic findings warrant subsequent surgical excision, it is helpful to perform the preoperative needle localization from the same approach as that used for the stereotactic biopsy. For example, if the lesion was approached from the lateral skin surface for the stereotactic biopsy, the localization can also be performed from a lateral approach. If the clip is 1–2 cm deep (i.e., medial) to the lesion, with the tip of the wire at the clip, the more proximal portion of the wire will pierce the lesion; if the clip is 1–2 cm superficial (i.e., lateral) to the lesion, the wire can be placed through and beyond the clip with the wire tip at the lesion site and the more proximal portion of the wire at the clip. If the clip is so remote from the biopsy site that its retrieval would require placement of a second wire and/or a separate incision, we do not recommend that the clip be excised, but few data address this issue.

Localizing the "Invisible" Lesion: What to Do If No Clip Was Placed

Occasionally, a patient is referred for surgical excision of a lesion that underwent prior percutaneous biopsy where the mammographic lesion was removed and no localizing clip was left in place. Several steps may help in such cases. First, the prebiopsy mammograms should be carefully reviewed to look for adjacent landmarks (e.g., fat lobules, distinctive areas of parenchyma, adjacent benign calcifications, etc.). Second, if a postbiopsy mammogram was obtained, it should be reviewed; if not, performance of a postbiopsy mammogram is helpful to ascertain if any of the lesion is still present and to analyze adjacent landmarks that may be helpful in performing localization. It is preferable to perform and review the postbiopsy mammogram prior to the day of surgery. Fong et al.[78] have suggested that sonography may be helpful to identify the fluid-filled biopsy cavity in such cases.

Brenner[79] reported preoperative needle localization in seven cases in which the mammographic lesion was removed without placement of a localizing clip with a freehand technique using orthogonal and reproducible mammographic landmarks to guide needle placement. Successful surgical excision was accomplished in all cases, as evidenced by similar histopathologic findings, fibrin bands or collagen, and visualization of the core needle biopsy tract at microscopy. In such cases, it is helpful to specifically ask the pathologist to seek evidence of a recent biopsy tract, which would provide supportive evidence that the biopsy cavity was excised at surgery. Although published small series indicate that localization can be successfully performed without clip placement,[78,79] it is prudent to place a localizing marker if all imaging evidence of the lesion is removed.

FUTURE DIRECTIONS

Although the progress in stereotactic biopsy over the past decade has contributed to a revolution in breast diagnosis, further work is needed. New tissue acquisition devices should be developed and studied with respect to their accuracy, safety, and cost-effectiveness. Additional follow-up studies are needed to assess the long-term outcome. Development of evidence-based algorithms is needed to optimize the choice of biopsy method for various lesions. With continued improvements in equipment and technique, stereotactic biopsy may afford more women a minimally invasive alternative to surgery for breast diagnosis.

REFERENCES

1. Bolmgren J, Jacobsen B, Nordenstrom B. Stereotaxic instrument for needle biopsy of the mamma. AJR 1977;129:121–125.
2. Liberman L. Percutaneous image-guided core breast biopsy: state of the art at the millennium. AJR 2000;174:1191–1199.
3. Pisano ED, Fajardo LL, Tsimikas J, et al. Rate of insufficient samples for fine-needle aspiration for nonpalpable breast lesions in a multicenter clinical trial: the Radiologic Diagnostic Oncology Group 5 study. Cancer 1998;82:678–688.
4. Parker SH, Lovin JD, Jobe WE, et al. Stereotactic breast biopsy with a biopsy gun. Radiology 1990;176:741–747.
5. Parker SH, Lovin JD, Jobe WE, Burke BJ, Hopper KD, Yakes WF. Nonpalpable breast lesions: stereotactic automated large-core biopsies. Radiology 1991;180:403–407.
6. Elvecrog EL, Lechner MC, Nelson MT. Nonpalpable breast lesions: correlation of stereotaxic large-core needle biopsy and surgical biopsy results. Radiology 1993;188:453–455.
7. Dronkers DJ. Stereotaxic core biopsy of breast lesions: correlation of stereotaxic large-core needle biopsy and surgical biopsy results. Radiology 1992;188:631–634.
8. Gisvold JJ, Goellner JR, Grant CS, et al. Breast biopsy: a comparative study of stereotaxically guided core and excisional techniques. AJR 1994;162:815–820.
9. Dowlatshahi K, Yaremko ML, Kluskens LF, Jokich PM. Nonpalpable breast lesions: findings of stereotaxic needle-core biopsy and fine-needle aspiration cytology. Radiology 1991;181:745–750.
10. Jackman RJ, Nowels KW, Rodriguez-Soto J, Marzoni FA, Finkelstein SI, Shepard MJ. Stereotactic, automated, large-core needle biopsy of nonpalpable breast lesions: false-negative and histologic underestimation rates after long-term follow-up. Radiology 1999;210:799–805.
11. Lee CH, Philpotts LE, Horvath LJ, Tocino I. Follow-up of breast lesions diagnosed as benign with stereotactic core-needle biopsy: frequency of mammographic change and false-negative rate. Radiology 1999;212:189–194.
12. Jackman RJ, Marzoni FA. Needle-localized breast biopsy: why do we fail? Radiology 1997;204:677–684.
13. Liberman L, Fahs MC, Dershaw DD, et al. Impact of stereotaxic core biopsy on cost of diagnosis. Radiology 1995;195:633–637.
14. Lee CH, Egglin TIK, Philpotts LE, Mainiero MB, Tocino I. Cost-effectiveness of stereotactic core needle biopsy: analysis by means of mammographic findings. Radiology 1997;202:849–854.
15. Hillner BE, Bear HD, Fajardo LL. Estimating the cost-effectiveness of stereotaxic biopsy for nonpalpable breast abnormalities: a decision analysis model. Acad Radiol 1996;3:351–360.
16. Liberman L, Sama M. Cost-effectiveness of stereotactic 11-gauge directional vacuum-assisted breast biopsy. AJR 2000;175:53–58.
17. Liberman L. Clinical management issues in percutaneous core breast biopsy. Radiol Clin North Am 2000;791–807.
18. American College of Radiology. Breast imaging reporting and data system (BI-RADS), 2nd ed. Reston, VA: American College of Radiology, 1995.
19. Liberman L, Abramson AF, Squires FB, Glassman J, Morris EA, Dershaw DD. The breast imaging reporting and data system: positive predictive value of mammographic features and final assessment categories. AJR 1998;171:35–40.
20. Orel SG, Kay N, Reynolds C, Sullivan DC. BI-RADS categorization as a predictor of malignancy. Radiology 1999;211:845–850.
21. Liberman L, Dershaw DD, Rosen PP, Cohen MA, Hann LE, Abramson AF. Stereotaxic core biopsy of impalpable spiculated breast masses. AJR 1995;165:551–554.
22. Liberman L, LaTrenta LR, Van Zee KJ, Morris EA, Abramson AF, Dershaw DD. Stereotactic core biopsy of calcifications highly suggestive of malignancy. Radiology 1997;203:673–677.
23. Sickles EA. Periodic mammographic follow-up of probably benign lesions: results of 3,184 consecutive cases. Radiology 1991;179:463–468.
24. Varas X, Leborgne F, Leborgne JH. Nonpalpable, probably benign lesions: role of follow-up mammography. Radiology 1992;184:409–414.
25. Parker SH, Jobe WE, Dennis MA, et al. US-guided automated large-core breast biopsy. Radiology 1993;187:507–511.
26. Rubin E, Dempsey PJ, Pile NS, et al. Needle-localization biopsy of the breast: impact of a selective core needle biopsy program on yield. Radiology 1995;195:627–631.
27. Liberman L, Feng TL, Dershaw DD, Morris EA, Abramson AF. Ultrasound-guided core breast biopsy: utility and cost-effectiveness. Radiology 1998;208:717–723.
28. Catterall W, Mackie K. Local anesthetics. In Hardman JG, Limbird LE, Molinoff PB, Ruddon RW, Gilman AG (eds) Goodman & Gilman's The Pharmacological Basis of Therapeutics. New York: McGraw-Hill, 1996;331–347.
29. Liberman L, Dershaw DD, Morris EA, Abramson AF, Thornton CM, Rosen PP. Clip placement after stereotactic vacuum-assisted breast biopsy. Radiology 1997;205:417–422.
30. Burbank F, Forcier N. Tissue marking clip for stereotactic breast biopsy: initial placement accuracy, long-term stability, and usefulness as a guide for wire localization. Radiology 1997;205:407–415.
31. Philpotts LE, Lee CH, Horvath LJ, Tocino I. Canceled stereotactic core-needle biopsy of the breast: analysis of 89 cases. Radiology 1997;205:423–428.
32. Hendrick RE, Parker SH. Principles of stereotactic mammography and quality assurance. In Parker SH, Jobe WE (eds) Percutaneous Breast Biopsy. New York: Raven Press, 1993;49–59.
33. Welle GJ, Clark M, Loos S, et al. Stereotactic breast biopsy: recumbent biopsy using add-on upright equipment. AJR 2000;175:59–63.
34. Dershaw DD, Fleming ID, Liberman L. Use of digital mammography in needle localization procedures. AJR 1993;161:559–562.
35. Parker SH, Dennis MA, Jobe WE, Hendrick RE. Clinical efficacy of digital stereotaxic mammography. Radiology 1993;189(P):326.
36. Meyer JE, Smith DN, DiPiro PJ, et al. Stereotactic breast biopsy of clustered microcalcifications with a directional, vacuum-assisted device. Radiology 1997;204:575–576.

37. Jackman RJ, Burbank F, Parker SH, et al. Accuracy of sampling microcalcifications by three stereotactic breast biopsy methods (abstract). Radiology 1997;205(P):325.

38. Reynolds HE, Poon CM, Goulet RJ, Lazaridis CL. Biopsy of breast microcalcifications using an 11-gauge directional vacuum-assisted device. AJR 1998;171:611–613.

39. Burbank F. Stereotactic breast biopsy of atypical ductal hyperplasia and ductal carcinoma in situ lesions: improved accuracy with a directional, vacuum-assisted biopsy instrument. Radiology 1997;202:843–847.

40. Jackman RJ, Burbank F, Parker SH, et al. Atypical ductal hyperplasia diagnosed at stereotactic breast biopsy: improved reliability with 14-gauge, directional, vacuum-assisted biopsy. Radiology 1997;204:485–488.

41. Jackman RJ, Burbank F, Parker SH, et al. Atypical ductal hyperplasia diagnosed by 11-gauge, directional, vacuum-assisted breast biopsy: how often is carcinoma found at surgery? Radiology 1997;205(P):325.

42. Meyer JE, Smith DN, Lester SC, et al. Large-core needle biopsy of nonpalpable breast lesions. JAMA 1999;281:1638–1641.

43. Jackman RJ, Burbank F, Parker SH, et al. Stereotactic breast biopsy of nonpalpable lesions: determinants of ductal carcinoma in situ underestimation rates. Radiology 2001;218:497–502.

44. Melotti MK, Berg WA. Core needle breast biopsy in patients undergoing anticoagulation therapy: preliminary results. AJR 2000;174:245–249.

45. Parker SH, Burbank F, Jackman RJ, et al. Percutaneous large-core breast biopsy: a multi-institutional study. Radiology 1994;193:359–364.

46. Dershaw DD, Caravella DA, Liberman L, Abramson AF, Cohen MA, Hann LE. Limitations and complications in the utilization of stereotaxic core biopsy. Breast J 1996;2:1–6.

47. Dershaw DD, Morris EA, Liberman L, Abramson AF. Nondiagnostic stereotaxic core breast biopsy: results of rebiopsy. Radiology 1996;198:323–325.

48. Meyer JE, Smith DN, Lester SC, et al. Large-core needle biopsy: nonmalignant breast abnormalities evaluated with surgical excision or repeat core biopsy. Radiology 1998;206:717–720.

49. Philpotts LE, Shaheen NA, Carter D, Lange RC, Lee CH. Comparison of rebiopsy rates after stereotactic core needle biopsy of the breast with 11-gauge vacuum suction probe versus 14-gauge needle and automatic gun. AJR 1999;172:683–687.

50. Jackman RJ, Nowels KW, Shepard MJ, Finkelstein SI, Marzoni FA. Stereotaxic large-core needle biopsy of 450 nonpalpable breast lesions with surgical correlation in lesions with cancer or atypical hyperplasia. Radiology 1994;193:91–95.

51. Liberman L, Cohen MA, Dershaw DD, Abramson AF, Hann LE, Rosen PP. Atypical ductal hyperplasia diagnosed at stereotaxic core biopsy of breast lesions: an indication for surgical biopsy. AJR 1995;164:1111–1113.

52. Liberman L, Drotman MB, Morris EA, et al. Imaging-histologic discordance at percutaneous breast biopsy. Cancer 2000;89:2538–2546.

53. Kaye MD, Vicinanza-Adami CA, Sullivan ML. Mammographic findings after stereotaxic biopsy of the breast performed with large-core needles. Radiology 1994;192:149–151.

54. Burbank F. Mammographic findings after 14-gauge automated needle and 14-gauge directional, vacuum-assisted stereotactic breast biopsies. Radiology 1997;204:153–156.

55. Lamm RL, Jackman RJ. Mammographic abnormalities caused by percutaneous stereotactic biopsy of histologically benign lesions evident on follow-up mammograms. AJR 2000;174:753–756.

56. Meyer JE, Lester SC, Frenna TH, White FV. Occult breast calcifications sampled with large-core biopsy: confirmation with radiography of the specimen. Radiology 1993;188:581–582.

57. Liberman L, Evans WP III, Dershaw DD, et al. Radiography of microcalcifications in stereotaxic mammary core biopsy specimens. Radiology 1994;190:223–225.

58. Berg WA, Jaeger B, Campassi C, Kumar D. Predictive value of specimen radiography for core needle biopsy of noncalcified breast masses. AJR 1998;171:1671–1678.

59. Liberman L, Dershaw DD, Rosen PP, Abramson AF, Deutch BM, Hann LE. Stereotaxic 14-gauge breast biopsy: how many core biopsy specimens are needed? Radiology 1994;192:793–795.

60. Parker SH. Stereotactic large-core breast biopsy. In Parker SH, Jobe WE (eds) Percutaneous Breast Biopsy. New York: Raven, 1993;61–79.

61. Liberman L, Smolkin JH, Dershaw DD, Morris EA, Abramson AF, Rosen PP. Calcification retrieval at stereotactic 11-gauge vacuum-assisted breast biopsy. Radiology 1998;208:251–260.

62. Hann LE, Liberman L, Dershaw DD, Cohen MA, Abramson AF. Mammography immediately after stereotaxic breast biopsy: is it necessary? AJR 1995;165:59–62.

63. Liberman L, Hann LE, Dershaw DD, Morris EA, Abramson AF, Rosen PP. Mammographic findings after stereotactic 14-gauge vacuum biopsy. Radiology 1997;203:343–347.

64. Parker SH, Klaus AJ. Performing a breast biopsy with a directional, vacuum-assisted biopsy instrument. RadioGraphics 1997;17:1233–1252.

65. Burbank F. Stereotactic breast biopsy: comparison of 14- and 11-gauge mammotome probe performance and complication rates. Am Surg 1997;63:988–995.

66. Brem RF, Askin FB, Gatewood OMB. Selection of core biopsy specimens for pathologic evaluation of targeted microcalcifications. AJR 1999;173:901–902.

67. Freeman HP. Racial injustice in health care. N Engl J Med 2000;342:1045–1047.

68. Liberman L, Dershaw DD, Glassman J, et al. Analysis of cancers not diagnosed at stereotactic core breast biopsy. Radiology 1997;203:151–157.

69. Liberman L. Stereotactic breast biopsy: difficult cases. MammoMatters 1999;6:35–43.

70. Soo MS, Walsh R, Patton J. Prone table stereotactic breast biopsy: facilitating biopsy of posterior lesions using the arm-through-the-hole technique. AJR 1998;171:615–617.

71. Helvie MA, Chan HP, Adler DD, Boyd PG. Breast thickness in routine mammograms: effect on image quality and radiation dose. AJR 1994;163:1371–1374.

72. Parker SH, Burbank F. A practical approach to minimally invasive breast biopsy. Radiology 1996;200:11–20.

73. Bober SE, Russell DG. Increasing breast tissue depth during stereotactic needle biopsy. AJR 2000;174:1085–1086.

74. Liberman L, Dershaw DD, Rosen PP, Morris EA, Cohen MA, Abramson AF. Core needle biopsy of synchronous ipsilateral breast lesions: impact on treatment. AJR 1996;166:1429–1432.

75. Rosenblatt R, Fineberg SA, Sparano JA, Kaleya RN. Stereotactic core needle biopsy of multiple sites in the breast: efficacy and effect on patient care. Radiology 1996;201:67–70.

76. Liberman L, Dershaw DD, Rosen PP, Morris EA, Abramson AF, Borgen PI. Percutaneous removal of malignant mammographic lesions at stereotactic vacuum-assisted biopsy. Radiology 1998;206:711–715.

77. Rosen EL, Vo TT. Metallic clip deployment during stereotactic breast biopsy: retrospective analysis. Radiology 2001;218:510–516.

78. Greenlee RT, Hill-Harmon MB, Murray T, Thun M. Cancer statistics, 2001. CA Cancer J Clin 2001;51:15–36.

79. Brenner RJ. Lesions entirely removed during stereotactic biopsy: preoperative localization on the basis of mammographic landmarks and feasibility of freehand technique—initial experience. Radiology 2000;214:585–590.

CHAPTER 6

Ultrasound-Guided Core Breast Biopsy

Linda R. LaTrenta

Percutaneous image-guided core biopsy with either stereotactic or sonographic guidance has been shown to be an economical, accurate alternative to the surgical biopsy of suspicious breast lesions.[1–17] In 1993 Parker et al. first described the use of ultrasound-guided core biopsy in a study of 181 lesions sampled with a 14-gauge automated needle.[4] In the 49 lesions that underwent subsequent surgical excision, there was 100% histopathologic correlation with core biopsy results. In the remaining 132 lesions yielding benign results, no carcinomas were identified at follow-up (range 12–36 months). Although no subsequent study specifically addresses the false negative rate of ultrasound-guided core biopsy, clinical studies of stereotactic 14-gauge automated core needle biopsy demonstrate an average false negative rate of 2.8%,[18,19] which is comparable to the 2.0% frequency of missed carcinoma at needle localization and surgical biopsy.[20] Therefore, ultrasound-guided core biopsy can accurately diagnose benign lesions without surgery and facilitate preoperative planning for malignant lesions. In a study of 151 consecutive nonpalpable masses that underwent ultrasound-guided core biopsy, a surgical procedure was obviated in 85%, and the cost of diagnosis was estimated to decrease by 56% relative to surgical biopsy.[21]

ADVANTAGES

Besides a lower cost of diagnosis, percutaneous image-guided biopsy has several advantages over surgical biopsy. It does not cause cosmetic deformity or scarring visible on mammography,[22,23] can be performed the same day as the diagnostic mammogram, uses local anesthe-

sia, and can provide estrogen/progesterone receptor status in patients with concurrent stage IV disease when therapeutic breast surgery is not indicated.

Ultrasound-guided core biopsy also has several advantages over stereotactic biopsy. The necessary equipment is widely available, is less expensive, and does not require additional radiation exposure to the breast. Procedure time is reportedly as low as 20 minutes.[4] Patients who are unable to lie prone on a stereotactic table due to spinal arthritis or recent abdominal surgery can usually lie in the supine or supine-oblique position for an ultrasound-guided procedure. Because the patient is recumbent instead of seated as with some stereotactic units, vasovagal reactions rarely occur. Moreover, the breast is not compressed during ultrasound, which may increase patient comfort. Lesions that are not amenable to stereotactic biopsy because of their inability to be positioned in the stereotactic field of view because of their close proximity to the chest wall are easily biopsied with sonographic guidance, when they can be visualized sonographically. Because the breast is not compressed during sonographically guided biopsy, the inability to perform a biopsy because the breast is too thin to accommodate the throw of the needle or the length of the tissue acquisition chamber is obviated in sonographically guided procedures. This also applies to situations where the lesion is in a thin area of the breast, such as behind the nipple.

Because of the limited volume of the axilla and the presence of the large, axillary vascular and neural structures, tissue sampling in the axilla is frequently done as fine-needle aspiration. However, if an axillary mass is large enough to accommodate the throw of the needle safely, ultrasound guided biopsy of the axilla can be performed. Because of the difficulty of positioning the axilla in the stereotactic device, these biopsies usually cannot be done under stereotactic guidance. Ultrasound may also be helpful for percutaneous biopsy of mammographically subtle lesions that are better seen with sonography. Of course, it is the only appropriate method for biopsy of those lesions only seen with sonography.

DISADVANTAGES/COMPLICATIONS

The major limitation of ultrasound-guided core biopsy is that a small subset of solid masses are isoechoic with breast parenchyma and not sonographically evident. In addition, although biopsy of calcifications under ultrasound guidance has been reported,[24,25] stereotactic biopsy is the preferred method, as calcifications are not reliably identified under sonography. Masses smaller than 5 mm are problematic, as biopsy can obscure or remove the lesion making subsequent localization difficult. The vacuum-assisted ultrasound-guided biopsy probe (Mammotome, Biopsys/Ethicon Endo-surgery, Cincinnati, OH) enables placement of a metallic localizing clip through the 11-gauge needle and may be an alternative in these cases. Radiologists are often reluctant to perform ultrasound-guided core biopsy in patients with breast implants because of concern about rupturing the implant and therefore prefer fine needle aspiration. The vacuum-assisted biopsy probe may be an alternative in these patients as it is not fired in the breast, thereby decreasing the probability of implant penetration. However, this method requires expensive dedicated equipment and may have a higher rate of bleeding complications than conventional 14-gauge automated biopsy.[26]

Ultrasound-guided biopsy is not ideal for patients who cannot cooperate with positioning, as they are not immobilized by breast compression and must maintain their position for 20–30 minutes. Contraindications common to all percutaneous large-core needle procedures include allergy to local anesthetics and a history of a bleeding diathesis. We request that patients avoid aspirin-containing medications for 1 week and nonsteroidal antiinflammatory medications (NSAIDs) for 3–5 days before the procedure. Some authors have reported successful performance of ultrasound-guided biopsy while the patient is on warfarin.[27] However, because these are not emergency procedures, if possible we request that the patient discontinue her warfarin for 1 week prior to biopsy. It has been suggested that in women in whom discontinuation is medically contraindicated, performance of the breast biopsy under sonographic rather than stereotactic guidance, when possible, is advantageous because of the greater ease in applying manual compression to the breast during sonographically guided procedures.[27] The performance of core biopsy in lactating women has been reported to be complicated by subsequent formation of milk fistula in some cases.[28]

Major complications are unusual, with infection or hematoma in approximately 0.2% of patients.[7] Minor complications, occurring in up to 50% of patients, include bruising, breast tenderness, and psychological stress.[29] In a study of 67 consecutive patients who underwent vacuum-assisted ultrasound-guided core breast biopsy, 5 (7%) had bleeding for longer than 10 minutes, suggesting a higher risk of bleeding complications.[26] Pneumothorax is also a theoretical complication of ultrasound-guided core biopsy if the needle is fired into the chest wall during the procedure. In a large multiinstitutional study, Parker et al. found no cases of seeding of carcinoma along the needle tract.[7]

EQUIPMENT REQUIREMENTS

All breast ultrasound procedures should be performed with a high frequency linear transducer of at least 7.5 MHz. The room should have adjustable lighting and the table or stretcher positioned to allow accessibility to all quadrants of the breast. A small portable table can serve as a flat surface for a sterile field (Figure 6.1). A needle disposal system should be maintained in the room for safe discard of sharps.

A wide variety of guns and needles are commercially available for performing ultrasound guided core biopsies (see Chapter 4). Ultrasound-guided core biopsy requires needles that are larger gauge than those used for aspiration to ensure that samples can be adequately analyzed histopathologically. Studies have shown that 14-gauge needles retrieve the most diagnostic specimens with no significant increase in complications or cost relative to 16- or 18-gauge needles.[30]

The most common biopsy guns utilize a spring mech-

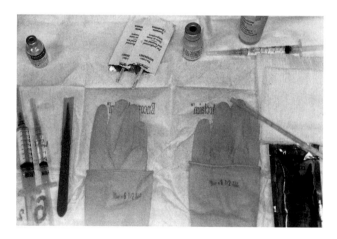

FIGURE 6.1. Biopsy tray. Small sterile field containing sterile gloves, two iodine swabs, sterile coupling gel, 1% lidocaine, 3 cc syringe with 25-gauge needle, 10 cc syringe with 22-gauge needle, 4 × 4 sterile gauze, no. 11 scalpel blade, 10 cc syringe of sterile saline with 22-gauge needle, 14-gauge biopsy needle.

anism to advance the inner and outer parts of a needle through the breast. The inner needle has a notch to trap tissue. After the inner needle fires, the outer needle advances over it to cut off the tissue sample within the notch. The entire needle is removed from the breast, and the outer needle is withdrawn over the inner needle to expose the sample. After the core is removed, cocking the gun retracts the inner needle prior to reinsertion into the breast for further sampling. Long-throw (22 mm) guns are preferable to short-throw (15 mm) guns because of better tissue acquisition.[31]

PREPARATION AND POSITIONING

It is worthwhile to review all films 1–2 days prior to the scheduled biopsy to ensure that the location of the lesion is clearly marked on the films and there is no uncertainty as to the indication for biopsy or site(s) to be biopsied. During diagnostic ultrasound examinations, it is helpful to record the lesion site on the film as the clock position and centimeters from the nipple to facilitate localization of the lesion during subsequent interventional procedures. On the day of the biopsy the case can be reviewed by the radiologist performing the biopsy to ensure that any clinical questions the patient has regarding the need for biopsy can be addressed.

Before the patient enters the biopsy suite, the table and ultrasound machine should be arranged to optimize access to the biopsy site. Positioning the patient incorrectly can lead to an awkward stance for the operator and can significantly impede performance of the procedure. For outer quadrant masses, the patient should be positioned so that the quadrant containing the lesion is on the same side of the table as the radiologist. The ultrasound unit is positioned so that the radiologist can scan with the left, or nondominant, hand and sample with the dominant hand while facing the screen. For inner quadrant lesions, depending on how far medial the lesion is, it may be easier to reach across the patient so that the lesion can be accessed from the medial side of the breast. In these cases, the breast should be positioned on the opposite side of the table from the radiologist. One should avoid positioning that requires the operator to twist his or her body to see the screen.

Before the patient is on the table, it should be confirmed that the patient has not recently taken anticoagulant medications and has no allergy to local anesthetics. Informed consent should be obtained. For lateral lesions, the supine oblique position with the ipsilateral arm raised above the head is recommended. This position flattens the breast against the chest wall, thereby reducing breast mobility and facilitating sound penetration by decreasing breast thickness. A pillow or wedge can be placed under the patient's shoulder to help her maintain this position comfortably. For medial lesions, the supine position has the same effect.

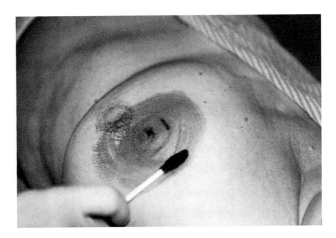

FIGURE 6.2. Patient marking. The straight line indicates the leading edge of the transducer, and the X marks the skin entry site. Note that the skin entry site is a short distance away from the transducer to facilitate an angle of approach parallel to the chest wall. The skin is cleansed with an iodine swab by concentric circular motions starting at the skin entry site.

The notation on all images should include the facility performing the biopsy, date of the procedure, patient's name, patient's identifying number (medical record number, social security number, or birth date), laterality (right or left), location of the lesion within the breast indicated by clock position/centimeters from the nipple, and the initials of the radiologist performing the procedure. Preliminary pictures should be obtained that include orthogonal images of the lesion to be sampled with measurements. At this time one can determine the approach to the lesion that is the most comfortable for the operator, optimizes lesion visualization, and maintains an approach parallel to the chest wall. The needle approach should always be along the long axis of the transducer to ensure that the needle can be visualized in its entirety during the procedure. A nonpermanent marker can be used to draw lines indicating the leading edge of the transducer and the expected needle entry site (Figure 6.2). Unlike aspiration, the needle entry site for core biopsy should be at least 1 cm away from the transducer so that the needle approach is nearly parallel to the chest wall. For deep lesions, it may need to be more than 1 cm away so that the needle is not angled toward the chest wall on approach.

TECHNIQUE

The nonsterile coupling gel is then removed and the skin cleansed with Betadine (Purdue Frederick Company, Norwalk, CT). The transducer should be wiped with alcohol. Sterile gloves should be donned, and a minimal amount of sterile coupling gel applied. Excessive gel can complicate the procedure by overflowing onto the skin entry site, and making the transducer slippery. Alcohol or Betadine can also be used as a coupling agent.

Anesthesia should be given near the lesion, along the biopsy tract, and at the skin entry site. Usually it is the subcutaneous injection of anesthetic that is the most painful. Therefore, the instillation of deep anesthesia first can be helpful in numbing the skin before anesthetic is injected subcutaneously. This may be more comfortable for patients. For deep anesthesia 1% lidocaine is injected through a 22-gauge needle, giving 3–10 cc. This should be done under direct sonographic visualization to be certain that the target lesion and the needle path are not obscured by anesthetic. This also makes it possible to do a practice approach to the lesion before the large core needle is placed in the breast. Before the needle is completely removed, 2–3 cc of anesthetic can be injected subcutaneously (Figure 6.3), sparing the patient a second needling. The addition of bicarbonate has been reported to be helpful in reducing the stinging sensation of the injected lidocaine. Besides providing anesthesia for the patient, the optimal approach to the lesion can be confirmed at the time of injection. For lesions close to the chest wall, injection of anesthetic underneath the lesion can elevate it and facilitate subsequent biopsy. In dense breast tissue that is resistant to the movement of a large gauge needle, injection of anesthetic in the needle path can be useful in separating tissues, making them less resistant to the movement of the biopsy probe. Care should be taken to eliminate air from the syringe as it may compromise further imaging. For subtle hypoechoic lesions, care should also be taken not to obscure the lesion during injection.

Although anesthetic will numb the breast to pressure and most pain, some patients will feel a pulling sensation in their breast, probably due to the cutting needle pulling on fibrous elements, perhaps those attached to the skin. It is very difficult, often impossible, to eliminate this sensation with anesthetic. Fortunately, this is not a problem for most women. Because the needle throws beyond the target lesion, sometimes there is a sensation of pain beyond the lesion. In order not to obscure the lesion, in-

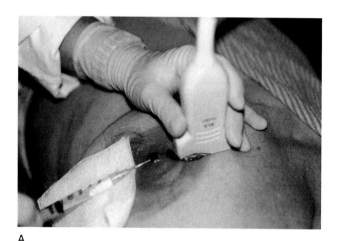

A

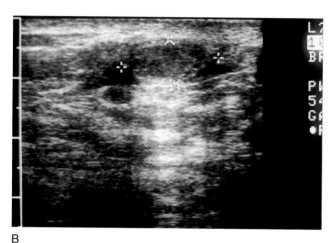

B

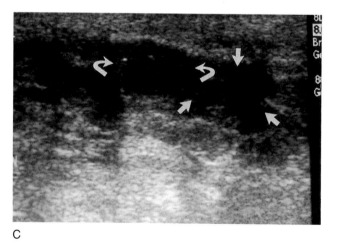

C

FIGURE 6.3. Local anesthesia. (A) Lidocaine 1% (2–3 cc) is injected into the skin entry site with a 25-gauge needle to raise a skin wheel. (B, C) Injection of anesthestic should be done with care and under sonographic visualization. Air should be purged from the syringe before the injection. Both air and the anesthestic can obscure the target. (B) Targeted lesion is shown in the prebiopsy scout scan surrounded by x marks of the electronic calipers. (C) After injection of 3 cc of anesthetic a pseudo-mass (straight arrows) has been created adjacent to the target (curved arrows).

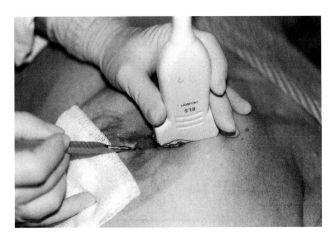

FIGURE 6.4. Scalpel incision. A small incision is made with a no. 11 scalpel to facilitate entry of the 14-gauge biopsy needle. Note the placement of a 4 × 4 gauze pad inferior to the site for patient comfort.

jection of anesthetic deep to and beyond the lesion can be helpful in eliminating this source of discomfort, when necessary.

A small skin incision is made with a No. 11 scalpel blade to facilitate entry of the 14-gauge biopsy needle (Figure 6.4). A sterile 4 × 4 gauze should be placed on the chest wall next to the skin entry site as the sensation of local anesthetic or blood dripping on the skin can be unpleasant. This is also helpful in clearing blood from the incision site so that it is more easily seen. The noise made by the sampling gun should be demonstrated by firing it out of the patient's visual range prior to the initial insertion. References to "firing the gun" should be avoided as some patients find this language upsetting. "Taking the sample" or a similar phrase is less anxiety provoking for the patient. Just prior to obtaining each sample, the patient should be warned that she will hear the noise to prevent a startle response.

Sonographically guided procedures require manual dexterity because one must coordinate scanning with one hand while maneuvering the needle with the other. Most people prefer to scan with their nondominant hand and sample with their dominant hand. Regardless of the method used, an absolute necessity for the technical success of the procedure is keeping the lesion within the focal plane of the transducer at all times. The transducer should be kept parallel to the table and the needle precisely aligned with the long axis of the transducer to allow visualization of the entire needle (Figure 6.5). Constant visualization of the tip is necessary to minimize complications such as pneumothorax. It may help to have an assistant manually support the transducer cord, thereby reducing tension on the transducer.

Under direct sonographic visualization, the needle should be inserted at a slightly acute angle aiming for the inferior third of the lesion. Once the tip is at the leading

edge of the lesion, the needle can be rocked superiorly so that it is parallel to or pointing away from the chest wall (Figure 6.6). The needle should never be fired toward the chest wall. If at any time the needle is not im-

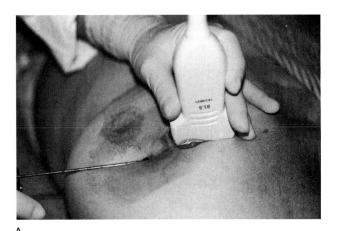

A

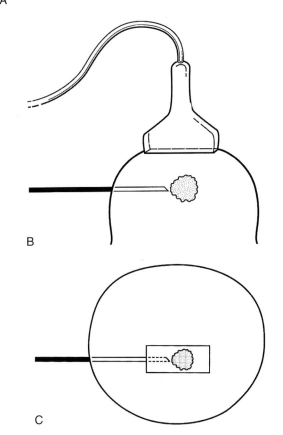

B

C

FIGURE 6.5. Needle position. (A) The long axis of the needle must remain aligned with the long axis of the transducer to ensure visualization of the entire needle during the procedure. Note that the transducer is held perpendicular to the skin surface. (B) Schematically, the prefire alignment of the transducer, target, and cutting needle are shown. The target should be near the middle of the transducer. The cutting needle is positioned parallel to the long axis of the transducer, along the center of the transducer. (C) Prefire alignment of transducer, cutting needle, and target are shown from above.

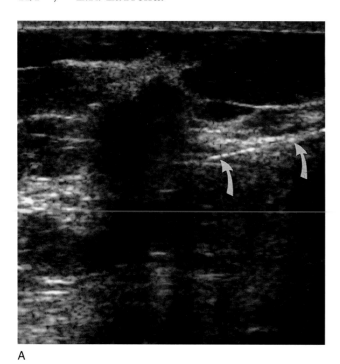
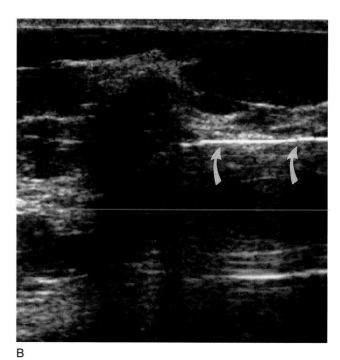

A   B

FIGURE 6.6. Needle position on approach. (**A**) The needle (arrows) is inserted at a slightly acute angle aiming for the inferior third of the lesion. (**B**) The needle (arrows) is rocked superiorly to ensure it is parallel to the chest wall in the prefire position. This method of targeting the lesion is especially important when the lesion is near the chest wall. So long as the cutting needle is aimed away from the chest wall, the danger of pneumothorax is eliminated.

aged in its entirety, one should swivel the transducer to elongate the image on the needle and determine its position. Without moving the needle, one can then swivel the transducer to image the lesion. Using this method, the relative position of the needle and mass can be determined; the needle is withdrawn slightly and then reinserted in the appropriate direction.

Penetration of dense breast tissue when approaching a lesion is usually best performed with short jabbing motions with counterpressure on the opposite side of the transducer with the fourth and fifth fingers of the scanning hand. This prevents sudden giving way of tissue that can occur during constant vigorous pressure. Generous injection of local anesthetic along the anticipated biopsy tract can also make needle insertion easier. Occasionally, in an extremely dense breast or fibrous lesion the inner needle may fire, but the outer needle fails to close. This is usually heralded by a dull thud instead of a sharp click.[32]

Images should be obtained in the pre- and postfire positions for each pass and labeled "precore #1," "postcore #1," and so on (Figure 6.7). The position of the needle tip should be included on the post-fire image to document needle placement. Often air is introduced along the tract of the needle during sampling. This appears on subsequent images as a hyperechoic linear focus within the mass (Figure 6.8). This can be used to identify sites that have undergone biopsy to direct further sampling to a different portion of the mass.

After firing the gun, the needle is removed from the breast and the core extracted from the inner needle using the scalpel blade (Figure 6.9). If one encounters resistance to removing the needle from a dense breast after firing, counterpressure against the skin on both sides of the needle by the technologist can be helpful. A syringe containing sterile saline with a sterile 22-gauge needle can assist in removing adherent samples from the scalpel. Cores are placed in a jar of 10% formalin that is prelabeled with the patient's name, identifying number, date of the procedure, and site of the biopsy (e.g., right breast 9 o'clock). While extracting the sample from the needle, someone should apply pressure to the biopsy site (not the skin entry site) with the transducer or sterile gauze. The needle should not be dipped into the formalin until the end of the procedure.

Although the optimal number of cores for ultrasound-guided biopsy has not been studied, extrapolations can be made from the data on stereotactic biopsies. In a study by Liberman et al.[33] of 14-gauge automated core biopsies of nonpalpable masses with stereotactic guidance, the first core had a diagnostic yield of 84%. Obtaining an additional two cores increased the diagnostic yield to 98%. Based on these data it is reasonable to obtain at least three to five cores, preferably from different areas of the mass. Real-time imaging can assess the adequacy of needle placement within the lesion. The adequacy of the samples can be assessed visually based on size and consistency. Cancers and fibrous solid lesions often yield stiff,

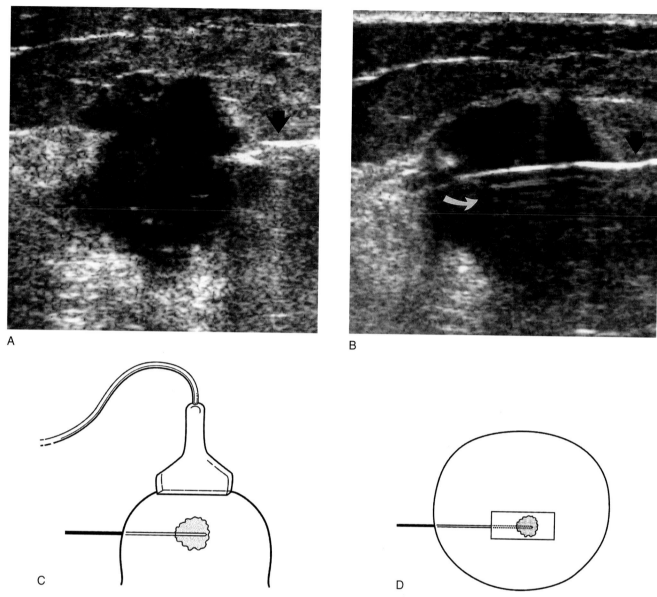

FIGURE 6.7. Documentation of tissue sampling. (**A**, **B**) Images should be obtained in the prefire (**A**) and postfire (**B**) positions for each pass and annotated appropriately (black arrow indicates the needle). Note the ring-down artifact from the 14-gauge needle (curved white arrow). (**C**, **D**) Alignment of the transducer, needle, and target to obtain postfire images, looking from the side (**B**) and from above (**C**). As in Figure 6.5, the needle is positioned along the center of the long axis of the transducer and parallel to it. The target is in the central third of the image. The needle tip should be near the far edge of the lesion or beyond it, documenting sampling of tissue from the area of interest.

white samples. Fragmented, short fatty cores may correlate with poor needle positioning within the mass and indicate the need for further sampling.

VACUUM-ASSISTED BIOPSY PROBE

For the vacuum-assisted ultrasound-guided biopsy probe (Mammotome, Biopsys/Ethicon Endo-surgery, Cincinnati, OH), the procedure is similar except that the needle is not fired in the breast. It must be positioned deep to

the lesion because the posterior acoustic shadowing from the 11-gauge probe will otherwise obscure the target (Figure 6.10). Injection of anesthetic underneath the lesion can facilitate placement of the probe by elevating the mass away from the chest wall. Once the probe is in position posterior to the mass, the apparatus can be locked into place by an articulating arm attached to the examination table. The inner needle is retracted to expose the aperture which is then centered on the lesion. Samples are taken anterior to the probe by rotating the aperture to different clock positions similar to those used during a

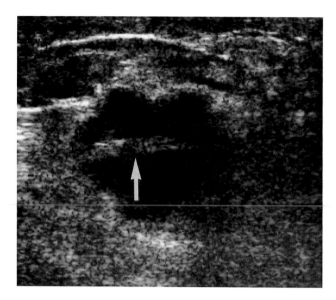

FIGURE 6.8. Visualization of the biopsy tract. Air introduced by sampling is visualized as a hyperechoic linear area within the mass (arrow) and can be used to direct further sampling to different areas of the mass.

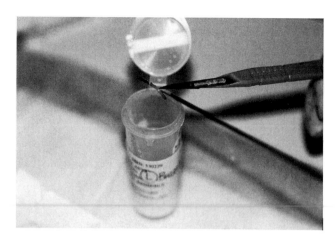

FIGURE 6.9. Extracting the sample. The scalpel blade can be used to transfer the sample from the inner needle to the prelabeled jar of 10% formalin. The needle or scalpel should not be dipped in formalin during the procedure. A syringe of sterile saline can facilitate removal of adherent samples from the scalpel.

vacuum-assisted stereotactic biopsy procedure.[34] Accurate sampling of the lesion can be observed in real time.

A major advantage of this procedure is that a metallic localizing clip can be left at the biopsy site after sampling small masses (<5 mm) that may be either obscured or removed by conventional ultrasound core biopsy (Figure 6.11). It may also be preferable for biopsy of lesions close to the chest wall or to an implant because the nee-

dle is not fired in the breast, reducing the chance of chest wall or implant penetration. The disadvantages are a potentially higher rate of bleeding[26] and higher cost of the dedicated equipment and biopsy needles.

MULITPLE, SYNCHRONOUS BIOPSIES

If there are multiple, suspicious areas in the breast that require biopsy, these can be done during the same procedure. The first biopsy should be completely finished,

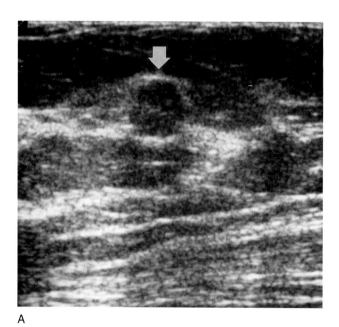

A

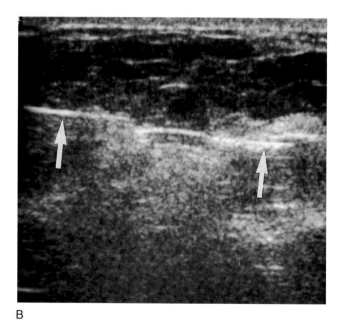

B

FIGURE 6.10. Vacuum-assisted biopsy probe. **(A)** Preprocedure image documenting an indeterminate 6 mm mass (white arrow). **(B)** The 11-gauge probe (arrows) must be inserted posterior to the mass or acoustic shadowing from the probe will obscure the lesion.

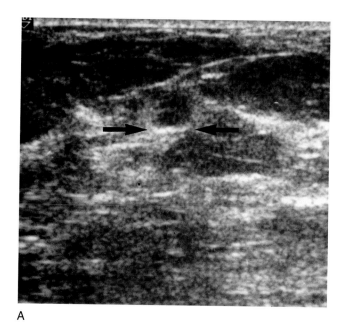

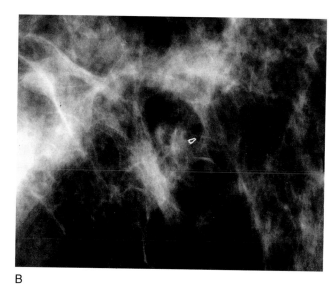

A   B

FIGURE 6.11. Localizing clip placement. (A) Postprocedure picture demonstrating that the mass has been obscured or removed during sampling. A localizing clip (arrows) has been inserted at the biopsy site through the 11-gauge probe. (B) Post-biopsy mammogram demonstrates the localizing clip in place with no mammographically evident lesion at the biopsy site.

including establishing hemostasis and putting Steri-Strips on the skin incision, before biopsy of the second lesion is begun. If a third biopsy is to be performed, the same procedure should be followed.

The assumption should be made that the first biopsy was of a malignant lesion, and the second is of a benign site. Equipment should be completely changed before the second procedure is done. This includes changing gloves.

Care should be take to label the two specimens so that it is easy to identify which lesion yielded which diagnosis. It may be worthwhile to state on the pathology requisition that two specimens from the same breast of the same patient are being submitted.

It is also possible to perform bilateral imaging guided breast biopsies or sonographically and stereotactically guided biopsies of the same or both breasts on the same date. The decision about which biopsy to perform first may depend upon a variety of factors. It may be appropriate to perform the biopsy first that is most easily tolerated by the patient; then she may be more willing to undergo a second procedure. If the results from one site are more likely to change patient management than those from another, biopsy of that site first may be appropriate. For example, if there is an obvious cancer and an indeterminate lesion, if biopsy of the indeterminate lesion shows a second cancer, mastectomy may be performed rather than lumpectomy. If the patient desires mastectomy if only one is malignant, biopsy of the more suspicious lesion first would be indicated.

POSTPROCEDURE CARE AND REPORTING

Once adequate samples have been obtained, the area is cleansed with alcohol, and pressure is applied for 5–10 minutes to achieve hemostasis. Holding pressure with ice can help establish hemostasis. To bandage the site, Steri-Strips are applied and covered with sterile gauze to prevent staining of the patient's bra or clothing by oozing from the puncture wound (Figure 6.12). The patient should be given oral and written postbiopsy instructions. These should include care of the biopsy site and how she will receive biopsy results. If possible, specimens should be hand delivered to the pathology laboratory. Histologic results should be carefully correlated with the imaging findings to identify discordance that necessitates surgical excision.

The report of the procedure should include the location of the lesion, the amount and volume of anesthetic given, the type of biopsy needle used, and the number of cores obtained. Communication of instructions for postbiopsy care and delivery of the specimen to the pathology laboratory should also be included. When the pathology results become available, it is worthwhile to add this information to the report of the procedure. The communication of these results to the patient and/or her referring physician and the recommendation for follow-up care, whether this is routine screening, short-term follow-up, repeat biopsy, treatment, or some other recommendation, should be included also.

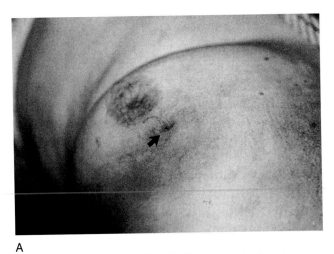
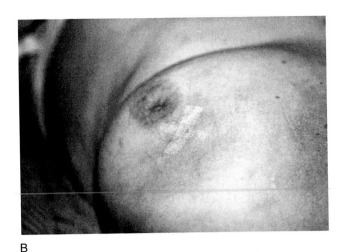

A   B

FIGURE 6.12. Postprocedure. **(A)** The incision site (arrow) following biopsy with a 14-gauge needle. **(B)** Steri-Strips are applied to the biopsy site after it is cleansed with alcohol.

PROBLEMS DURING THE PROCEDURE

As with any interventional procedure, unexpected problems can be encountered during these biopsies. They are best managed with calm, logic, and an understanding of the equipment being used. Some of the more common problems that may be encountered include:

- *Moving target.* On the postfire image it may be evident that the targeted lesion has moved away from the needle as it traveled through the breast. This is most common with dense, firm lesions, such as fibroadenomas, in fatty breasts. The target can be wedged against the chest wall with pressure from the transducer. The transducer can be slightly angled so that the far edge of the transducer (farther from the needle) is closer to the chest wall. It may also be helpful to skewer the lesion with the needle so that the needle tip is in the target before the gun is fired.

- *Needle does not completely fire.* This may be the result of dense, fibrous tissue. To remove the needle from the breast, it can be taken out of the gun and the outer, cutting needle manually moved fully over the inner needle. The biopsy probe can then be removed from the breast. For more effective biopsy, another needle can be tried or the target can be sampled at its edge, where it may be commingled with less resistant tissue.

- *Lesion near the chest wall.* These lesions can be intimidating to biopsy because of the danger of pneumothorax. Anesthetic can be injected deep to the mass, elevating it somewhat away from the chest wall. The needle can be positioned behind the mass and then angled up away from the chest wall before it is fired. When this is done, it is sometimes helpful to position the needle tip beyond the mass, angle the needle upward, and then pull the needle back, catching the mass

on the needle tip before it is fired. If it seems too dangerous to do the biopsy in this fashion, fine needle aspiration or surgical excision with preoperative needle localization can be done.

- *Difficulty getting the needle posterior enough in a thin breast or in thin areas of the breast.* Because of the curvature of the chest wall and because the needle is positioned very anteriorly in some guns, it can be difficult to get the cutting needle posterior enough in the breast in some patients. This situation can be improved by rotating the gun 180° so that the top of the gun is now against the chest wall, placing the needle against the chest wall. Because the target can be approached from any direction, it is also helpful sometimes to change the direction of approach, taking advantage of the curvature of the chest wall to get the needle entry site closer to the target.

- *Fragmented, hemorrhagic specimens.* With repeated biopsy of a small volume of the breast, the specimens retrieved become increasingly hemorrhagic and fragmented when a gun–needle probe is used to perform the biopsy. Therefore, it is important to try to obtain good specimens in the first two or three passes into the targeted lesion. If this situation is felt to be likely during a biopsy and if vacuum-suction probes are available, they can obviate this problem as they do not cause repetitive puncturing of the same volume of breast tissue.

- *Lesion becomes difficult to see.* Once the lesion becomes sonographically inapparent, continued biopsy is not possible. This situation is best avoided by being aware of the circumstances that cause it to develop. Anesthetic should be purged of all air before it is injected. Injection of anesthetic into the breast should be done under sonographic guidance to be certain that the target is not obscured. Anesthetic can be injected near, not at, the site of the target lesion. With repetitive biopsy, air is introduced to the site of the target and hemorrhage occurs, often obscuring the target. Therefore, the best opportunity to visualize the lesion and the needle is during the first one or two passes. All effort should be made to successfully biopsy the lesion during these first passes. Because the lesion becomes increasingly difficult to see during the biopsy, optimum sonographic technique is important. The TGC curve should be appropriately set, the ultrasound beam should be focused at the level of the target lesion, and adequate amounts of coupling agent should be placed between the transducer and the skin of the breast.

REFERENCES

1. Parker SH, Lovin JD, Jobe WE, et al. Stereotactic breast biopsy with a biopsy gun. Radiology 1990;176:741–747.
2. Parker SH, Lovin JD, Jobe WE, et al. Nonpalpable breast lesions: stereotactic automated large-core biopsies. Radiology 1991;180:403–407.
3. Dowlatshahi K, Yaremko ML, Kluskens LF, et al. Nonpalpable breast lesions: findings of stereotaxic needle-core biopsy and fine-needle aspiration cytology. Radiology 1991;181:745–750.
4. Parker SH, Jobe WE, Dennis MA, et al. US-guided automated large-core biopsy. Radiology 1993;187:507–511.
5. Elvecrog EL, Lechner MC, Nelson MT. Nonpalpable breast lesions: correlation of stereotaxic large-core needle biopsy and surgical biopsy results. Radiology 1993;188:453–455.
6. Jackman RJ, Nowel KW, Shepard MJ, et al. Stereotaxic large-core needle biopsy of 450 nonpalpable breast lesions with surgical correlation in lesions with cancer or atypical hyperplasia. Radiology 1994;193:91–95.
7. Parker SH, Burbank F, Jackman RJ, et al. Percutaneous large-core breast biopsy: a multi-institutional study. Radiology 1994;193:359–364.
8. Rubin E, Dempsey PJ, Pile NS, et al. Needle-localization biopsy of the breast: impact of a selective core needle biopsy program on yield. Radiology 1995;195:627–631.
9. Liberman L, Cohen MA, Dershaw DD, et al. Atypical ductal hyperplasia diagnosed at stereotaxic core biopsy of breast lesions: an indication for surgical biopsy. AJR 1995;164:1111–1113.
10. Liberman L, Fahs MC, Dershaw DD, et al. Impact of stereotaxic core breast biopsy on cost of diagnosis. Radiology 1995;195:633–637.
11. Dershaw DD, Morris EA, Liberman L, et al. Nondiagnostic stereotaxic core breast biopsy: results of rebiopsy. Radiology 1996;198:323–325.
12. Brenner RJ, Fajardo L, Fisher PR, et al. Percutaneous core biopsy of the breast: effect of operator experience and number of samples on diagnostic accuracy. AJR 1996;166:341–346.
13. Liberman L, LaTrenta LR, Dershaw DD, et al. Impact of core biopsy on the surgical management of impalpable breast cancer. AJR 1997;168:495–499.
14. Kaye MD, Vicinanza-Adami CA, Sullivan ML. Mammographic findings after stereotaxic biopsy of the breast performed with large-core needles. Radiology 1994;192:149–151.
15. Lindfors KK, Rosenquist CJ. Needle core biopsy guided with mammography: a study of cost effectiveness. Radiology 1994;190:217–222.
16. Lee CH, Egglin TK, Philpotts L, et al. Cost-effectiveness of stereotactic core needle biopsy: analysis by means of mammographic findings. Radiology 1997;202:849–854.
17. Fajardo LL. Cost-effectiveness of stereotaxic breast core needle biopsy. Acad Radiol 1996;3:521–523.
18. Jackman RJ, Nowels KW, Rodriguez-Soto J, et al. Stereotactic, automated, large-core needle biopsy of nonpalpable breast lesions: false-negative and histologic underestimation rates after long-term follow-up. Radiology 1999;210:799–805.
19. Lee CH, Philpotts LE, Horvath LJ, et al. Follow-up of breast lesions diagnosed as benign with stereotactic core-needle biopsy: frequency of mammographic change and false-negative rate. Radiology 1999;212:189–194.
20. Jackman RJ, Marzoni FA. Needle-localized breast biopsy: why do we fail? Radiology 1997;204:677–684.
21. Liberman L, Feng TL, Dershaw DD, et al. US-guided core breast biopsy: use and cost-effectiveness. Radiology 1998;208:717–723.
22. Kaye MD, Vicinanza-Adami CA, Sullivan ML. Mammographic findings after stereotaxic biopsy of the breast performed with large-core needles. Radiology 1994;192:149–151.
23. Burbank F. Mammographic findings after 14-gauge automated needle and 14-gauge directional vacuum-assisted stereotactic breast biopsies. Radiology 1997;204:153–156.
24. Mester J, Eisen CS, Keating DM, et al. The role of ultrasound for biopsy of microcalcifications. AJR 2000;174 (suppl):47–48.
25. Weinstein SP, Conant EF, Patton J, et al. Targeting and core biopsy of breast microcalcifications under ultrasound using acoustic resonance. Radiology 1999;213 (suppl):371–372.
26. Simon JR, Kalbhen CL, Cooper RA, et al. Accuracy and complications rates of US-guided vacuum-assisted core breast biopsy: initial results. Radiology 2000;215:694–697.
27. Melotti MK, Berg WA. Core needle breast biopsy in patients undergoing anticoagulation therapy: preliminary results. AJR 2000;174:245–249.
28. Schackmuth EM, Harlow CL, Norton LW. Milk fistula: a complication after core biopsy. AJR 1993;161:961–962.
29. Dershaw DD, Caravella BA, Liberman L. Limitations and complications in the utilization of stereotaxic core breast biopsy. Breast J 1996;2:13–17.
30. Nath ME, Robinson TM, Tobon H, et al. Automated large-core needle biopsy of surgically removed breast lesions: comparison of samples obtained with 14-, 16-, and 18-gauge needles. Radiology 1995;197:739–742.
31. Parker SH. When is core biopsy really core? Radiology 1992;185:641–642.
32. Liberman L, Dershaw DD, Glassman JR, et al. Analysis of cancers not diagnosed at stereotactic core biopsy. Radiology 1997;203:151–157.
33. Liberman L, Dershaw DD, Rosen PP, et al. Stereotaxic 14-gauge breast biopsy: how many core biopsy specimens are needed? Radiology 1994;192:793–795.
34. Parker SH, Klause AJ. Performing a breast biopsy with a directional, vacuum-assisted biopsy instrument. RadioGraphics 1997;17:1233–1252.

CHAPTER 7

Magnetic Resonance Imaging Guided Localization and Biopsy

Elizabeth A. Morris

The strength of breast magnetic resonance (MR) imaging lies in its ability to detect invasive and preinvasive ductal breast carcinomas not seen on conventional imaging. The use of breast MR imaging in the detection and diagnosis of breast cancer is growing. One of the reasons for this is its high sensitivity for invasive breast cancer detection that approaches 100%.[1–4] In situations where there is a high probability of cancer, such as preoperative staging and high risk screening, use of MR imaging can be extremely helpful.

Although the sensitivity is high, specificity ranges from 37% to 97%.[1–4] Intense investigation into improving specificity with particular attention to morphologic and kinetic parameters has been performed. Although it has improved specificity, there is the realization that overlap between benign and malignant lesions exists regardless of the method of analysis.[5] As it is likely that specificity of breast MR imaging will never be perfect, the ability to biopsy MR imaging-detected lesions is essential. Since MR imaging will detect both invasive and preinvasive carcinomas not seen on conventional imaging, breast intervention under MR guidance needs to be an integral part of any breast MR imaging program.

At the time of this writing, intervention of the breast under MR guidance is performed primarily at institutions that perform a large number of MR examinations. Because of a need to biopsy and localize lesions seen only on MR imaging and, until recently, the lack of biopsy systems that were MR compatible and commercially available, many institutions designed their own systems. As a result, there are many different types of intervention systems using different approaches that are described in the literature.[6–17] In this chapter a commercially available device is described for those who are interested in performing this procedure.

EQUIPMENT

Magnets

Systems that have been validated for MR intervention are the 1.5 T closed magnets, as they allow a high signal-to-noise ratio and high resolution, making possible the visualization of small lesions.[18] The aim of MR imaging is to detect nonpalpable lesions that are not seen on conventional imaging. Therefore, for the purposes of MR intervention, MR imaging systems that allow visualization of small lesions with high enough spatial resolution are needed, so that a needle can be placed accurately. Similarly, MR imaging systems that perform rapidly are needed so that dynamic data can be obtained in addition to morphologic information; this is important in characterizing lesions and determining the need for biopsy.

Closed magnets are more ubiquitous than open magnets and have been the only magnets thus far validated for high quality diagnostic examinations, as the field strength is higher. Therefore, a system for MR-guided biopsy must incorporate the possibility of performing a biopsy in a closed system, requiring that the patient be removed from the bore of the magnet, in order to gain access to the breast to perform an interventional procedure.

Open magnets are of lower field strength than closed magnets and have poorer homogeneity. However, they are advantageous from the point of view that they can offer access to the breast from all angles. Open-access systems also allow interactive real-time needle visualization allowing accurate needle placement, possibly advantageous in the placement of fibers for MR-guided treatment of tumors. Real-time imaging provides frequent updates about the change in anatomy and is able to give feedback on the procedure as it is happening, possibly advantageous for margin assessment during tumor ablation. Of all the imaging modalities, breast MR imaging has the most potential for guiding, monitoring, and controlling therapy.[19,20]

Techniques

Interventional procedures can be performed free hand or by using guidance systems, such as compression grid systems that allow coordinates to be obtained. Open systems that allow real-time imaging lend themselves to the free-hand approach,[21] as repositioning of the needle can be performed and confirmed in a matter of seconds. The free-hand technique is advantageous as the needle is not in a fixed orientation and can be angled as desired to reach the target.[22,23] In a closed system, the free-hand approach is potentially disadvantageous because of long examination time secondary to repeat imaging, if multiple repositionings are required, as the patient needs to be removed and replaced in the bore of the magnet. Therefore, in a closed system, grid systems that allow more controlled initial needle placement are preferred.

SYSTEMS FOR LOCALIZATION AND BIOPSY

The basic design of breast MR localization/biopsy systems incorporates many of the same techniques used for mammographic localization or stereotactic biopsy. To accomplish this, the breast is immobilized, and all parts of the breast are made accessible. The breast lesion that is to be localized or biopsied must be visualized and needle placement must be verified. Because the material used in these systems needs to be MR-compatible, most systems are designed with plastic.

Patient Position

Intervention of the breast under MR guidance can be performed with the patient in a supine or prone position. Prone positioning is generally preferred as the breast is pendant and away from the chest wall; the needle direction is generally parallel to the chest wall, although some groups have obtained success with supine positioning.[7,24] In addition, dedicated breast coils may be used in the prone position (Figure 7.1). Some investigators have found that placing the patient in the prone oblique position facilitates access to the axillary tail and posterior breast tissue.[14]

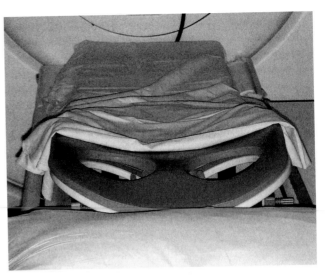

FIGURE 7.1. Bilateral breast coil (MRI Devices, Waukesha, WI) provides imaging of the entire breast, axillary tail, and excellent penetration to the chest wall. Multiple coil elements surround the breast. The coil can be used for either unilateral or bilateral imaging with high signal-to-noise ratio. Open architecture facilitates examination of very large breasts.

Breast Stabilization

Fixing the breast in the prone position has many advantages, including decreased movement of the breast when placing a needle. As MR-compatible needles have traditionally not been as sharp as their non-MR counterparts, fixation of the breast is an important consideration. Fixation of the breast can be achieved by a thermoplastic mesh[25,26] or by immobilization between two compression plates.[8,9,14,17] In addition to immobilizing the breast, mild compression requires fewer sagittal slices for complete breast coverage, thereby decreasing acquisition time.

Immobilization of the breast tissue for most systems is performed in the mediolateral plane between compression plates. However, some systems, which are not currently commercially available, also allow compression in the craniocaudad direction.[6,14] The compression plates used allow access to the breast from whatever direction compression is obtained. A variety of compression plates have been manufactured. Compression plates with perforated holes to accommodate needles have been described,[4] as well as flexible movable horizontal bands.[27] A limitation in the use of lateral compression plates is that they have allowed needle placement only from the lateral aspect of the breast. However, some investigators have developed a new prototype that allows both lateral and medial access, as well as allowing needle angulations.[16]

Two commercially available localization and biopsy devices are currently manufactured by MRI Devices (Waukesha, WI) and USA Instruments (Aurora, OH). At our institution we use a compression plate consisting of

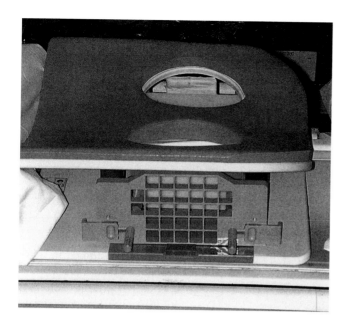

FIGURE 7.2. Breast coil with lateral compression grid plate of a commercially available dedicated biopsy compression device (Biopsy-System No. NMR NI 160; MRI Devices, Waukesha, WI) fits into the breast coil base.

a grid into which a needle guide is inserted in order to direct the needle in a horizontal fashion (Figure 7.2). These compression plates provide immobilization of the breast, as well as a guide that acts as a coordinate system to enable accurate targeting of the lesion. One disadvantage of a grid system or a perforated hole system is that small lesions may lie in an area that is not accessible through the holes. If needle localization is being performed, this is usually not a problem, as the holes are not more than a few millimeters apart. However, if a biopsy is being performed of a small lesion, the inaccuracy of a few millimeters can prove crucial.

Access to the breast from more than one approach is desirable so that the shortest distance to the lesion is used for interventional procedures. Access to medial lesions may be challenging with most breast biopsy devices, as the needle can be placed from the lateral side but not from the medial side because the grid designs permit only lateral access. This is suboptimal for medial lesions requiring that the needle and wire traverse a longer distance. To compensate for this limitation in approaching medial lesions, the patient can be positioned in a prone oblique position rather than straight prone. For example, to localize a lesion in the medial left breast, the left breast can be placed in the right breast coil, making the medial aspect of the left breast accessible. The prone oblique position is most successful for women who are healthy and relatively thin; hip problems may make the oblique position less comfortable, and obesity may limit body access to the magnet in this position. The MR imaging technologist must be aware that the left breast is being imaged

within the right breast coil so that the images can be properly acquired and annotated.

Some investigators have experienced problems with contrast uptake when the breast is compressed.[14] Therefore, it is advisable to immobilize the breast rather than compress it. Yet, there are other groups that use compression without problems in contrast uptake. Although controversial, this appears to represent a small number of cases.

A potential problem with MR image-guided localizations results from wire deployment with the breast in compression parallel to the direction of needle placement. This allows for an "accordion effect" described by Liberman[28]: During compression, structures that were far apart are brought close together, and when compression is released, structures that were close together move farther apart. Any error in the depth direction (parallel to the axis of needle placement) can therefore be exaggerated when compression is released. Keeping compression to the minimum necessary to achieve immobilization can minimize the accordion effect.

Needle Guidance/Fiducial Markers

To place a needle at the desired location in the breast, the position of the lesion must be identified in relationship to the overlying grid system. One way to accomplish this is to place a fiducial marker on the grid system (usually close to the suspected location of the underlying lesion). The fiducial marker can be a vial filled with gadolinium-DTPA or copper sulfate ($CuSO_4$)[10] inserted into one of the grid holes or a vitamin E capsule taped to the grid and skin. The fiducial marker is visualized as a high signal on the initial postcontrast image, and the exact insertion site over the lesion can be determined by measuring the lesion location relative to the fiducial marker. The depth of the lesion from the level of the grid and skin surface can be calculated by multiplying the number of sagittal slices by the slice thickness.

In order to introduce the needle into the breast, an opening in the compression plate is needed. This can be accomplished in several ways. A large opening with freehand guidance can be used. However, because compression is suboptimal and accuracy of placement suffers, this is less desirable than other methods. A grid system allows some compression to be maintained and allows a needle guide (Figure 7.3) to be inserted into the desired grid hole to facilitate needle placement. Alternatively, the compression plate itself can be perforated with multiple holes at fixed intervals, which guide needle placement.[10] The guides are advantageous in that they allow the needle to remain relatively straight and horizontal to the chest wall.

At this time, needle access is performed in the horizontal direction parallel to the chest wall without the benefit of angulation. The flexible rib system potentially avoids these pitfalls, though breast immobilization may suffer.

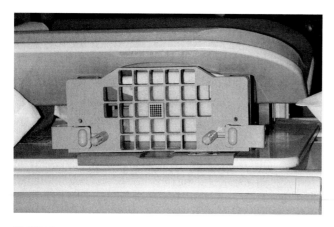

FIGURE 7.3. Compression grid plate with needle guide (Biopsy-System No. NMR NI 160; MRI Devices, Waukesha, WI).

MR Compatible Needles

There are a limited number of materials from which localization and biopsy needles can be manufactured for use in MR imaging. Conventional ferromagnetic needles and biopsy guns cannot be used because of the high magnetic field. Nonferromagnetic materials, such as stainless steel, produce severe artifacts. However, certain alloys and ceramic materials are ideal materials to be used in an MR environment. Increased nickel content alloys, such as iconel, and other high nickel and low susceptibility alloys reduce artifacts. Several MR-compatible needles are commercially available from Daum (Schwerin, Germany) and E-Z-M (Glen Falls, NY) that contain a high nickel stainless steel alloy. Other options include the Homer wire that is a J-shaped wire (Medex, Germany) made out of nitinol alloy; however, the needle that is sold with the wire is not MR-compatible and cannot be used. A Lufkin needle can be used with the Homer wire if need be. Titanium wires and needles have fewer artifacts but are difficult to manufacture and are much less rigid than the alloys. Nonmetallic substances such as plastics and ceramics are being investigated, and these materials seem to produce even less artifact. Although artifacts can be a nuisance on MR images, visualization of artifacts can be used to recognize the presence and position of the wire or needle.[29,30]

Material used for wires and needles needs to be strong, sharp, and able to produce enough spring force to adequately biopsy. In addition, there should be no deflection within the breast or possibility of heating during scanning. Ideally, the needles for breast procedures should be scored along the length so that the depth of insertion can be determined. The trajectory of the needle should be completely seen from the entry point where the needle enters the breast up to the tip of the needle.

For localization, there are choices in wires (Figure 7.4). Some wires are designed with reinforced portions

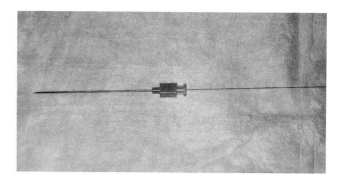

FIGURE 7.4. Commercially available MR compatible needle and localization wire.

that may be desirable for surgeons accustomed to these types of wires for localizations done mammographically or sonographically. Ideally, when performing a biopsy, the needle should allow multiple samples to be taken without needle removal and repeated targeting. If this feature is not available, strong spring-loaded devices of at least 14 gauge should be used to provide adequate specimens for histologic analysis and to diminish the chance of underestimation of a heterogeneous lesion such as ductal carcinoma in situ (DCIS) commingled with invasive carcinoma or ductal atypia commingled with ductal carcinoma.

At the time of this writing, the largest available MR compatible needles are 14 gauge. Current problems facing MR biopsy include the need for multiple needle insertions, hemorrhagic specimens, underestimation, and the inability to place a localizing marker. Eleven-gauge directional vacuum-assisted devices have been shown to decrease atypia and DCIS underestimation[28] and are advantageous in that the probe is inserted once and a localizing clip may be placed. No MR compatible version is available at the time of this writing. One investigator[31] has used a non-MR-compatible vacuum device with success in 100 cases. Future investigation into this area is crucial, in order to offer biopsy for small MR-only detected lesions.

INDICATIONS FOR MR IMAGING INTERVENTION

MRI-Only Detected Lesion

Any suspicious lesion seen only on MR imaging should be a candidate for MR intervention. These would include lesions that on MRI have characteristics like those mammographically graded as Breast Imaging Reporting and Data System (BIRADS) category 4 or 5 lesions. The BIRADS classification of lesions includes these categories: 0, needs additional imaging evaluation; 1, normal; 2, benign; 3, probably benign, recommend 6-month follow-up MR imaging; 4, suspicious; 5, highly suggestive of malignancy. Lesions suspicious or highly suggestive of malignancy have morphologic features that include spiculated or irregular margins, heterogeneous or rim enhancement or clumped enhancement in a linear or segmental distribution. Tiny (1 mm) foci of enhancement or a pattern of stippled enhancement are morphologic features that should not prompt biopsy. Similarly, masses with smooth borders and homogeneous enhancement are generally not considered suspicious. Classification of suspicious lesions also relies on kinetic features, particularly for lesions with morphologic features considered to be "probably benign." Lesions that are clearly benign or probably benign are inappropriate for MR intervention.

MRI interventional procedures can sometimes be avoided if the lesion is seen reliably on another modality. For lesions interpreted as suspicious or highly suggestive of malignancy at MRI, correlative sonography can be performed to determine if the lesion is sonographically evident. If this is the case, these lesions are amenable to tissue sampling under sonographic guidance. Any MR identified lesion that is reliably visualized on sonography or mammography can be biopsied under the guidance of those imaging modalities. Breast intervention with mammography or sonography is less expensive, more available, more comfortable, and generally more expeditious. Importantly, small lesions can be biopsied percutaneously with stereotactic or sonographic guidance without having to send the patient to surgery because a clip can be deployed if the lesion is removed. To date, small lesions detected only by MRI require surgery, as the possibility of complete removal after percutaneous MR biopsy is a real concern. Current technology does not allow placement of an MR-compatible clip. It should be stressed that the lesion should be biopsied by alternate means only if lesion conspicuity is not compromised.

Lesion Size

Because MR imaging will identify small lesions not seen on conventional imaging studies, biopsy systems must provide accurate localization and sampling of small lesions. With currently available systems, biopsy of lesions >10 mm should be possible. Biopsy should not be done on lesions <1 cm because of severe needle artifacts, tissue shift during the intervention, fast equalization of contrast enhancement in lesions and surrounding tissue, and the possibility of complete removal without the benefit of placement of a clip.[27,31]

The problem with lesions smaller than 10 mm is twofold. First, these lesions are difficult to target. Second, even if successfully biopsied, there is the potential of complete removal without the benefit of clip placement. Currently, there are limited alternatives when a small lesion is detected. In our practice most of these patients undergo needle localization and surgical biopsy. Clearly, as with mammography, the best solution would be a directional vacuum-assisted device that is MR compatible. Such a system would be more forgiving of less accurate targeting and enable larger volumes of tissue to be removed. It would also make it possible to deploy a localizing clip at the biopsy site. Ideally, all standard needle configurations, including vacuum-assisted needle compatibility, should be available for use in MR systems.[18]

ACCURACY OF NEEDLE PLACEMENT FOR LOCALIZATION AND BIOPSY

The targeting accuracy of breast lesions in multiple series[32,33] has been shown to be high with one series demonstrating 100% accuracy in 20 patients. In another series, of 137 lesions, 98% were successfully excised,[34] and 100 lesions <1 cm were successfully biopsied with directional vacuum-assisted biopsy.[31] Clearly, the accuracy of needle placement for both localization and biopsy is high and is not significantly different from that reported in the mammographic literature.[35,36] Published experience is shown in Tables 7.1 and 7.2. Although accuracy was favorable in most series, many investigators found certain lesions close to the chest wall and nipple to be difficult to access.

TABLE 7.1. *MRI localizations*

Study	Year	No.	Needle (gauge)	Size (cm)a	DIST (lesion/wire) (mm)	Accuracy (%)	Diagnosis (%)			
							MG	IFDC	DCIS	ADH/LCIS
Orel[8]	1994	10	18	0.3–2.0 (0.9)	0–5 (1.6)	100	40	20	20	10
Fischer[13]	1995	15	n/a	n/a	0–15 (0.4)	100	33	33	0	0
Kuhl[14]	1997	97	n/a	0.4–2.0 (0.9)	0–6	98b	54	43	11	5
Daniel[21]	1998	19	20/21	0.3–6.0	0–9 (3.8)	100	42	26	16	11
Fischer[33]	1998	132	n/a				48			
Orel[34]	1999	137	20	0.3–7.0 (1.2)		98c	43	30	13	
Morris	2001	115	20	0.2–8.0 (1.1)	0–34 (10)	100	31	16	15	9

DIST, distance; MG, malignant; IFDC, infiltrating ductal carcinoma; DCIS, ductal carcinoma in situ; ADH, atypical ductal hyperplasia; LCIS, lobular carcinoma in situ; n/a, not applicable.
aResults in parentheses are means.
bIncludes two cases of suspected needle migration (fibroadenoma, infiltrating ductal carcinoma).
cReasons not given.

TABLE 7.2. *MRI biopsies*

Study	Year	No. of lesions	System	Needle	Sufficient (%)	Size (mm)	Malignant (%)
Fischer[7]	1994	8	Supine	19.5G FNA	n/a	n/a	50
Fischer[13]	1995	11	Prone	19.5G FNA	82[a]	n/a	27
		12	Supine	19.5G FNA	100	n/a	33
Döler[24]	1996	2	Supine	14G	100	n/a	50
Wald[42]	1996	18	Prone	22G FNA	61[b]	18	11
Kuhl[14]	1997	5	Semiprone	16G	75[c]	n/a	80
Fischer[33]	1998	31		FNA	90[d]		26
		4		Core			
Heywang-Kobrunner[31]	1999	100	Prone	11G vacuum	99[e]	All < 10 (27% < 5)	25
Kuhl[37]	2001	78	Semiprone	14G core	98[f]	6–30 (mean 15)	35

n/a = not applicable; FNA, fine-needle aspiration; G, gauge.
[a]Two lesions could not be aspirated due to posterior location.
[b]Includes four lesions that were too posterior and three lesions that were located too anteriorly to be accessed.
[c]Insufficient material obtained in one case.
[d]Insufficient material obtained in three cases.
[e]One failure due to incorrect usage of vacuum probe.
[f]Insufficient material obtained in one case.

Additionally, it was noted in several series that the performance of MR-compatible biopsy equipment could be problematic, and insufficient material for diagnosis was an infrequent but possible result. Blunt needles can push tissue and displace the target lesion. During the time required for these procedures, the lesion can become less visible as contrast washes out. Second injections in one series[37] were necessary in 49 of 78 (63%) cases due to the "vanishing" target. The 14-gauge needles used in this series often delivered empty samples, requiring up to 12 passes per lesion to obtain sufficient material for analysis. Clearly, there is a need for improved MR-compatible biopsy needles.

Verification of the accuracy of needle localization and tissue retrieval is difficult to prove absolutely as no specimen image can be obtained. Knowledge of MR appearances of breast diseases as well as comfort with issues of concordance and discordance should help the imager assess whether the appropriate area was biopsied. As with mammographic needle localization, there exists the potential for wire movement during and after these procedures. Careful close follow-up may help. Routine follow-up MR examinations following a benign biopsy might catch any false negative biopsies. However, this approach has yet to be validated.

MR INTERVENTION PROCEDURE

MR needle biopsies and localizations are an essential part of a breast MR imaging program. The learning curve is short for breast imagers who are used to performing this type of intervention, as the technique is essentially the same as that used for imaging-guided interventions done under mammographic or sonographic guidance. How-

ever, as the procedures are performed with a new modality, there are special considerations. Speed becomes more important with this procedure, as the contrast agent stays only temporarily in the breast. Generally, the contrast agent remains in the breast long enough to do the procedure in question. If the contrast agent vanishes and washes out, the patient may be safely re-injected in order to see the lesion. Importantly, accuracy is essential as there is no specimen radiograph that can be obtained with the contrast agent within the lesion once it has been removed from the patient.

When performing interventions with MR imaging, it is best to work efficiently and rapidly. There is limited time following the contrast injection to perform the procedure and verify needle placement because of the transient nature of contrast enhancement on MRI. Continued lesion visibility is an issue, and most lesions do not remain visible for more than 10–20 minutes following injection.

Technical support with the interventional procedure as well as with the imaging will speed up the process. At our institution a technologist trained in MR imaging sets up the sequences so that time is used efficiently. A second technologist skilled at mammographic intervention helps with the intervention procedure in the magnet. A tray that can be wheeled into the MR suite is prepared ahead of time (Figure 7.5).

For all procedures, the patient has had a recent MR examination performed at our institution. If there is a finding on an outside examination that may represent a benign or probably benign finding, we will repeat the MR examination prior to scheduling the patient for an MR procedure. Therefore, when the patient arrives for a procedure, the lesion is almost always visible. Before the patient arrives in the MR suite, the films are reviewed, the

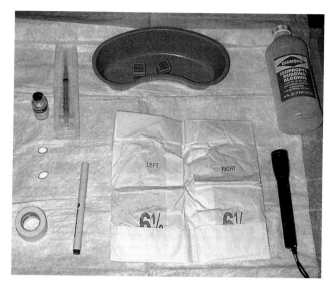

FIGURE 7.5. Preparation tray includes gloves, felt-tip marker, 1% lidocaine HCl (Xylocaine; Astra USA, Westborough, MA), needle, tape, vitamin E capsules, alcohol, needle guides, and flashlight (in order to better visualize the area undergoing intervention).

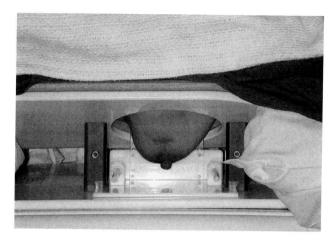

FIGURE 7.6. Breast is placed centrally in the breast coil and is pulled away from the chest wall.

approach is chosen, and the depth of the lesion is estimated from the diagnostic MR examination.

Because there is usually a complete examination performed at our institution, the procedure sequence is designed to be as fast as possible. The entire breast may not be imaged, and the field of view is tailored to the area of interest in the breast. The grid of the interventional system and the breast tissue between the grid and the suspicious lesion are always included in the field of view. Also, the entire estimated needle path beyond the target is included. Because MR interventional procedures require efficiency, the time to perform these procedures is not excessively long.

Pulse Sequences

Pulse sequences are chosen to be rapid so that the abnormality can be identified, followed immediately by intervention to localize or biopsy the lesion. Optimal systems should allow fast acquisition and display of images with high enough spatial resolution and precise interventional device localization. Ideally, sufficient anatomic detail and lesion contrast can allow identification of the lesion after contrast has washed out, if the procedure takes longer than expected. Subtraction imaging is less desirable because of time constraints and possible misregistration due to patient motion and tissue movement during needle placement. The ability to rotate the imaging plane in the plane of the path of the needle may be helpful so that visualization of a linear low signal identifies the precise location of the needle.

An intravenous line is put in the patient before she is placed in the magnet. The breast is placed in the center of a dedicated breast coil (MRI Devices, Waukesha, WI) and positioned so that the posterior tissue near the chest wall is maximally brought into the coil (Figure 7.6). The lateral grid plate of the dedicated biopsy compression device contains a grid-localizing system that is a commercially available model (Biopsy-System No. NMR NI 160, MRI Devices, Waukesha, WI). This is securely placed so that the breast is immobilized, minimizing tissue movement when the needle is inserted. Positioning of the breast is accomplished by first positioning the medial aspect of the breast flush against a compression plate. A vitamin E capsule is then taped over the estimated location of the lesion (Figure 7.7), based on review of the prior diagnostic MR examination.

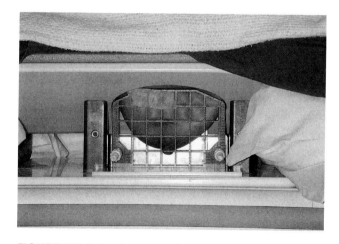

FIGURE 7.7. Lateral compression grid plate is firmly placed against the lateral breast to immobilize it so that tissue movement is minimal when the needle is placed. The medial aspect of the breast is first positioned flush against the compression plate. Vitamin E fiducial marker is taped over the expected needle entrance site.

The first sequence for an MR intervention procedure that is acquired is a postcontrast image. Gadopentetate dimeglumine (Magnevist; Berlex, Wayne, NJ), 0.1 mmol/L/kg of body weight, is injected intravenously as a rapid bolus injection through the indwelling intravenous catheter. The precontrast image has already been performed on the diagnostic examination and does not add information to the procedure. The imaging sequence used at our institution is a fat suppressed 3D gradient echo T1-weighted image (TR 17.1/TE 2.4, angle 35°, matrix 256 × 192, 1 NEX, 2 mm slice thickness without gap, frequency anterior/posterior direction) obtained in the sagittal plane to allow visualization of enhancing lesions (Figure 7.8). Sagittal slices are obtained and the grid is visualized laterally because of the impression that it makes on the skin. The vitamin E marker is clearly visualized at the level of the grid where it is taped to the skin (Figure 7.9). A cursor is then placed over the lesion in the breast, and sequential sagittal sequences are scrolled through on the console in order to identify the location on the grid that overlies the lesion. The skin en-

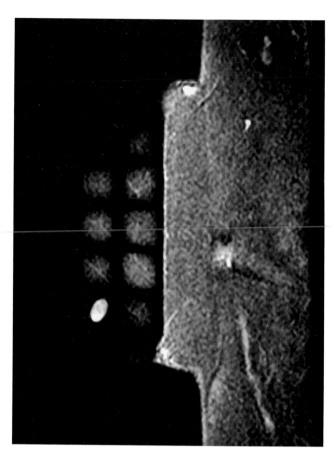

FIGURE 7.9. Sequential sagittal fat suppressed 3D FSPGR echo image of grid and vitamin E capsule, taped on the breast (in a different patient than in Figure 7.8). Coordinates of the lesion within the grid hole overlying the lesion are identified by placing a cursor over the lesion, then scrolling from lesion to grid (keeping the cursor visible). The cursor location of the lesion in the *x* and *y* planes relative to the grid plate and vitamin E marker is used to identify the needle entry site.

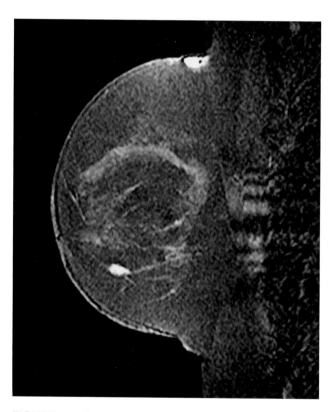

FIGURE 7.8. Contrast-enhanced sagittal 3D FSPGR image of breast demonstrates lesion to be localized. Gadopentetate dimeglumine (Magnevist; Berlex, Wayne, NJ), 0.1 mmol/L/kg body weight, is injected intravenously as a rapid bolus injection through an indwelling intravenous catheter. Imaging is performed using sagittal fat suppressed 3D FSPGR echo T1-weighted image (17.1/2.4, 35°, 259 × 192, 1 NEX, 2 mm slice thickness without gap, frequency A/P direction).

try site is determined based on visual assessment of the location of the lesion with respect to the grid lines, using the vitamin E capsule as a reference. The depth is calculated by multiplying the number of slices scrolled through by the slice thickness. Approximately 2 cm is added to the depth to account for the width of the needle guide (1 cm) and the fact that the tip ideally should be no more than 1 cm beyond the lesion.

Prior to placement of the needle, the skin is marked over the area with a felt tip pen. The skin is cleansed with alcohol and anesthetized with 1–2 cc 1% lidocaine HCl (Xylocaine, Astra USA, Westborough, MA) (Figure 7.10). If a biopsy is performed, a small skin nick may need to be made to accommodate the needle. The needle guide is placed in the grid (Biopsy-System No. NMR NI 160, MRI Devices, Waukesha, WI) overlying the lesion (Figure 7.11) and is inserted into the breast to the previously calculated depth (Figure 7.12).

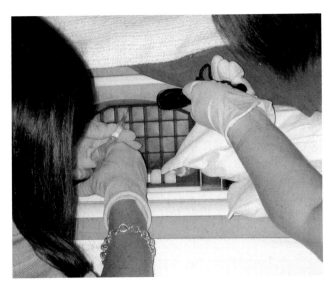

FIGURE 7.10. Once the location in the grid hole is identified, the skin is marked with a felt-tip pen, wiped with alcohol, and anesthetized with 1–2 cc 1% lidocaine HCl (Xylocaine, Astra USA, Westborough, MA). If biopsy is performed, a small skin nick may need to be made to accommodate the needle. A flashlight may aid in visualization if the room housing the magnet is not well lit.

After the needle has been inserted, the patient is reimaged in the same limited fashion with the same sequence as was used for the postinjection scanning to document accurate needle placement (Figure 7.13). There is the op-

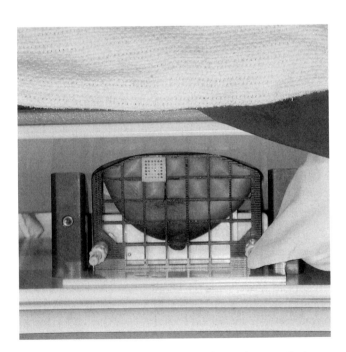

FIGURE 7.11. Needle guide is placed over the area that was anesthetized within the grid hole. Needle guides can be obtained in different gauges to accommodate localization and biopsy needles.

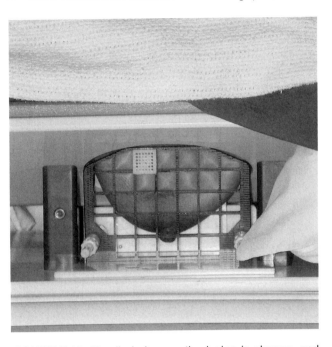

FIGURE 7.12. Needle hole over the lesion is chosen, and the needle is inserted to an appropriate depth (calculated by multiplying the number of slices by slice thickness and adding the depth of the needle guide and the desired distance that the tip of the needle be placed beyond the lesion).

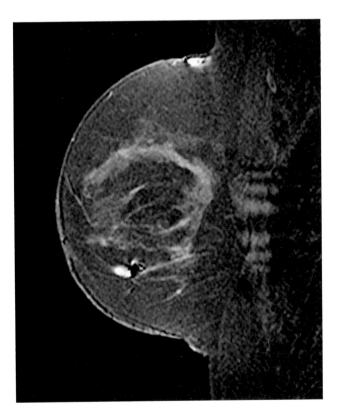

FIGURE 7.13. Repeat MR examination after needle placement demonstrates the needle (arrow) adjacent to the lesion. Needle is passively visualized owing to artifact.

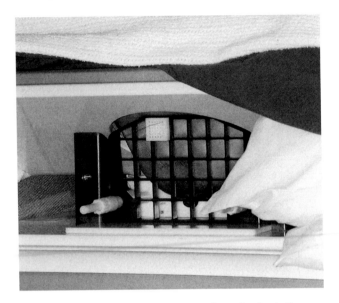

FIGURE 7.14. Once the needle is confirmed to be in the correct location, the needle is removed, and a wire remains in place. Confirmatory final MRI documents accurate wire placement. A mammogram is obtained to document wire placement and demonstrate the relationship of the wire to the lesion for the surgeon. The patient then goes to the operating room.

tion of acquiring images in the axial plane so that the needle trajectory can be visualized in its entirety rather than sequentially. Once the needle is verified to be in the correct location, localization or biopsy is performed. Figure 7.14 shows the breast after needle removal with the wire in place. After the procedure, the patient is then re-imaged a final time to either document placement of the wire for needle localization or evaluate the biopsy cavity. Following MR imaging localization, a mammogram is performed to document wire position before the patient goes to the surgical suite.

Number of Wires

An ideal system would allow the placement of multiple wires or the performance of multiple biopsies in suspected cases of multifocal or multicentric disease. Bracketing of suspicious areas for surgical biopsy using more than one wire should pose no problem and should be encouraged for large lesions where an attempt at breast conservation is made.

In practice, because biopsy procedures take longer to perform, multiple skin incisions and multiple needle insertions may be difficult to achieve before the contrast vanishes from within the lesion. Therefore, when planning the procedure, administration of a second bolus should be considered in order to visualize a second lesion, if this is required. If this is not feasible, the patient

might need to be brought back another day. Hopefully, not more than two sites would need to be sampled within the same breast, a task that should be accomplished within one setting in most cases.

As MRI intervention is currently not well suited for multiple sites or multiple samples from the same site because of the issue of contrast enhancement, the same may be true for bilateral breast biopsy procedures. When performing biopsies in both breasts, additional contrast will likely be needed unless landmarks can be relied upon. As with any biopsy procedure, the more suspicious lesion should undergo intervention first, in case the second site is not visualized or the patient is unable to tolerate further imaging. In contrast, bilateral needle localization procedures can generally be performed with one dose of contrast if a bilateral breast compression device is used.

Verification of Biopsy

During the biopsy procedure, verification of the biopsy results can be performed in real time. If the biopsy is performed in a closed system, a repeat MR scan after the procedure will usually document the biopsy cavity, and assessment of the adequacy of tissue sampling is possible. If there is discordance between the pathologic and imaging findings, a postbiopsy MR to assess the biopsy site may be indicated. In the immediate postbiopsy period, residual disease can be seen if it is separate from the biopsy cavity or if it is large enough that the postbiopsy enhancement from granulation tissue does not obscure the residual disease. It needs to be remembered that postsurgical inflammation around the biopsy cavity can obscure small residual disease. A postoperative MRI after surgery should be obtained in any case where imaging and pathologic discordance arises.

Confirmation of lesion retrieval when surgery is performed is difficult, as contrast enhancement within the lesion cannot be used to identify it. Once the lesion is removed, routine specimen radiography is usually not helpful, as the lesion is generally occult mammographically. MRI of the specimen has met with limited success and is generally not feasible because the lesion does not enhance ex vivo. Although specimen MRI techniques are not yet developed, several potentially useful methods have been proposed. Contrast agents that are retained in the tumor for long periods may be identified on specimen X ray. MR spectroscopy may play a role in the verification of lesion removal. Other alternatives include carbon or a dye.[38,39] Liberman et al.[28,40] have suggested the placement of a localizing clip at the site of the biopsy to use as a marker to confirm lesion retrieval.

A technique of marking the lesion or biopsy site that is visible on mammography or sonography would potentially serve several purposes. If the lesion is marked with a substance that did not diffuse, biopsy or localization could theoretically be performed outside the MR suite under mammographic or ultrasonographic guidance. Additionally, if the patient is having a surgical procedure, a substance that marked the lesion site could verify lesion removal at specimen radiography.

PITFALLS

Lesions Near the Chest Wall and Axillary Tail

Lesions within the posterior breast can be difficult for MRI-guided intervention. In these cases positioning the patient by mammography technologists may improve visualization of the area of interest because of their experience with positioning the breast for diagnostic mammography as well as a variety of interventional breast procedures (including stereotactic biopsy with the patient prone). If a lesion cannot be included in the grid because of its extreme posterior location, the radiologist can place a localization needle within the grid as close to the lesion as possible and confer with the surgeon. The surgeon can then excise the tissue posterior to the needle (extending from the wire toward the pectoral muscle), as is our practice for mammographically guided needle localizations of extremely posterior lesions. Alternatively, a "freehanded" technique may be used to attain closer proximity to the lesion by placing the needle posterior to the grid (Figure 7.15). Regarding biopsy of posterior lesions, if the needle cannot be placed within the lesion in question, surgical excision with preoperative MRI needle localization would be appropriate.

Access to lesions near the chest wall and axillary tail may be improved by using angled grid holes in the grid hole system and angled approaches used by biopsy systems that can be programmed by the software.[41]

Artifacts

Signal void on MR can be caused by MR needles, proton poor calcifications, surgical clips, air, fibrous tissue, magnetic susceptibility effects of blood breakdown products, and flow phenomena (high flow void/dephasing due to turbulence). Several MRI equipment manufacturers are developing titanium alloy needles that produce low susceptibility artifact. However, there is a trade-off with needle strength and sharpness. When imaging, the use of pulse sequences with high bandwidth can help to reduce artifacts.

Knowledge of artifact produced by the chosen needle is important when estimating the depth of insertion, as different needles in different MR systems with different pulse sequences will produce varying artifacts. The best way to study this problem is with a phantom in the mag-

net before commencing an interventional program and each time a new needle type is used. The needle should be placed at least 5 mm beyond the lesion for a needle localization procedure and should be placed at the lesion for a biopsy procedure.

Needle artifact can obscure the lesion, particularly if small (Figure 7.16). Therefore, it can be helpful to review landmarks to ensure accurate placement.

CONTRAINDICATIONS TO MR INTERVENTION

Lesions that are posterior in location along the chest wall or in the axillary tail where access is difficult may be inappropriate for MR intervention. Similarly, superficial lesions, lesions near the nipple, and thin breast compression may be difficult for core biopsy procedures, although these should pose no problem for localization procedures.[42]

The patient's inability to cooperate with the procedure due to her inability to lie prone or claustrophobia should be apparent at the diagnostic MR examination. Bleeding diathesis or anticoagulation are contraindications for breast intervention procedures as well. Contraindications to MR imaging in general include cardiac pacemakers, aneurysmal clips, cochlear implants, and some tissue expanders.

POTENTIAL FUTURE DEVELOPMENTS

Areas of investigation for breast MR imaging include the potential for therapeutic intervention.[43–48] MRI intervention can provide direct visualization of the entire breast anatomy while the procedure is performed, allowing real time percutaneous treatment. The ability of MR imaging to provide three-dimensional data[49] enhances the visibility of the biopsy site and possibly in the future treatment of the operative site. MR imaging can also define the margins of lesions that can aid in targeting for biopsy or surgical resection. By virtue of the enhancement of tumor identified on MRI, the most active area of the tumor could be targeted for percutaneous biopsy, a consideration in larger tumors that may contain partially necrotic areas. MRI has the potential to monitor thermal ablations using temperature-sensitive sequences. MRI-guided interstitial laser therapy, cryotherapy, and radiofrequency-induced thermal ablative treatment can replace some open tumor surgeries. Temperature-sensitive imaging is necessary to avoid the heating of normal structures. MRI can monitor continuously the heating or freezing of tissue. However, it is unknown if the changes seen on MR correspond to irreversible cell death. Complete removal of the mammographic lesion does not ensure complete excision of the carcinoma. It is uncertain whether the same is true

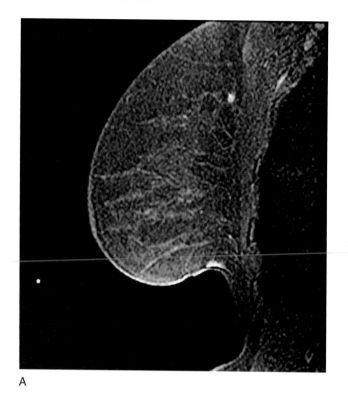

A

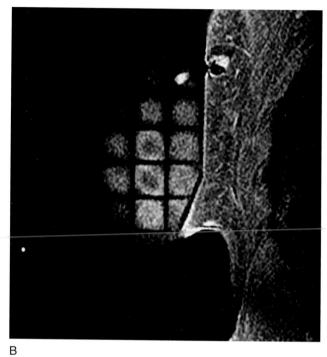

B

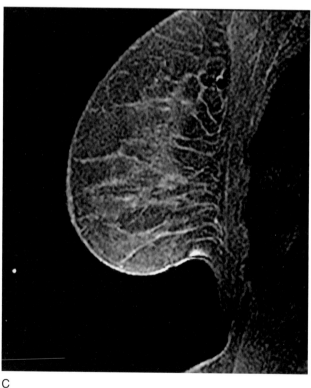

C

FIGURE 7.15. Needle localization of posterior lesions. **(A)** Posterior lesion seen on the initial examination is found to be located posterior to the grid. The needle can be placed using a needle guide so the needle is anterior to the lesion. Close communication with the surgeon should indicate that tissue posterior to the wire should be removed. **(B)** Alternatively, the needle can be placed posterior to the grid with a freehand approach over the estimated lesion location, realizing that angulation of the needle may occur. **(C)** MRI after needle placement demonstrates that the needle is placed directly through the lesion.

for MRI, and further investigation is essential. Focused ultrasound treatment, an additional therapy that can be administered under MR direction, can avoid tissue damage outside the focal volume of treated tissue and has great potential in this regard.[50]

Development of rapid and dynamic sequences for tar-

geting and monitoring therapy are under investigation. This may involve a shift in medical imaging from diagnosis to treatment, making the breast imager more involved in the treatment of the patient. Intravascular contrast agents that remain in the tumor for a prolonged period of time are necessary for long MR-guided proce-

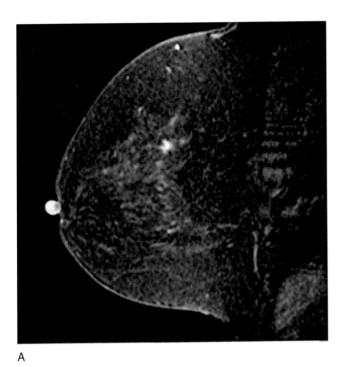
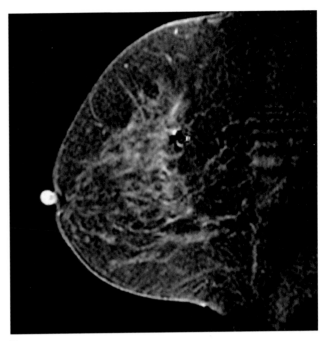

A   B

FIGURE 7.16. Needle localization of a small lesion. (**A**) Small (4 mm) irregular mass is proven to represent invasive ductal carcinoma seen on the initial diagnostic MR examination. (**B**) Same sagittal MR image obtained after needle placement demonstrates that the needle obscures the lesion owing to artifact. For small lesions obscured by the needle, confirmation of accuracy can be obtained from surrounding adjacent landmarks.

dures and need to be developed if advancement in MR intervention can be expected.

CONCLUSIONS

Intervention of the breast under MR guidance is an exciting, emerging technology that has been shown to be extremely robust despite current limitations. In order to develop and maintain a breast MR program, intervention under MR guidance is an essential component. As some carcinomas will be identified only with MRI, the ability to localize and biopsy is imperative. Future developments appear promising with the potential of MR guided therapies.

REFERENCES

1. Heywang SH, Wolf A, Pruss E, Hilbert T, Eiermann W, Permanetter W. MR imaging of the breast with Gd-DTPA: use and limitations. Radiology 1989;171:95–103.
2. Kaiser WA, Zeitler E. MR imaging of the breast: fast imaging sequences with and without Gd-DTPA. Radiology 1989; 170:681–686.
3. Harms SE, Flamig DP, Hesley KL, et al. MR imaging of the breast with rotating delivery of excitation off resonance: clinical experience with pathologic correlation. Radiology 1993; 187:493–501.
4. Orel SG, Schnall MD, LiVolsi VA, Troupin RH. Suspicious breast lesions: MR imaging with radiologic-pathologic correlation. Radiology 1994;190:485–493.
5. Schnall MD. MR-guided breast biopsy. In Lufkin RB (ed) Interventional MRI. St. Louis: Mosby, 1999.
6. Hussman K, Renslo R, Phillips JJ, et al. MR mammographic localization: work in progress. Radiology 1993;189:915–917.
7. Fischer U, Vosshenrich R, Keating D, et al. MR-guided biopsy of suspect breast lesions with a simple stereotaxic add-on device for surface coils. Radiology 1994;192:272–273.
8. Orel SG, Schnall MD, Newman RW, Powell CM, Torosian MH, Rosato EF. MR imaging-guided localization and biopsy of breast lesions: initial experience. Radiology 1994;193: 97–102.
9. Heywang-Kobrunner SH, Huynh AT, Viehweg P, Hanke W, Requardt H, Paprosch I. Prototype breast coil for MR-guided needle localization. J Comput Assist Tomogr 1994;18:876–881.
10. Schnall MD, Orel SG, Connick TJ. MR guided biopsy of the breast. Magn Reson Imaging Clin N Am 1994;2:585–589.
11. Fischer U, Vosshenrich R, Doler W, Hamadeh A, Oestmann JW, Grabbe E. MR imaging-guided breast intervention: experience with two systems. Radiology 1995;195:533–538.
12. Orel SG, Schnall MD, Powell CM, et al. Staging of suspected breast cancer: effect of MR imaging and MR-guided biopsy. Radiology 1995;196:115–122.
13. Fischer U, Vosshenrich R, Bruhn H, Keating D, Raab BW, Oestmann JW. MR-guided localization of suspected breast lesions detected exclusively by postcontrast MRI. J Comput Assist Tomogr 1995;19:63–66.

14. Kuhl C, Elevelt A, Leutner CC, Gieseke J, Pakos E, Schild HH. Interventional breast MR imaging: clinical use of a stereotactic localization and biopsy device. Radiology 1997;204:667–675.

15. Daniel BD, Birdwell RL, Black JW, Ikeda DM, Glover GH, Herfkens RJ. Interactive MR-guided, 14-gauge core-needle biopsy of enhancing lesions in a breast phantom mode. Acad Radiol 1997;4:508–512.

16. Heywang Kobrunner SH, Kolem H, Henig A, et al. A new design for a breast biopsy device suitable for MR application (abstract). Eur Radiol 1997;7(suppl):243.

17. Schneider E, Rohling KW, Schnall MD, Giaquinto RO, Morris EA, Ballon D. An apparatus for MR-guided breast lesion localization and core biopsy: design and preliminary results. J Magn Reson Imaging 2001;14:243–253.

18. Technical Report of the International Working Group on Breast MRI. J Magn Reson Imaging 1999;10:980–981.

19. Mumtaz H, Harms SE. Biopsy and Intervention Working Group report. J Magn Reson Imaging 1999;10:1010–1015.

20. Goldberg SN, Gazelle GS, Mueller PR. Thermal ablation therapy for focal malignancy: a unified approach to underlying principles, techniques, and diagnostic imaging guidance. AJR 2000;174:323–331.

21. Daniel BL, Birdwell RL, Ikeda DM, et al. Breast lesion localization: a freehand, interactive MR imaging-guided technique. Radiology 1998;207:455–463.

22. Brenner RJ, Shellock FG, Rotherman BJ, Giuliano A. Technical note: magnetic resonance imaging-guided pre-operative breast localization using a "free hand technique." Br J Radiol 1995;68:1095–1098.

23. Coulthard A. Magnetic resonance imaging-guided preoperative breast localization using a free hand technique. Br J Radiol 1996;69:482–483.

24. Döler W, Fischer U, Metzger I, Harder D, Grabbe E. Stereotaxic add-on device for MR-guided biopsy of breast lesions. Radiology 1996;200:863–864.

25. DeSouza NM, Kormos DW, Krausz T et al. MR-guided biopsy of the breast after lumpectomy and radiation therapy using two methods of immobilization in the lateral decubitus position. J Magn Reson Imaging 1995;5:525–528.

26. De Souza N, Coutts G, Puni R, Young I. Magnetic resonance imaging guided breast biopsy using a frameless stereotactic technique. Clin Radiol 1996;51:425–428.

27. Heywang-Kobrunner SH, Heinig A, Pickuth D, Alberich T, Spielmann RP. Interventional MRI of the breast: lesion localization and biopsy. Eur Radiol 2000;10:36–45.

28. Liberman L. Centennial dissertation: percutaneous imaging-guided core breast biopsy: state of the art at the millennium. AJR 2000;174:1191–1199.

29. Shellock FG. Metallic marking clips used after stereotactic breast biopsy: ex vivo testing of ferromagnetism, heating, and artifacts associated with MR imaging. AJR 1999;172:1417–1419.

30. Lewin JS, Duerk JL, Jain VR, Petersilge CA, Chao CP, Haaga JR. Needle localization in MR-guided biopsy and aspiration: effects of field strength, sequence design, and magnetic field orientation. AJR 1996;166:1337–1345.

31. Heywang-Kobrunner SH, Schaumloeffel-Schulze U, Heinig A, Beck RM, Lampe D, Buchmann J. MR-guided percutaneous vacuum biopsy of breast lesions: experiences with 100 lesions (abstract). Radiology 1999;213(P):289.

32. Gorczyca DP, DeBruhl ND, Sullenberg PC, Farria D, Sinha S, Bassett LW. Wire localization of breast lesions before biopsy: use of an MR-compatible device in phantoms and cadavers. AJR 1995;165:835–838.

33. Fischer U, Kopka L, Grabbe E. Magnetic resonance guided localization and biopsy of suspicious breast lesions. Top Magn Reson Imaging 1998;9:44–59.

34. Orel SG, Schnall MD, Czerniecki B, Lawton T, Reynolds C. MRI-guided needle localization: Indications and clinical efficacy (abstract). Radiology 1999;213(P):454.

35. Dershaw DD. Nonpalpable, needle-localized mammographic abnormalities: pathologic correlation in 219 patients. Cancer Invest 1986;4:1–4.

36. Proudfoot RW, Mattingly SS, Stelling CB, Fine JG. Nonpalpable breast lesions: wire localization and excisional biopsy. Am Surg 1986;52:117–122.

37. Kuhl CK, Morakkabati N, Leutner CC, Schmiedel A, Wardelmann E, Schild HH. MR imaging-guided large-core (14-gauge) needle biopsy of small lesions visible at breast MR imaging alone. Radiology 2001;220:31–39.

38. Mullen DJ, Eisen RN, Newman RD, Perrone PM, Wilsey JC. The use of carbon marking after stereotactic large-core-needle breast biopsy. Radiology 2001;218:255–260.

39. VanSlyke MA, Mazurchuk RV, Stomper PC. A technique for specimen magnetic resonance imaging of excisional breast biopsies. Breast Dis 1994;7:139–142.

40. Liberman L, Dershaw DD, Morris EA, Abramson AF, Thornton CM, Rosen PP. Clip placement after stereotactic vacuum-assisted breast biopsy. Radiology 1997;205:417–422.

41. Heywang-Kobrunner SH, Heinig A, Schaumloffel U, et al. MR-guided percutaneous excisional and incisional biopsy of breast lesions. Eur Radiol 1999;9:1656–1665.

42. Wald DS, Weinreb JC, Newstead G, Flyer M, Bose S. MR-guided fine needle aspiration of breast lesions: initial experience. J Comput Assist Tomogr 1996;20:1–8.

43. Harms SE. MR-guided minimally invasive procedures. Magn Reson Imaging Clin N Am 2001;9:381–392.

44. Singletary SE. Minimally invasive techniques in breast cancer treatment. Semin Surg Oncol 2001;20:246–250.

45. Mumtaz H, Hall-Craggs MA, Wotherspoon A, et al. Laser therapy for breast cancer: MR imaging and histopathologic correlation. Radiology 1996;200:651–658.

46. Gazelle GS, Goldberg SN, Solbiati L, Livraghi T. Tumor ablation with radiofrequency energy. Radiology 2000;217:633–646.

47. McGahan JP, Griffey SM, Schneider PD, Brock JM, Jones CD, Zhan S. Radio-frequency electrocautery ablation of mammary tissue in swine. Radiology 2000;217:471–476.

48. Lai LM, Hall-Craggs MA. MR-guided laser breast treatment. In Lufkin RB (ed) Interventional MRI. St. Louis: Mosby, 1999.

49. Lufkin R, Teresi L, Hanafee W. A technique for MR-guided needle placement. AJR 1988;151:193–196.

50. Hynyen K, Pomeroy O, Smith DN, et al. MR imaging-guided focused ultrasound surgery of fibroadenomas in the breast: a feasibility study. Radiology 2001;219:176–185.

CHAPTER 8

Fine-Needle Aspiration and Cyst Aspiration

Handel E. Reynolds and D. David Dershaw

FINE-NEEDLE ASPIRATION BIOPSY

The first report of a stereotactic device for fine-needle aspiration biopsy (FNAB) of nonpalpable breast lesions appeared in the medical literature in 1977.[1] A decade later, this device was on the leading edge of a revolution in the management of small, nonpalpable abnormalities detected at mammography. The increasing application of screening mammography led to an increase in the number of breast biopsies. Stereotactic FNAB provided a cheaper, less invasive biopsy option for these small, mammographically detected abnormalities. At around the same time, the technique of ultrasound-guided FNAB for nonpalpable breast masses was described.[2] The early experience with imaging guided FNAB revealed some of the limitations of the technique. Foremost among them were high rates of specimen inadequacy.[3–6] Partly to overcome this weakness, large-gauge core needle biopsy (LGCNB) was introduced in 1990.[7] This was associated with a reduction in specimen inadequacy rates and provided other advantages. Core needle specimens allowed routine histologic processing so there was no requirement for cytopathology expertise. In addition, core material allowed differentiation between in situ and invasive carcinoma, a distinction usually not possible with FNAB. A vacuum-assisted needle biopsy (VNB) device was introduced in 1994. The much larger specimens provided by this device allowed more efficient sampling of microcalcifications and more reliable diagnosis of atypical hyperplasia and ductal carcinoma in situ.[8,9] Currently, the VNB technique has all but replaced FNAB and LGCNB for stereotactically guided procedures. All three techniques are currently in use, however, for procedures done under ultrasound guidance. This chapter deals exclusively with ultrasound guided FNAB and cyst aspiration.

Advantages of FNAB

FNAB, LGCNB, and VNB share some important advantages over surgical biopsy including being less invasive with minimal to no scarring and no effect on subsequent mammography, high patient acceptance, cost-effectiveness, and avoidance of a two-stage surgical procedure in cases of malignant disease. FNAB has some unique advantages, however. The most significant of these is the potential for determination of the adequacy of tissue sampling and the possibility of offering an immediate diagnosis. If the procedure is performed by or with a cytopathologist in attendance, a preliminary diagnosis may be rendered on the spot. This allows the patient to receive immediate counseling regarding her disease and facilitates expeditious treatment planning, if indicated. A second, albeit minor, unique advantage of FNAB is that it is incrementally less invasive than the other options. LGCNB and VNB use larger caliber needles and typically require a small skin incision. FNAB does not require an incision and so typically does not produce any cutaneous scarring.

Disadvantages of FNAB

As already noted, a significant limitation of FNAB is the issue of specimen insufficiency. Rates of insufficient specimens of up to 54%, far higher than those for LGCNB and VNB, have been reported.[3–6,10,11] Increased operator experience is associated with lower rates of specimen insufficiency.[12]

Another limitation of the technique is its dependence on cytopathology expertise. High interpretive accuracy requires extensive training and experience in the technique. Expert cytopathologists have higher sensitivity and specificity rates than do nonexperts.[13] In many smaller communities, this expertise may not exist. In such settings, the options are either to prepare the slides locally and ship them to a cytopathology laboratory elsewhere or to perform LGCNB or VNB. Local pathologists can then evaluate the resulting histologic material.

Requirements for a Successful FNAB Program

There are two important requirements for a successful FNAB program. The first is adequately trained personnel. It is essential that the individuals involved in the procedure have the necessary training and experience in aspiration techniques, smear preparation, and cytologic interpretation. The second is a multidisciplinary environment. In this setting, the radiologist, surgeon, and cytopathologist work collaboratively to ensure the best possible outcome for the patient. This includes ensuring that the appropriate patients are referred for the procedure, that the procedure is performed in a manner that maximizes yield and accuracy, and that patients are appropriately managed after the procedure.

Indications for FNAB

The indications for FNAB are no different from the indications for breast biopsy in general. Although the least invasive biopsy option, FNAB is a biopsy technique nonetheless. As such, its use should be limited to situations where a biopsy is clearly necessary. The main indication is the presence of a suspicious breast mass. This includes palpable and nonpalpable lesions that are categorized as "suspicious" or "highly suggestive of malignancy" by the American College of Radiology's Breast Imaging Reporting and Data System Lexicon.[14] Nonpalpable masses are biopsied with imaging guidance, while palpable ones can be biopsied in the clinic without imaging assistance. In some cases, for example when it is adjacent to a breast implant or close to the chest wall, it may be prudent to use imaging guidance even though the mass is palpable. In these instances, sonography makes it possible to accurately determine the position of the needle so that the possibility of rupture of the implant or penetration of the chest wall can be minimized. As is the case when other biopsy techniques are being considered, masses judged to be "probably benign" based on imaging features are best managed with short-term imaging follow-up. There are, however, occasional cases where the patient and/or her physician are uncomfortable with this management strategy, and a biopsy is requested. This is usually the case when the patient is extremely anxious about the possibility of malignancy and will not tolerate short-term follow-up or when she is not reliable to return

for repeat imaging in 6 months. Otherwise, routine biopsy of "probably benign" lesions by any technique should be avoided.

As with any needling procedure, it is desirable to obtained informed consent from the patient before the procedure is done. The advantages of this are more fully discussed in Chapter 11.

Technique

Equipment

FNAB can be successfully performed with 21- to 25-gauge needles. The distance of the lesion from the site where the skin will be punctured dictates the required needle length. Ten or 20 ml syringes provide adequate suction. These may be handheld or placed within a syringe holder, depending on the preference of the physician. Alcohol is needed to cleanse the skin at the puncture site. A bandage is used to cover the wound (Figure 8.1). Some physicians use connecting tubing between the needle and the syringe, with the technologist or other assistant applying suction while the needle is moved in the lesion to obtain cells. Scanning should be performed with a high resolution (at least 7.5 MHz) linear array transducer.

Preparation

Patient positioning depends on the location of the lesion to be biopsied. For lesions in the medial hemisphere, the patient is often best positioned supine. For lateral lesions a contralateral posterior oblique position may be best. This places the lateral breast in a roughly horizontal orientation, more amenable to needle insertion. This position can be achieved most comfortably by placing a pillow or foam wedge under the ipsilateral upper body. For example, if a right medial lesion is to be biopsied, the pa-

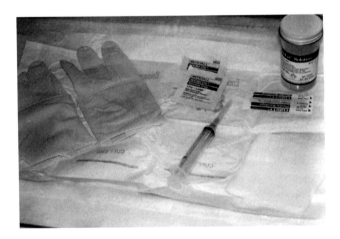

FIGURE 8.1. Performance of aspiration procedures requires minimal equipment. Gloves, a 10- or 20-cc syringe, needle of appropriate length and gauge, alcohol swabs, bandage, and specimen container are needed.

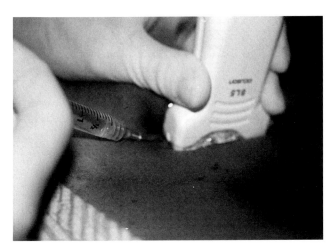

FIGURE 8.2. Sonographic visualization of the needle and injected bolus of anesthetic is recommended during instillation of local anesthetic. Although not necessary for cyst aspirations requiring a single needlestick, local anesthetic can decrease the pain associated with aspirations requiring multiple needle insertions.

tient is often best positioned supine. If a left lateral lesion is targeted, the patient may be best positioned in the right posterior oblique position with a pillow or wedge under her left side.

The area of interest is scanned in order to identify the lesion and plan an appropriate needle approach. The skin is then cleansed. An alcohol swab can be used to clean the needle site, as would be done for any needle punc-

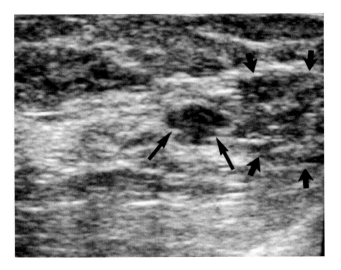

FIGURE 8.3. Care should be taken to be certain that the injected anesthetic bolus does not obscure the target. In this patient, injected anesthetic (short arrows) is near the targeted lesion (long arrows). If unmonitored at the time of injection, the anesthetic can be injected so that it envelops the target and obscures it. Also, injected air in the needle tract can make it impossible to sonographically visualize the needle while it is being inserted.

ture. Some prefer a more elaborate preparation with a sterile field defined. As the ultrasound (US) transducer is not at the puncture site, it does not necessarily need to be sterile. However, it should be cleaned. Some prefer to place the US transducer in a sterile sheath, while others simply clean it with alcohol or surgical soap. A noncontaminating coupling agent should be used. This can be sterile gel, alcohol, or surgical soap. It has been suggested that it might be preferable to use a small quantity of surgical soap as a US coupling agent rather than US transmission gel as the latter is a potential cause of a cytologic artifact resembling cellular necrosis.[15,16] Even though not always necessary, administration of a local anesthetic is extremely reassuring to the patient and should be performed routinely (Figure 8.2). One of the authors administers 5 ml of a 4:1 mixture of 1% lidocaine HCl and sodium bicarbonate. The sodium bicarbonate neutralizes the pH of the lidocaine solution and makes administration more comfortable. A small amount of the anesthetic is administered intradermally, then, under direct US guidance, the remainder is administered in the vicinity of the mass, being careful not to inject directly into the mass. The other author prefers 10 ml of 1% lidocaine, injecting first deeply and as the needle is withdrawn administering the subcutaneous injection. Using this technique, the more painful site of injection, the subcutaneous site, is frequently at least partially anesthetized by the preceding deep injection. The injection of anesthetic should be done under sonographic visualization to be certain that the targeted lesion and the needle tract are not obscured by the injected anesthetic (Figure 8.3). Lidocaine administration in the vicinity of the mass does not interfere with cytological interpretation.[17]

Needle Placement

In general, the needle is placed using a freehand technique in which the transducer is held in the operator's nondominant hand, and the needle is placed with the dominant hand. Although the freehand approach allows limitless angles of approach, these can be reduced to a basic three: oblique, horizontal, and vertical. The approach chosen depends on the location of the lesion and the preference of the operator. In the oblique approach, the skin entry is approximately 1 cm from the end of the transducer, and the needle intersects the US beam at an angle of approximately 30°–60° (Figure 8.4). This allows a relatively short approach to the lesion and good visualization of the needle throughout its course. The vertical approach involves piercing the skin adjacent to the midpoint of the transducer and advancing the needle directly down into the mass (Figure 8.5). As one might expect, the needle is not seen until it is actually within the mass. This allows the shortest approach of the three techniques. In the horizontal approach the skin entry is farther from the end of the transducer and is selected to allow a needle

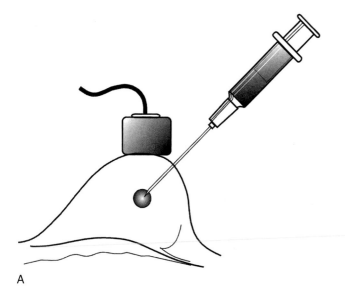

A

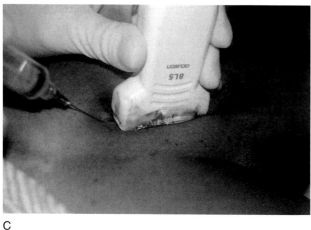

C

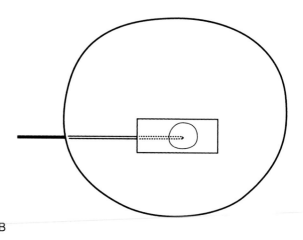

B

FIGURE 8.4. A variety of angulations of the aspirating needle can be used. (**A**) In the oblique approach the needle is usually angled at 30°–60°. (**B**) The needle should be introduced at the midline of the leading edge of the transducer (rectangle) and inserted along the long axis of the transducer, positioning it within the ultrasound beam so that it is visible. The target (small circle) is positioned in the middle or distal third of the field of view. This makes it possible to visualize the needle as it approaches the target so that its course can be adjusted as needed to successfully puncture the lesion. (**C**) After the transducer is positioned over the lesion, the needle is inserted at the center of the leading edge of the transducer, parallel to its long axis. This is most easily accomplished by not moving the transducer once it is well positioned and then visually aligning the needle appropriately with the transducer. Proper alignment is best achieved by the physician watching the relationship of the needle to the transducer on the patient rather than on the sonography screen.

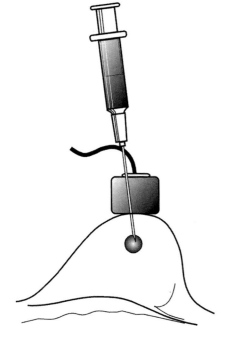

FIGURE 8.5. In the vertical approach the needle is directed toward the chest wall and inserted adjacent to the lateral aspect of the transducer at the level of the sonographically identified lesion. The needle tip becomes visible only when the needle intersects the ultrasound beam. Because of the difficulty visualizing the needle and the danger of violating the chest wall, this technique should be used with caution.

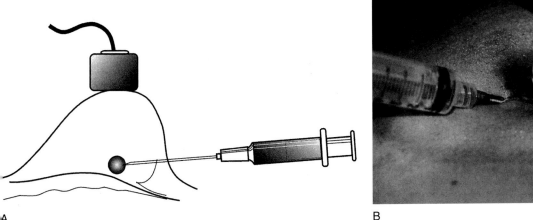
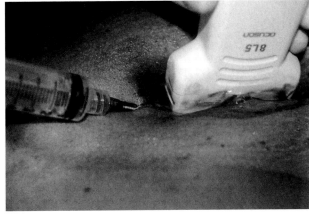

A   B

FIGURE 8.6. (A) Using a horizontal approach, the needle is introduced into the breast parallel to the chest wall. This technique minimizes the possibility of penetrating the chest wall during needle insertion. **(B)** Except for the difference in needle angulation, the orientation of the needle to the transducer is the same as with the oblique approach.

path that is perpendicular to the US beam and parallel to the chest wall (Figure 8.6). This technique is preferred for lesions situated on the chest wall or next to an implant. If the skin entry site is beyond the leading edge of the transducer, the needle will not be seen until it reaches the transducer. However, using this approach, visualization of the needle is optimized because it is perpendicular to the sound beam (Figure 8.7). Also, if the target lesion is in the middle or distant third of the field of view, there is sufficient distance to correct the course of the needle as it approaches the lesion so that it can intersect the target. When it is possible to use this approach, the horizontal orientation of the needle often provides the best visualization and control of the needle and is there-

fore generally preferred. Regardless of the approach employed, US images documenting the needle tip within the mass should be acquired.

Sampling

Using one of the above techniques, the needle is advanced to the edge of the mass. For FNA the needle tip may be best positioned near the far edge of the lesion but within the mass. When the needle tip is good position, the plunger is then pulled back to create suction of 5–10 ml. The suction is maintained as the needle is moved through the mass multiple times at slightly different angles, fanning throughout the volume of the mass (Figure 8.8). In addition to this

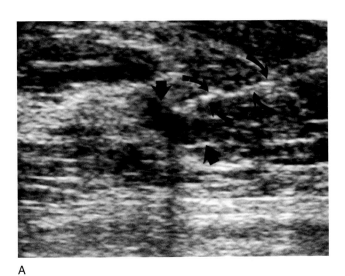
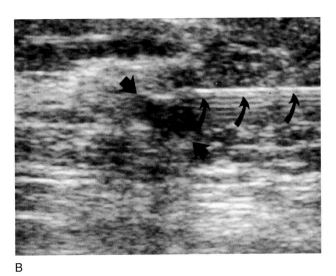

A   B

FIGURE 8.7. The conspicuity of the needle can change with its orientation to the sound beam. **(A)** The needle (curved arrows) approaches the target lesion (short arrows) at a 30° angle and is poorly seen. **(B)** After changing the angle of the needle (curved arrows) so that it is parallel to the transducer, its reflectivity is improved, and it is now easily seen.

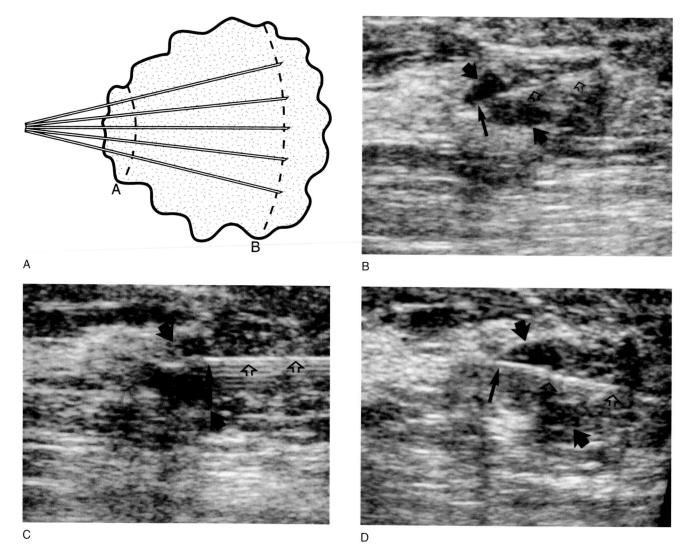

FIGURE 8.8. **(A)** Sampling a solid mass with fine-needle aspiration is best accomplished by initially positioning the needle near the far edge of the mass (line B), drawing it back to the near edge (line A), and moving it back and forth between these lines while fanning throughout the mass. This practice samples cells from throughout the volume of the mass. Negative pressure should be applied during this motion and released before the needle tip is withdrawn from the mass. A corkscrew motion of the needle also assists in dislodging cells. **(B)** The position of the needle (open arrows) tip (long arrow) at the far edge of a mass (short arrows) is seen at the beginning of fine needle aspiration. Negative pressure is applied with the needle tip at this site. **(C)** While suction is applied, the most proximal position of the needle (open arrows) tip (long arrow) is at the near edge of the mass (short arrows). The needle tip does not leave the volume of the mass while negative pressure is applied. **(D)** Angulation of the needle (open arrows; tip indicated by the long arrow) is altered during aspiration to sample cells throughout the volume of the mass (short arrows).

to and fro movement in and out of the mass, some recommend that simultaneously rotating the needle along its long axis helps to dislodge tissue from the mass.[18] While negative suction is applied and the needle tip is fanned and rotated within the targeted lesion, the needle tip should remain within the mass (Figure 8.9). With this positioning, only cells from within the target will be sampled. As soon as a drop of fluid or tissue specimen is noted in the hub of the needle (Figure 8.10) or after 10–15 needle excursions within the mass, if no sample is seen the suction is released

completely and the needle withdrawn. It is especially important to avoid or limit contamination of the specimen with blood. Even small quantities of blood may cause microscopic clots that impair cytologic interpretation. Therefore, if blood appears in the needle hub, sampling should be stopped, the specimen from that sampling prepared as described below, and a new specimen obtained.

An alternative approach, termed fine needle capillary (FNC) sampling, uses no suction at all. The needle, minus the syringe, is passed into the mass multiple times at

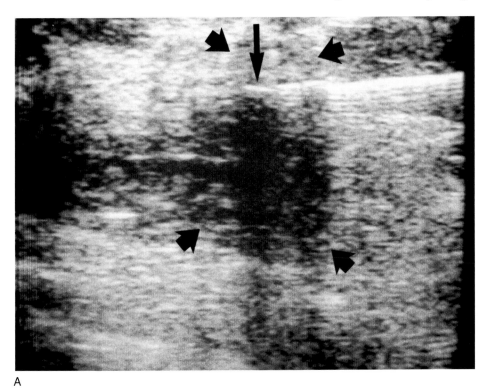

A

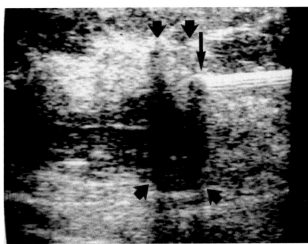

B

FIGURE 8.9. Aspiration of an irregular mass (short arrows) is performed with the needle (tip indicated by the long arrow) excursion from the far edge (**A**) to the near edge (**B**) of spicules on the upper portion of this carcinoma.

different angles in the same manner as in the suction technique. Cells enter the needle by capillary action. Some authors have reported good results using this method.[19–21] It may be particularly useful in reducing blood contamination in vascular lesions. Its main disadvantage is that it tends to produce material that is less cellular than the aspiration technique.[19,20]

Using either method, at least three to five samples, obtained from different portions of the mass, should be acquired. Larger masses may require more passes for adequate sampling. If the sample can be assessed at the time of FNA, then sampling can be stopped when an adequate specimen for diagnosis has been obtained. Otherwise,

multiple samples must be procured to minimize the likelihood of insufficient sampling for diagnosis.

Slide Preparation

Slides should be prepared as soon as possible following specimen acquisition. In an ideal multidisciplinary environment, slides are prepared by a cytotechnologist and immediately reviewed by a cytopathologist who are both in attendance at the procedure. This allows immediate feedback regarding specimen adequacy to the radiologist performing the aspiration. In less ideal settings, the radiologist or other radiology personnel may be required

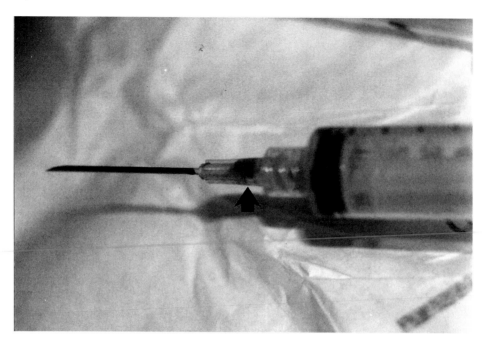

FIGURE 8.10. For each needle insertion, sampling is complete when material appears at the hub of the needle (arrow) or 10–15 excursions have been made through the target.

to perform this function. In such situations, it is very important that the involved individuals receive adequate training to ensure that high quality slides are consistently produced.

The aspirated material is carefully expelled near the frosted end of one or more slides, depending on the quantity of material. Slides are prepared by one of several direct smear techniques (Figure 8.11). With one of these techniques a glass slide (smearing slide) makes contact with the aspirated material and is held at an angle of approximately 45° as it is quickly advanced down the length of the specimen-bearing slide (specimen slide). Another technique involves placing the smearing slide at right angles to the specimen slide and drawing the former down the length of the latter. In the third technique, the smearing slide is placed directly on top of the specimen slide and the two are quickly drawn apart.

A variety of staining options are available. The method(s) used will largely depend on the preferences of the cytopathologist. The most common techniques are Diff-Quik, Papanicolaou, and hematoxylin and eosin staining. The Diff-Quik method uses air-dried slides and is used for immediate diagnosis or assessment of specimen adequacy. The Papanicolaou and hematoxylin and eosin methods use alcohol-fixed material and are used for routine diagnosis. It is important that slides that are to be alcohol-fixed be submerged in or sprayed with alcohol as soon as they are prepared, since drying will degrade the diagnostic quality of the material.

After the aspirate from each pass has been expelled onto slides (or instead of slide preparation), any residual cellular material (or the entire specimen) can be dispersed into an appropriate rinse solution by flushing the needle (Figure 8.12). In the cytopathology laboratory this material will be spun in a centrifuge, and the resulting precipitant used to produce cytospin smears.

Following the procedure, the biopsy site is dressed with an adhesive bandage, and the patient is given a telephone number to call if she has any concerns during the ensuing days. She is informed about how she will obtain the results of the aspiration. If needed, acetaminophen-containing over-the-counter analgesics are sufficient to control any postprocedure discomfort.

Interpretation of Results and Patient Management

In 1996, the National Cancer Institute sponsored a conference on breast FNAB, the purpose of which was to standardize the approach to cytologic evaluation of breast disease. This conference included experts from all the relevant medical specialties and resulted in the publication of a comprehensive document that covered all aspects of the procedure, from indications to practitioner credentials, procedure technique, reporting terminology, and patient management.[22] One of the most important results of this effort was the establishment of a standard system for reporting breast FNAB results. Prior to this conference, there was little consistency among laboratories in the way

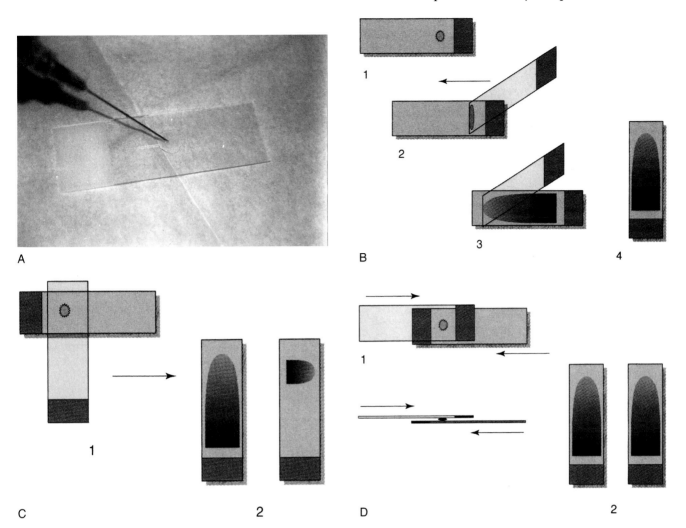

FIGURE 8.11. (A) Slides can be prepared using several techniques. In all cases a small volume of aspirate should be expelled onto a glass slide. **(B)** In one technique the smearing slide is drawn down the specimen slide at a 45° angle. **(C)** Slides can also be prepared by placing the smearing slide directly on top of the specimen slide; the two are drawn apart at a 90° angle. **(D)** Using another technique, the smearing slide is placed directly on top of the specimen slide, and the slides are drawn apart. (B, C, D: *From* Zakhour H, Wells C. *Diagnostic Cytopathology of the Breast,* with permission. Churchill Livingston, 1999, London.

results were reported. FNAB results are to be reported using one of the following five categories:

1. *Benign.* There is no evidence of malignancy. If possible, a specific diagnosis or further description should be given.
2. *Atypical/intermediate.* The cellular findings are not diagnostic. There may be changes of atypical hyperplasia versus low-grade carcinoma.
3. *Suspicious/probably malignant.* Findings are highly suggestive of malignancy.
4. *Malignant.* Findings are diagnostic of malignancy. The specific type of malignancy should be indicated, if possible.
5. *Unsatisfactory (because of):*

    a. scant cellularity;
    b. air-drying or distortion artifact;
    c. obscuring blood/inflammation;
    d. other.

As with any needle biopsy technique, benign FNAB results should be evaluated in the context of the lesion's imaging and clinical (if palpable) features. If the imaging (or clinical) features are highly suggestive of malignancy, the FNAB results should be considered discordant, and a core needle or excisional biopsy considered. If the imaging features are less suspicious (e.g., a mass with circumscribed margins) the FNAB results (especially if a specific diagnosis, such as fibroadenoma, is given) may be considered concordant, and periodic or

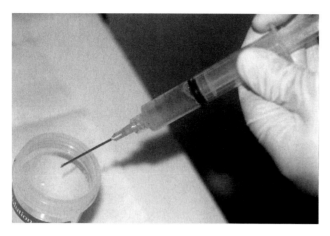

FIGURE 8.12. Specimens not submitted on slides should be placed in preservative. All needles and syringes should be flushed with preservative to extract all of the specimen for cytologic examination.

routine imaging (and clinical, if palpable) follow-up recommended. Specifically follow-up imaging is recommended by some at 12 and 24 months to ensure benignity by documenting stability or involution of the lesion. However, some deem the FNA adequate for definitive diagnosis with no further assessment necessary.

If the results are unsatisfactory or atypical/indeterminate, repeat biopsy is needed. This can be done with a variety of biopsy techniques, including a core needle biopsy or excisional biopsy. Suspicious/probably malignant results may need to be confirmed prior to definitive surgery at the surgeon's discretion. Patients with malignant results may proceed directly to definitive therapy.

CYST ASPIRATION

Cysts are the most common type of breast mass. Many are palpable; many more are detected at screening mammography as nonpalpable abnormalities. US is a reliable tool with which to make the diagnosis of a simple cyst. When the criteria of anechogenicity; thin, smooth walls; a well-defined posterior wall; and increased through sound transmission are present, the accuracy of US is essentially 100%.[23] In general, simple breast cysts require no intervention. Patients are simply reassured of the benign nature of the diagnosis and encouraged to continue age-appropriate breast cancer screening activities. There are circumstances, however, where cyst aspiration may be considered.

Indications

A common reason to recommend aspiration is that the lesion in question does not strictly fulfill all of the US criteria necessary for a diagnosis of simple cyst. The most frequent scenario is where a circumscribed mass contains a few internal echoes that appear to be more than rever-

beration artifact. Such lesions may represent complicated cysts or solid masses (Figure 8.13). US-guided aspiration is necessary to distinguish between these two possibilities. Less commonly, the patient or her physician may request aspiration of a lesion that is clearly a simple cyst. This may be because of the lesion's size, associated discomfort, or emotional distress.

Technique

Equipment

The authors' preference is for an 18-gauge needle. However, some perform these aspirations using 21-gauge needles. Although most cysts can be aspirated using smaller-caliber needles, cysts undergoing aspiration often contain thick, inspissated material. This is commonly found in those cysts that undergo diagnostic aspiration because the thick fluid produces internal echogenicity. The use of a larger gauge needle during the initial aspiration attempt obviates multiple cyst punctures with increasingly larger needles in an effort to aspirate the thick cyst contents. The length of the needle depends on the location of the cyst and the needle approach to be employed. A 10 ml syringe is adequate for most cysts.

Preparation and Needle Placement

Patient positioning and local anesthetic administration are the same as for FNAB. The same needle approach options apply here as well. Because only a single needle puncture is needed for most cyst aspirations, the advantage of local anesthesia may be less pronounced. The pain of the single needlestick for the aspiration procedure may be comparable to the pain of the needlestick for the injection of anesthetic.

Aspiration

Under direct US guidance, the needle is advanced to the edge of the mass. The cyst wall is then pierced, sometimes requiring a firm, brisk jab, particularly if the wall is thickened by inflammation. Cyst walls are sometimes very fibrous and resist penetration if this jabbing technique is not utilized. The needle should be positioned at the center of the cyst. As the cyst collapses with the removal of fluid, positioning in the center of the cyst will keep the needle tip within the cyst, avoiding puncture of the cyst wall. Once inside the lesion, a preaspiration US image should be acquired for the patient's permanent record. This should be labeled preaspiration with needle. Suction should then be applied and the syringe carefully observed for aspirated fluid. More than one approach has been described for proceeding with the aspiration once fluid is obtained. For many the aspiration proceeds to complete evacuation of the cyst or removing as much fluid as possible whatever the appearance of the retrieved fluid. However, for others, as soon as fluid is seen, the

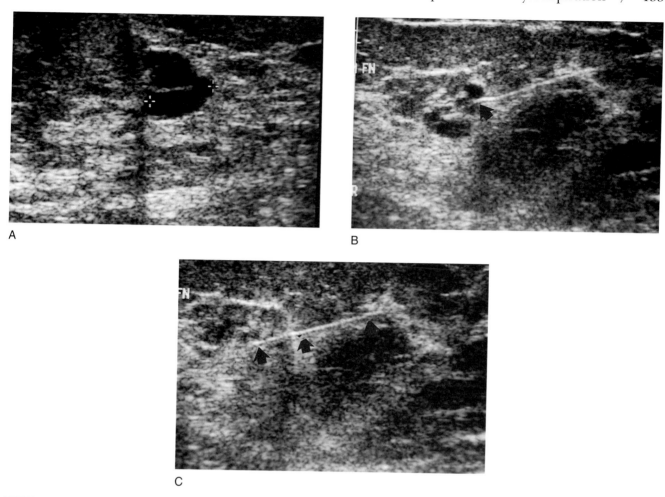

FIGURE 8.13. (**A**) Aspiration was performed to confirm the impression that this complex, largely cystic mass was a septated simple cyst. (**B**) Aspiration began with positioning a needle tip (arrow) in the center of the upper portion of the lesion. (**C**) After it was aspirated, the needle (arrows) was moved to the center of the lower portion of the mass. Complete disappearance of the mass helps confirm that it was due to a septated cyst. Contents were milky white, also consistent with benign cyst contents.

aspiration is briefly halted, and the fluid visually inspected. If it does not consist of dark blood, the aspiration is continued to completion. If the fluid appears to consist of dark blood, the procedure is terminated without completing the aspiration; the patient is advised to have more substantial tissue sampling, often surgical excision, because of the increased likelihood of an intracystic mass in this setting. However, others advocate completing the aspiration, believing that if the cystic mass is malignant, fluid will reaccumulate, making it possible to locate the malignancy within a short period of time after the aspiration. Also, many believe that if an intracystic lesion is present, sampling of the mass within the cyst by FNA of the solid component or core needle biopsy should be done, rather than aspiration of the fluid associated with the solid lesion. This will enable a more definitive diagnosis of the solid lesion to be made.

If the aspiration yields no fluid and proper needle placement is confirmed by orthogonal plane imaging, the patient is advised that the lesion is not a cyst but a solid mass. The aspiration can be converted to an FNAB, or a needle biopsy may be performed at the same visit.

At the conclusion of the procedure, postaspiration US images are recorded, and they are labeled as such. It is important to note the presence or absence of a residual mass on US or physical examination (if the lesion had been palpable). A postprocedure mammogram may be obtained if the lesion had been mammographically visible (Figure 8.14). A bandage is applied to the aspiration site. The patient is warned that she may have some bruising. Analgesia is almost never necessary; acetaminophen-containing agents can be used if needed. If a specimen is sent for cytologic analysis, the patient is informed how she will receive the results of this assessment. If a specimen is sent to cytology, the results of this analysis should be included in the final report, as well as documentation of how results were communicated to the patient and/or referring physician and what patient management is appropriate.

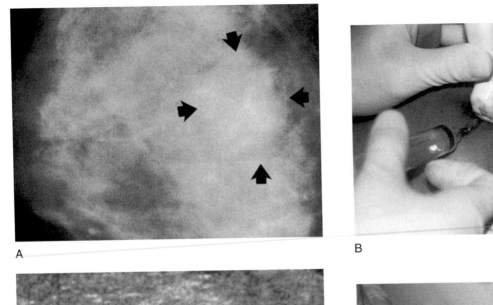

A

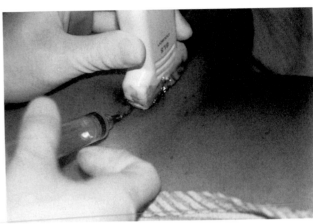

B

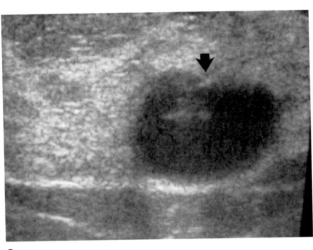

C

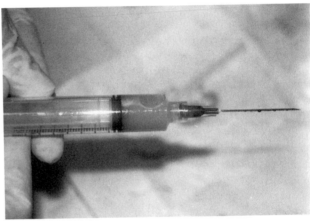

D

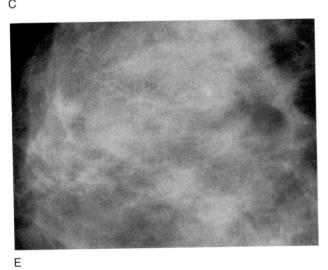

E

FIGURE 8.14. (A) Mammography demonstrated the presence of a new mass (arrows) on routine screening. **(B)** Sonography suggested a cyst, and aspiration was performed to confirm this diagnosis. **(C)** Sonographic image shows the aspirating needle puncturing the cyst wall (arrow). **(D)** Aspiration yielded several cubic centimeters of turbid, nonbloody fluid, typical of benign cyst contents. **(E)** A postaspiration mammogram shows that the mammographic lesion has resolved, confirming that the mass was the simple cyst.

Fluid Disposition and Patient Management

Normal, benign cyst fluid varies in color from milky to clear, amber, or shades of green. Its consistency varies from thin and watery to very thick (toothpaste-like). The presence of bright red blood usually indicates aspiration-related trauma, whereas dark blood may indicate the presence of an intracystic tumor such as a papilloma or carcinoma or aspiration of the necrotic center of a solid tumor.

The appropriate disposition of fluid aspirated from breast cysts is controversial. Some advocate cytologic evaluation in all cases,[24] whereas others do it in cases where the aspirate is bloody.[25] Still others advise against cytology altogether.[26] In a series of 6872 consecutive aspirations where all the aspirates were subjected to cytologic evaluation, Ciatto et al. reported that among the 6747 nonbloody aspirates there were no cases of suspicious cytology.[25] Furthermore, no malignancies developed at the site of these cysts during an extended follow-up period. Thus, routine cytologic evaluation of nonbloody cyst fluid does not appear to be necessary. Among the 125 bloody aspirates, there was a single case of suspicious cytology that was found to represent a benign intracystic papilloma at excision.

It has been suggested that patient management after cyst aspiration is possible without the use of cytology. In this management algorithm, if the cyst fluid is nonbloody and there is no residual mass found by imaging or clinical examination, the patient is reassured that the lesion was a benign cyst, and she can continue routine, age-appropriate breast cancer screening. If there is a residual mass, the patient can be advised to consider a biopsy. If the aspirate contains dark blood, the patient can be advised to undergo a biopsy of the mass. Surgical excision is often the preferred biopsy technique for these cystic masses, as core needle biopsy may cause the lesion to disappear altogether or become very vague after one or two passes.

REFERENCES

1. Bolmgren J, Jacobson B, Nordenstrom B. Stereotaxic instrument for needle biopsy of the mamma. AJR 1977;129:121–125.
2. Fornage BD, Faroux MJ, Simatos A. Breast masses: US-guided fine needle aspiration biopsy. Radiology 1987;162:409–414.
3. Dowlatshahi K, Gent HJ, Schmidt R, et al. Nonpalpable breast tumors: diagnosis with stereotactic localization and fine needle aspiration. Radiology 1989;170:427–433.
4. Hann L, Ducatman BS, Wang HH, et al. Nonpalpable breast lesions: evaluation by means of fine needle aspiration cytology. Radiology 1989;171:373–376.
5. Ciatto S, Rosselli Del Turco M, Bravetti P. Nonpalpable breast lesions: stereotaxic fine needle aspiration cytology. Radiology 1989;173:57–59.
6. Lofgren M, Andersson I, Lindholm K. Stereotactic fine needle aspiration cytologic diagnosis of nonpalpable breast lesions. AJR 1990;154:1191–1195.
7. Parker SH, Lovin JD, Jobe WE, et al. Stereotactic breast biopsy with a biopsy gun. Radiology 1990;176:741–747.
8. Reynolds HE, Poon CM, Goulet RJ, et al. Biopsy of breast microcalcifications using an 11 gauge directional vacuum-assisted device. AJR 1998;171:611–613.
9. Darling ML, Smith DN, Lester SC, et al. Atypical ductal hyperplasia and ductal carcinoma in situ as revealed by large core needle breast biopsy: results of surgical excision. AJR 2000;175:1341–1346.
10. Helvie MA, Baker DE, Adler DD, et al. Radiographically guided fine needle aspiration of nonpalpable breast lesions. Radiology 1990;174:657–661.
11. Pisano ED, Fajardo LL, Caudry DJ, et al. Fine-needle aspiration biopsy of nonpalpable breast lesions in a multicenter clinical trial: results from the Radiologic Diagnostic Oncology Group V. Radiology 2001;219:785–792.
12. Lee, KR, Foster RS, Papillo JL. Fine needle aspiration of the breast: importance of the aspirator. Acta Cytol 1987;31:281–284.
13. Cohen MB, Rodgers RP, Hales MS, et al. Influence of training and experience in fine needle aspiration biopsy of breast: receiver operating characteristics curve analysis. Arch Pathol Lab Med 1987;111:518–520.
14. American College of Radiology. Illustrated Breast Imaging Reporting and Data System, 3rd ed. Reston, VA: American College of Radiology, 1998.
15. Sack MJ, Langer JE. Ultrasound transmission gel mimicking necrosis in ultrasound guided fine needle aspiration specimens. Diagn Cytopathol 1994;11:309–310.
16. Molyneux AJ, Coghill SB. Cell lysis due to ultrasound gel in fine needle aspirates; an important new artefact in cytology. Cytopathology 1994;5:41–45.
17. Daltrey IR, Lewis CE, McKee GT, et al. The effect of needle gauge and local anesthetic on the diagnostic accuracy of breast fine needle aspiration cytology. Eur J Surg Oncol 1999;25:30–33.
18. Pisano ED. Fine needle aspiration biopsy of breast lesions. In Dershaw DD (ed) Interventional Breast Procedures. New York: Churchill Livingstone, 1996;89–102.
19. Cajulis RS, Sneige N. Objective comparison of cellular yield in fine needle biopsy of lymph nodes with and without aspiration. Diagn Cytopathol 1993;9:43–45.
20. Ciatto S, Catania S, Bravetti P, et al. Fine needle cytology of the breast: a controlled study of aspiration versus nonaspiration. Diagn Cytopathol 1991;7:125–127.
21. Mair S, Dunbar F, Becker PJ, et al. Fine needle cytology: is aspiration suction necessary? A study of 100 masses in various sites. Acta Cytol 1989;33:809–813.
22. The uniform approach to breast fine needle aspiration biopsy. Diagn Cytopathol 1997;16:295–311.
23. Sickles EA, Filly RA, Callen PW. Benign breast lesions: ultrasound detection and diagnosis. Radiology 1984;151:467–470.
24. McSwain G, Valicenti J, O'Brien P. Cytologic evaluation of breast cysts. Surg Gynecol Obstet 1978;146:921–925.
25. Ciatto S, Cariaggi P, Bularisis P. The value of routine cytologic examination of breast cyst fluids. Acta Cytol 1987;31:301–304.
26. Kinnard D. Results of cytological study of fluid aspirated from breast cysts. Am Surg 1975;41:505–506.

CHAPTER 9

Specimen Radiography

Eva Rubin

Specimen radiography is a valuable tool for ascertaining the adequacy of surgical biopsy and removal of nonpalpable breast lesions.[1] It was originally intended primarily to document the excisional biopsy of indeterminate lesions. Since the widespread use of percutaneous needle biopsies for nonsurgical diagnosis, patients with nonpalpable benign lesions undergo needle localization biopsy with specimen radiography relatively less frequently than in the past.[2] Specimen radiography is now increasingly used to ascertain adequacy of excision for known malignant lesions.

Radiographs of mastectomy specimens performed by Salomon[3] in the late nineteenth century were the first indicators of the potential of radiographs to detect breast cancer and depict its extent. At that time, breast cancers were typically large, requiring mastectomy for adequate local control. Today, because improvements in breast cancer detection and diagnosis, specimen radiographs ideally reveal the results of a successful lumpectomy (i.e., the complete removal of a small, potentially curable breast cancer).

RATIONALE FOR SPECIMEN RADIOGRAPHY

Ensure Removal of Mammographically Suspicious Lesions

The primary reason for obtaining a specimen radiograph is to ensure that the area containing a suspicious lesion has been removed (Figure 9.1). Nowadays, many, if not most, lesions undergoing surgery for mammographically detected abnormalities have already been sampled percutaneously. Thus, most tissue that is radiographed after breast surgery contains a known malignancy. The objective of needle localized surgical biopsies has changed from minimal excision of breast tissue for *diagnosis* to complete removal of malignant breast tissue with an adequate margin of surrounding normal tissue for *treatment*.

Obtaining an optimal specimen radiograph begins with the needle localization procedure. When the objective of most of these procedures is to facilitate performance of a lumpectomy with negative margins, the localization procedure must result in (1) placement of a marker at the site of the known or suspected malignancy and (2) definition of the entire extent of the malignant process. Placement of multiple wires may be necessary to fully delineate an area of involvement.[4] Carcinomas with an extensive intraductal component or cases in which calcifications are linearly or segmentally distributed often require bracketing with two or more wires (Figure 9.2).

Document Removal of Any Inserted Foreign Bodies

The individual performing the needle localization procedure is required to demonstrate that any inserted needles, wires, or other metallic markers have been removed totally. The exception is that malpositioned percutaneous biopsy clips may be left in place. The radiologist must be careful to correlate the prebiopsy radiographs with those obtained postbiopsy in order to ensure that the clip corresponds to the site that needs to be localized.

Ensuring removal of needle localization wires or other objects is not problematic when intact wires are visible in the radiographed tissue. If documentation of complete removal of this hardware is required, wires pulled from the tissue by the surgeon should be submitted with the resected tissue so that their removal can be documented on the specimen radiography report. If the specimen radiograph suggests that the localizing wire has been un-

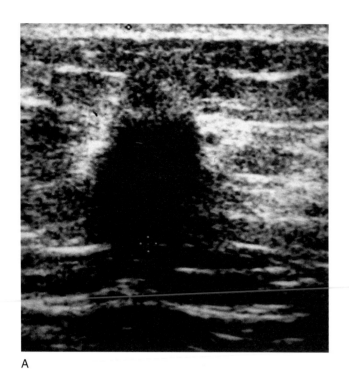

A

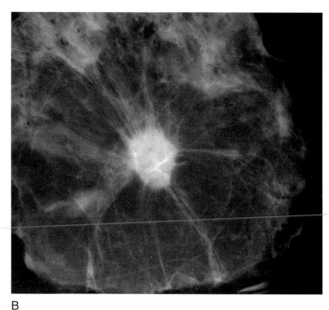

B

FIGURE 9.1. (**A**) A spiculated mass was found on mammography. An irregular, solid mass is demonstrated by sonography and underwent sonographically guided core biopsy. It was shown to be malignant and underwent localization and removal. (**B**) Specimen radiography shows that the carcinoma has been removed. Note that there is minimal lucency centrally in the carcinoma due to the needle biopsy. The specimen radiograph documents that the mass has been excised and directs the pathologist to the area of the specimen containing the lesion.

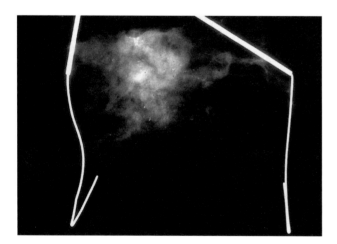

FIGURE 9.2. A broad area of calcifications with a central area of mass was biopsied and found to be malignant. To direct surgical excision of the carcinoma, wires were placed at the margins of the carcinoma to increase the likelihood that the surgeon could remove all of the mammographic evidence of the cancer. Bracketing of some lesions can require placement of more than two wires.

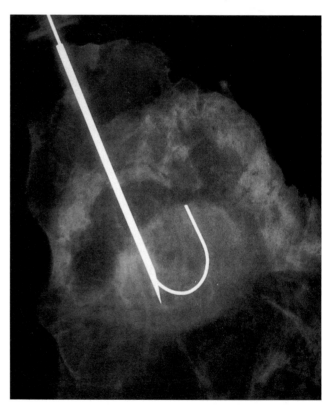

FIGURE 9.3. After removal of a carcinoma, a residual mass was present in the breast that was suspicious for carcinoma. A specimen radiograph of the localized and removed lesion shows that the mass is contained within the removed tissue. Residual mass was due to a postbiopsy hematoma.

160

expectedly transected, this should be communicated to the surgeon while the patient is still on the table, and this should be noted on the report.

Define the Size, Extent, and Nature of the Lesion

Although histopathologic findings are considered the gold standard for defining abnormalities within tissue, the visual information that is provided by a well-performed specimen radiograph may supplement the pathologic interpretation and should not be overlooked.

The presence and extent of malignant calcifications are more easily defined on specimen radiographs than on histologic sections. For the pathologist, the determination of the size of a malignant process manifest by calcifications is difficult. This may be estimated by reconstruction of the three-dimensional volume using a sequential series of slides.[5,6] However, specimen radiography may be as, or more, accurate in many cases. For areas of carcinoma that are evident radiographically and have intervening areas of normal breast tissue, the extent of the tumor and suspicion of residual disease within the breast can also be a difficult determination for the pathologist. The presence of multiple tumor nodules may be more apparent on specimen radiography than on the pathology slides. Therefore, this is more likely to be identified by the pathologist if the specimen radiograph is inspected by the pathologist prior to sectioning of the tissue.

It is important to recognize that the lesions undergoing needle localization after percutaneous biopsy may have been significantly altered by the percutaneous biopsy procedure. Postbiopsy hematomas are common and may obscure residual disease at the biopsy site or mimic the appearance of a carcinoma on the specimen radiograph (Figure 9.3). The distribution of calcifications is altered by their partial removal (Figure 9.4A). After complete removal has occurred, a percutaneously placed clip may be the only remaining indicator of the site of the original abnormality (Figure 9.5). In the case of mass lesions, the contour of the mass may be altered resulting in underestimation of tumor volume (Figure 9.6). Also, defects produced by the needle tracks may lead to "holes" within the tumor mass (Figure 9.1B). If sufficiently large, these defects can mimic the appearance of separate tumor foci.

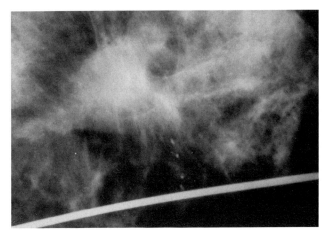

B

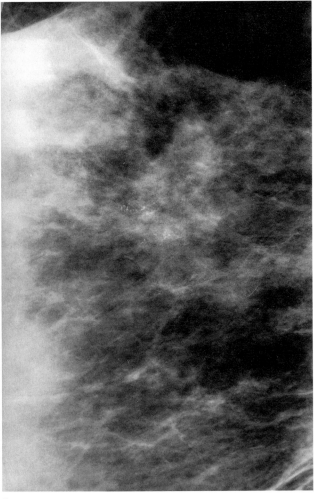

A

FIGURE 9.4. (A) An area of suspicious calcifications was found on mammography. These were biopsied percutaneously and found to be malignant. (B) Specimen radiography of the excised tissue shows how the area of calcifications has been modified by core biopsy.

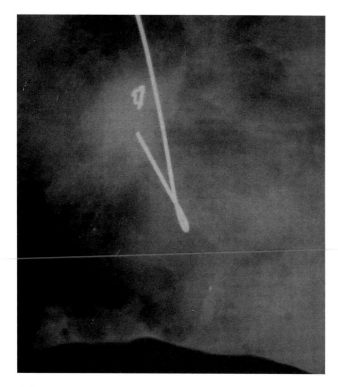

FIGURE 9.5. Lesions that are completely excised during core biopsy procedures should have the site of the lesion marked at the end of the procedure. The marker is used as the target for reexcision. This specimen radiograph shows removal of the clip placed as a marker at the completion of a stereotactic biopsy.

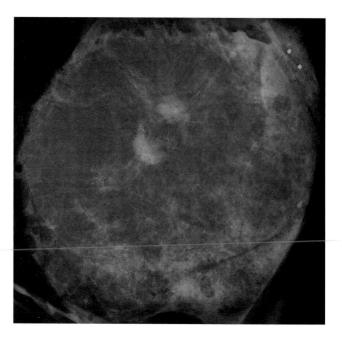

FIGURE 9.6. Specimen radiography of a mass-like carcinoma that has undergone core biopsy shows that the tumor has been bisected. Histopathologically, this can result in tumor staging by measuring two separate lesions rather than a single, larger mass. However, presence of histologic changes in the needle biopsy specimen should suggest to the pathologist that the tumor may have been transected by the needling procedure.

Guide the Pathologist in Orientation and Sectioning of the Specimen

Optimal correlation of the specimen radiograph and the histopathology requires communication among the physicians participating in the localization procedure—surgeon, radiologist, and pathologist—as well as their assistants. The surgeon should orient the specimen before submitting it for specimen radiography and histologic sectioning. This may be done with sutures, colored inks, or other techniques. Radiograph(s) of the specimen should be available in the surgical suite and the pathology department.

Histotechnologists are often responsible for cutting and embedding the specimens. They must be educated as to the information available on the specimen radiograph so that the information is not lost to the pathologist ultimately responsible for the interpretation of the histopathology.

Multiple tumor masses or foci of calcification may be readily apparent on the specimen radiograph; knowledge of the location of these areas allows them to be specifically sampled histologically. Placing grease pencil marks on the specimen radiograph to identify areas that should be individually analyzed may be helpful. Alternatively, needles or wires may be placed secondarily in the resected tissue at sites of specific interest. Care should be

taken if this method is used to ensure that those handling tissue specimens containing sharp objects are not subjected to the dangers of needle puncture. Alerting the pathology personnel to the presence of more than one lesion within the resected tissue, particularly if one is benign and the other malignant, may also avoid misdiagnosis by the pathologist (Figure 9.7).

Aid in Margin Assessment

The radiologist is >95% accurate when defining margin involvement in cases where tumor is transected and malignant calcifications extend to a margin of the specimen on specimen radiography (Figure 9.8). Unfortunately, the absence of these findings does not ensure negative margins.[7]

Assessment of margins from a single specimen radiograph is limited. Ideally, orthogonal views of tissue specimens should be obtained (Figure 9.9), but this is often difficult, if not impossible, to achieve. The resected tissue is usually wet, slippery, irregularly shaped, and of variable thickness. This makes it imperfectly compressible in orthogonal planes. In addition, the presence of wires or other metallic objects within the resected tissue may not allow orthogonal compression. Although orthogonal views of specimens are recommended, they have not yet become the standard of care.[8]

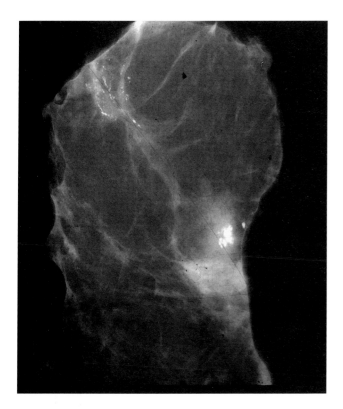

FIGURE 9.7. Excision was performed in this patient for a lesion containing calcifications. The specimen radiograph contains two calcified lesions, a carcinoma in the upper portion and a fibroadenoma in the lower portion. The pathologist should be advised that the specimen contains two separate calcified lesions and be directed to the one that was the reason for biopsy. Note also that the area of the carcinoma is very close to the resected margin, suggesting that tumor may have been transected surgically, leaving some carcinoma within the breast.

A much more precise assessment of gross specimen margin involvement can be obtained by breadloafing the specimen and radiographing each slice.[9,10] This facilitates the task of the pathologist in defining margins accurately and in defining multicentricity and multifocality of carcinomas.[11–13] Slicing the specimen and radiographing each contiguous slice is time-consuming and more expensive than standard methods. Logistically, this may also prove difficult unless the microtome and the specimen radiography unit are in the same location. However, this method is undobtedly worth the time and expense if more accurate diagnosis and appropriate treatment are the result.

Provide Resource for Quality Assurance and Education

In an unpublished study from our institution, six expert and nonexpert interpreters were asked to diagnose 220 randomly selected abnormalities as benign or malignant based on their appearance on specimen radiographs. Ap-

proximately 40% of the cases were malignant, and masses and calcifications were equally represented. For all interpreters, benign–malignant distinctions were more accurate when they were made on the basis of specimen radiographs performed at 2× magnification rather than on routine mammograms. One expert achieved an overall accuracy of 95%. As might be expected, accuracy was better for mass lesions than for calcifications.

The findings of this study suggest that if breast imagers had the quality of information available to them for standard or magnification mammography that is present in a magnified specimen radiograph, false-positive readings would be significantly decreased. A mammogram represents a composite image of multiple layers of breast tissue. A resected specimen contains less tissue around the area of abnormality. Therefore, pathology is less likely to be obscured by surrounding structure. In addition, patient

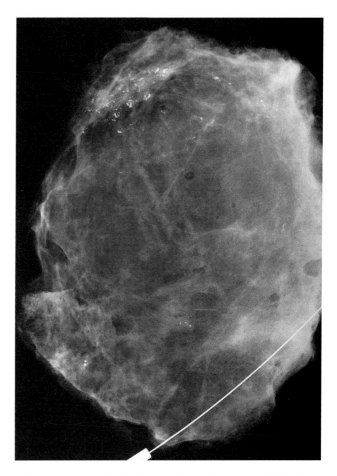

FIGURE 9.8. A calcified carcinoma is present in the upper portion of this specimen. Calcifications extend to the margin of the specimen. This suggests that residual carcinoma is present in the breast at this margin. At the time of this surgical procedure, the surgeon can reexcise this area of the lumpectomy bed based on the information contained in the specimen radiograph. This is helpful for decreasing the likelihood that the patient will need to return to surgery for reexcision because of positive margins.

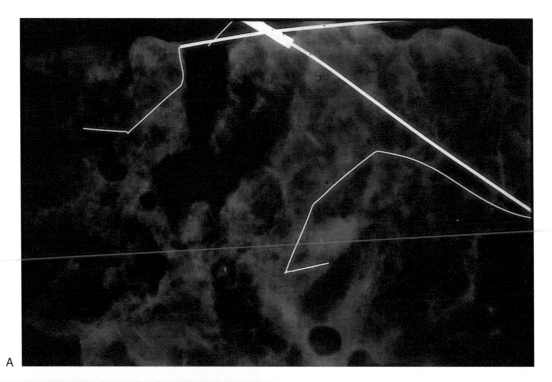

A

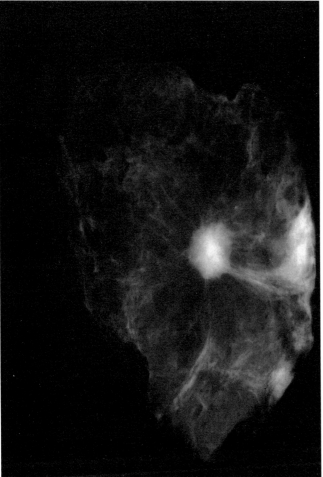

B

FIGURE 9.9. (**A**) Specimen radiography of a spiculated carcinoma shows on this single view that the tumor is centrally
positioned within the excised tissue. (**B**) An orthogonal view
of the same specimen demonstrates extension of a spicule
of carcinoma to the resected margin. Failure to obtain multiple views of the specimen can result in the inability to identify contamination of some margins by carcinoma.

motion and dose considerations are factors in the patient that compromise the ability to produce a diagnostic image. They are clearly not factors in ex vivo tissue.

The gross morphology of breast cancer is beautifully displayed in highly magnified specimen radiographs. Currently available technology allows specimen radiographs to be performed at 5× magnification or higher. Higher magnifications have the limitation that they require an area larger than that provided by standard mammography film cassettes, thereby requiring the specimen to be radiographed in sections. With the degree of resolution available on highly magnified specimen radiographs, depiction of margins and calcifications rivals that of low power photomicrographs.

The idea that specimen radiographs are only worthwhile for lesions manifest as calcifications[14] is not supported by analysis of high quality specimen radiography. With proper technique, true breast masses, even those without calcifications, are readily recognized. For the radiologist, there is no better way to learn the differences between benign and malignant diseases of the breast and to characterize their patterns of growth and distribution.

TECHNIQUE

Most specimen radiographs are performed on standard mammography equipment. Utilizing the smallest focal spot size (approximately 0.1 mm on most units), magnification factors of 1.5–2.0 are possible. Kilovoltage varies with tissue thickness and composition but most often is around 22 kV. Manually timed, rather than phototimed, exposure is common. A single emulsion film with a single-sided high-definition screen is most often used.

An alternative method of specimen radiography involves utilization of a tabletop magnification unit (Faxitron). These units have focal spots measuring 20–50 μm allowing 3–10× magnification. The available range of kilovoltage is from 10 to 35 kVp.

Digital specimen radiography is also available.[15] Such equipment may be placed in the surgical suite or in the pathology department, allowing rapid evaluation of the adequacy of the specimen. For optimal assessment, the digital image should also be made available to the breast imager.

Because of the nonuniform thickness of most resected tissue specimens, mild compression is often necessary to produce diagnostic image quality. Inadequate compression impedes detection of abnormalities, particularly when specimens are large (Figure 9.10). The degree of compression need only be sufficient to produce even thickness of the tissue such that exposure is adequate in all portions.

Although counterintuitive, motion artifact may occur during specimen radiography. Resected tissue may expand or contract, and wet tissue placed on a smooth sur-

face may slide during the time of the exposure. Compression also prevents artifacts caused by motion.

It has been proposed by some that overcompression of the specimen may have an adverse effect on margin assessment by causing the dyes used for margin definition to seep into deeper tissue. Such artifacts may lead to a diagnosis of margin involvement when none exists. In fact, any mishandling of the tissue, such as compression between forceps and other manipulations occurring during or after surgery, can compromise margin assessment.

It has also been suggested, although never demonstrated in a controlled study, that compression creates artifacts that result in an overdiagnosis of invasion. For these reasons, care should be taken that compression is not so vigorous as to disrupt the tissue.

PROBLEMS ASSOCIATED WITH SPECIMEN RADIOGRAPHY

Failure to Recognize

The lesion being localized may actually have been removed but may not be apparent in the radiograph obtained. Most often this is an imaging problem and can be rectified by altering the technique. Inadequate compression, improper choice of kV, overexposure or underexposure, and unfavorable orientation can all contribute to the inability to recognize that the lesion is present in the excised tissue. Reorienting the tissue and repeating the radiograph with altered technical factors may solve this problem.

The surgeon and radiologist should understand that some lesions that have been accurately localized, excised, and are included in the volume of tissue imaged on specimen radiography may not be appreciated on the specimen radiograph. This occurs most frequently after the localization of areas of asymmetry or architectural distortion. Asymmetric tissue may be impossible to appreciate ex vivo. Areas of architectural distortion can be obscured by the distortion resulting from the surgical procedure. When it is uncertain if these areas (or any other localized lesions) have been excised, postoperative mammography may be necessary to document excision of the suspicious area.

Areas that are only evident preoperatively by sonography or magnetic resonance (MR) imaging can also be inapparent on the specimen radiograph. For lesions that were found and localized with sonography, sonographic interrogation of the specimen may be necessary to document removal of the lesion. However, masses that are not appreciated on in vivo mammography can sometimes be seen on specimen radiography. Lesions localized under MR guidance present a greater problem. Because they are discovered by abnormal blood flow with contrast enhancement and because this enhancement cannot be dem-

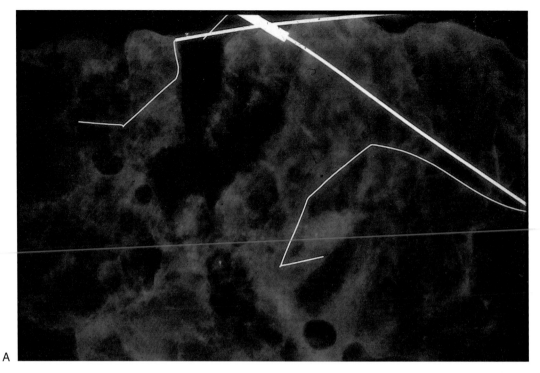

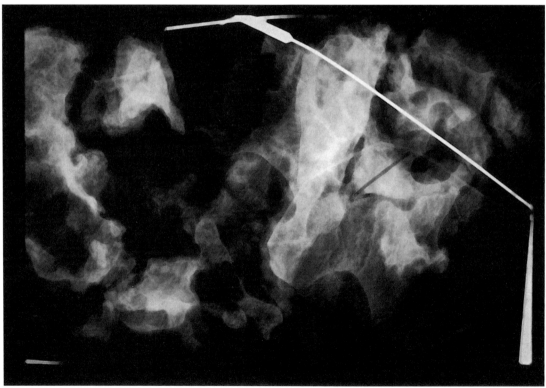

FIGURE 9.10. This large specimen contains multiple localizing wires. **(A)** When imaged under compression, a mass with a few microcalcifications is readily seen enclosed in the hook of the lower localizing wire. **(B)** When the same specimen is imaged without compression, this lesion is almost impossible to appreciate.

onstrated on excised tissue, it may be impossible to image the specimen so that removal of the area of interest can be documented. In these situations, if it is uncertain whether the suspicious area has been excised, postoper-

ative MR imaging of the breast may be necessary to ascertain if the suspicious area has been removed.

Lack of recognition by the pathologist can occur because of problems in the histologic assessment of the specimen. The explanation for the radiographic lesion may have been overlooked on examination of the prepared slides resulting in radiologic–pathologic discordance. This is easily solved by reexamination of the slides with appropriate attention to the information provided by the images. Pathologists are taught to focus on breast epithelium; lesions that are predominantly fibrous or fatty may fail to be described because they are considered irrelevant.

If reexamination of the prepared slides still fails to define the expected pathology, it may be necessary to cut deeper into the paraffin blocks and prepare additional slides. In addition, pathologists may not process the portions of excised tissue that are thought to contain only adipose tissue. Such fragments are often placed in formalin and discarded several days to weeks after the tissue diagnosis has been completed. Radiologists must ensure that the histopathologic evaluation is concordant with expected findings based on the radiologic appearance of the lesion. If radiologic–pathologic discordance is identified within a short period following the biopsy, appropriate steps can be taken to ensure that all tissue potentially containing the lesion of interest has actually been seen by the pathologist.

Failure to Remove the Lesion

Failure to remove the lesion has been reported to occur in 0.5% to 10% of needle localized biopsies. Higher numbers are reported from older series and likely do not reflect modern performance. Since most needle localizations now occur in the setting of known carcinoma, the absence of a malignant lesion in the resected tissue often indicates a failure to remove the lesion. If this is communicated to the surgeon in a timely fashion, additional tissue can be removed to salvage the procedure. Appropriate orientation of the resected tissue by the surgeon and/or the presence of identifiable anatomy within the tissue simplifies the radiologist's task of informing the surgeon as to what direction of additional resection is likely to yield the tissue of interest. If this fails, a second excisional biopsy may be necessary.

An exception to the scenario described above occurs in cases where the lesion has been totally excised during percutaneous biopsy. Again, communication regarding this possibility is critical to ensure that the patient receives a correct diagnosis and appropriate treatment. Also, histologic assessment of the excised specimen should document findings due to the needle tract. These include evidence of hemorrhage, tissue disruption consistent with needling, and post-biopsy inflammation.

Failure of Correlation

Failure to correlate the radiographic and histologic findings is a significant problem that may lead to over- or underdiagnosis. It is the responsibility of the breast imager to ensure that the histology corresponds to the diagnosis expected from the imaging findings. This presupposes that the imager has some method of correlating expected and actual results. The requirement for classifying mammographic lesions according to the Breast Imaging Reporting and Data System (BI-RADS™) assessment categories and the known results of percutaneous biopsy performed in many cases has made tracking discordant results much less complicated than in the past.

Nonetheless, failure of correlation remains a problem. If a distorted area is present on imaging, a benign result on percutaneous biopsy is usually considered discordant, and the patient will generally require an excisional biopsy for diagnosis. If distortion or spiculation is present on the specimen radiograph, there must be corresponding histology. This need not be malignant histology. Benign lesions such as radial scar, sclerosing adenosis, and fibrosis can be responsible for areas of distortion. Again, communication between the radiologist and pathologist is essential to ensure proper correlation and diagnosis.

More often than with masses, failure of correlation occurs in the setting of needle-localized biopsies performed for calcifications. Failure of the pathologist to describe calcifications should alert the radiologist to the possibility of a discordant result. Since pathologists tend to focus on alterations in epithelium, the presence of calcifications, particularly those located in benign tissue, may not be considered worthy of mention. If calcifications are identified histologically, their location and, when possible, their cause must be described. This avoids the error of inexperienced breast imagers who may assume that if cancer is identified in the tissue it is associated with the calcific focus. It is important for the pathologist to indicate whether calcifications are present in benign or malignant tissue or both. In addition, description of the size or extent of calcifications facilitates correlation.

Radiologists should be aware that pathologists are able to visualize calcifications that are beyond the resolution of mammography.[16] The simple acknowledgment of the presence of calcifications by pathologists does not ensure that they have looked at the area of radiographic concern (Figure 9.7).

It is possible for microcalcifications to be identified on the specimen radiograph and for none to be found on histologic examination. Calcifications may be lost during processing.[17] This is most likely to occur with calcifications present within a fluid-filled structure such as a duct or cyst that is evacuated during the biopsy or during sectioning of the tissue. Additionally, calcifications, especially macrocalcifications, may be shattered out of the tissue by the microtome. An astute pathologist may be alerted to this possibility by the identification of "holes" in the tissue corresponding to the site of the calcifications. Calcium oxalate calcifications, most often associated with benign pathology,[18] may not be visible on routine light microscopy. They are, however, easily identified with polarized light.

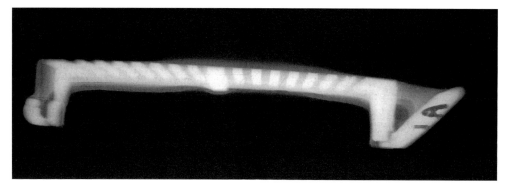

FIGURE 9.11. When the pathologist fails to identify calcifications present in the excised specimen on examination of the histopathologic slides, radiography of the paraffin block can determine if they have not been included in tissue sectioned for the slides but are in the remaining paraffin block. The failure to find them in the block indicates that they are present in the sectioned tissue and not appreciated by the pathologist or that they were lost during preparation of the tissue.

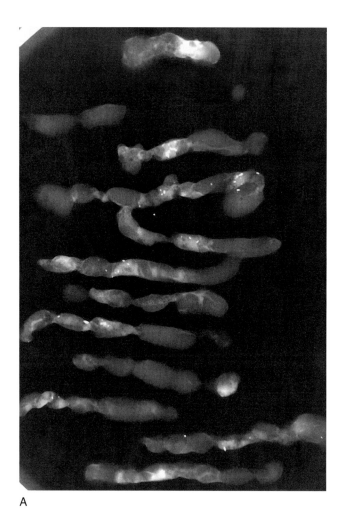

A

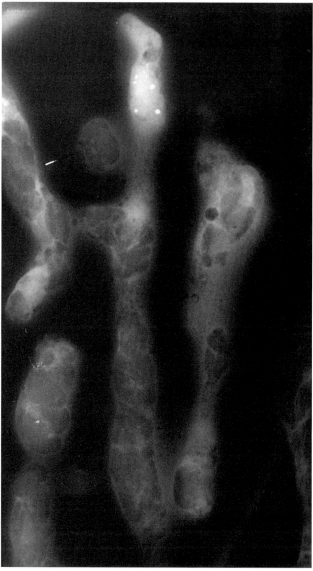

B

FIGURE 9.12. (A) Core biopsy procedures done to evaluate calcifications should include radiography of the tissue cores. It is usually helpful to the pathologist to separate cores containing calcifications from those without calcium. **(B)** Note that on core radiography it is possible to identify areas of fat, soft tissue density, and calcification within the removed tissue.

Finally, calcifications seen on the specimen radiograph but not identified histologically may not have been processed. In the preparation of slides from tissue blocks, <1% of the available tissue may be inspected by the pathologist. Typically, the initial slices from the paraffin block contain no tissue and are discarded. Once tissue is encountered, only one slice of a thickness of approximately 4 μm is prepared from each paraffin block.

If no calcifications have been described histologically but calcifications have been verified on specimen radiographs, the first option should be a review of the existing slides. The pathologist may simply have failed to describe calcifications that are actually present in the processed material. If review fails to identify calcifications, the paraffin blocks should be radiographed (Figure 9.11) and deeper sections should be performed on the blocks containing calcifications.[19,20] If no calcifications are present in the blocks, the unprocessed tissue should be radiographed.

SPECIMEN RADIOGRAPHY OF LARGE CORE TISSUE BIOPSIES

After any image-guided biopsy performed for diagnosis of a calcified lesion, the core fragments should be radiographed to ensure that calcifications have been retrieved (Figure 9.12). This may be done digitally[21] or with the techniques described for excisional biopsy specimens. Since the calcified fragments most often contain the pathology of interest,[22] identifying the fragments that contain calcification for the pathologist is recommended. The calcified fragments may be separated from the noncalcified fragments by placing them in histowrap, or the calcified fragments may be placed in one tissue cassette and the noncalcified fragments in another.

In cases where a soft tissue mass surrounded by adipose tissue has been biopsied, specimen radiographs of the cores may also provide assurance that the mass has been sampled. Core fragments containing soft tissue elements may be separated from those consisting of purely adipose tissue to facilitate pathologic identification and interpretation.

MEDICAL RECORD: THE REPORT AND THE FILMS

It is worthwhile to include a report of the specimen radiograph and correlation of the histopathologic diagnosis with the imaging pattern of the excised lesion in the medical record. The specimen radiograph can be reported separately or can be included in the report of (or as an addendum to) the localization procedure. If there is a suspicion that carcinoma has not been completely excised because tumor extends to the resected margin or if it is suspected that the worrisome area was missed during surgery, it is appropriate to personally communicate this to the surgeon and to document this communication in the specimen radiography report.

As is true for other images obtained during the preoperative localization, specimen radiography images should be maintained as part of the medical record. These images are important to document removal of the lesion and, for some patients, to compare with postoperative mammograms to ascertain if tumor calcifications have been completely excised. As noted above, they can also be valuable for teaching and studying mammographic patterns of various histopathologies.

CONCLUSIONS

Review of specimen radiographs is one of the best ways to learn the differences in the appearance of benign and malignant lesions of the breast. The size and extent of a malignant process may be better defined on specimen radiography than on histology. Margin assessment may be facilitated by specimen radiography; orthogonal views and radiographs of the sliced tissue should be encouraged. It is important for both radiologists and pathologists to understand which radiologic features are correlated with histologic findings in order that patients receive correct diagnoses and management tailored to the pathology found.

REFERENCES

1. Rubin E, Simpson J. Breast Specimen Radiography: Needle Localization and Radiographic Pathologic Correlation. Philadelphia: Lippincott-Raven, 1998.
2. Rubin E, Mennemeyer ST, Desmond RA, et al. Reducing the cost of diagnosis of breast carcinoma: impact of ultrasound and imaging-guided biopsies on a clinical breast practice. Cancer 2001;91:324–332.
3. Salomon A. Beitrage zur Pathologie und Klinik der Mammacarcinome. Arch Klin Chir 1913;101:573–668.
4. Silverstein MJ, Gamagami P, Colburn WJ. Coordinated biopsy team: surgical, pathologic, and radiologic issues. In Silverstein MJ (ed) Ductal Carcinoma in Situ of the Breast. Baltimore: Williams & Wilkins, 1997;333–342.
5. Lagios MD, Silverstein MJ. Outcomes and factors impacting local recurrence of ductal carcinoma in situ. Cancer 2000;89: 2323–2325.
6. Silverstein MJ, Lagios MD, Groshen S, et al. The influence of margin width on local control of ductal carcinoma in situ of the breast. N Engl J Med 1999;340:1455–1461.
7. Graham RA, Homer MJ, Sigler CJ, et al. The efficacy of specimen radiography in evaluating the surgical margins of impalpable breast carcinoma. AJR 1994;162:33–36.
8. Homer MJ, Berlin L. Radiography of the surgical breast biopsy specimen. AJR 1998;171:1197–1199.
9. D'Orsi CJ. Management of the breast specimen. Radiology 1995;194:297–302.

10. Gould EW, Robinson PG. The pathologist's examination of the "lumpectomy": the pathologists' view of surgical margins. Semin Surg Oncol 1992;8:129–135.

11. Holland R, Veling S, Mravunac M, Hendriks J. Histologic multifocality of Tis, T1–2 carcinomas: implications for clinical trials of breast-conserving surgery. Cancer 1985;56:979–990.

12. Holland R, Hendriks J, Verbeek A, et al. Extent, distribution, and mammographic/histological correlations of breast ductal carcinoma in situ. Lancet 1990;335:519–522.

13. Faverly DR, Hendriks JH, Holland R. Breast carcinomas of limited extent: frequency, radiologic-pathologic characteristics, and surgical margin requirements. Cancer 2001;91:647–659.

14. Rosen PP. Breast Pathology. Philadelphia: Lippincott-Raven, 1997;843–848.

15. Diekmann F, Grebe S, Bick U, et al. Intraoperative digital radiography for diagnosis of nonpalpable breast lesions. Rofo 2000;172:969–971.

16. Millis RR, Davis R, Stacey AJ. The detection and significance of calcifications in the breast: a radiological and pathological study. Br J Radiol 1976;49:12–26.

17. Stein MA, Karlan MS. Calcification in breast biopsy specimens: discrepancies in radiologic-pathologic identification. Radiology 1991;179:111–114.

18. Radi MJ. Calcium oxalate crystals in breast biopsies: an overlooked form of microcalcification associated with benign breast disease. Arch Pathol Lab Med 1989;113:1367–1369.

19. Rebner M, Helvie MA, Pennes DR, et al. Paraffin tissue block radiography: adjunct to breast specimen radiography. Radiology 1989;173:695–696.

20. Cardenosa G, Eklund GW. Paraffin block radiography following breast biopsies: use of orthogonal views. Radiology 1991;180:873–874.

21. Whitlock JP, Evans AJ, Burrell HC, et al. Digital imaging improves upright stereotactic core biopsy of mammographic microcalcifications. Clin Radiol 2000;55:374–377.

22. Liberman L, Evans WP III, Dershaw DD, et al. Radiography of microcalcifications in breast tissue. Radiology 1994;190:223–225.

CHAPTER 10

Histopathology of Needle Core Biopsy Specimens

P. Peter Rosen

There has been a rapid increase in the use of needle core biopsies for the diagnosis of breast lesions. This diagnostic method is especially attractive with the availability of image-guided biopsy instrumentation in conjunction with mammography and ultrasonography. The specimen consists of multiple cylindrical fragments, or cores, of tissue which can be used to make paraffin sections and imprint cytology preparations (Figure 10.1). One survey reported that most pathologists questioned had more experience in examining tissue sections, and they therefore found interpretation of needle core biopsies to be easier than the evaluation of fine-needle aspiration (FNA) cytology specimens.[1]

The increasing reliance on image-guided needle core biopsy has resulted in histological samples from a growing number of nonpalpable, radiographically detected lesions.[2–4] In many centers, needle core biopsy has replaced FNA cytology as the method of choice for evaluating nonpalpable lesions, and in a substantial number of cases it is the only diagnostic procedure.[5] The sensitivity and specificity of core biopsy are each generally reported to be at least 90%.[6]

Many mammographically detected nonpalpable lesions present the pathologist with challenging diagnostic problems when excised intact and viewed in context with surrounding tissues. The interpretation of incomplete portions of these lesions in disrupted needle core biopsy samples can be substantially more difficult. At the same time, clinical expectations for a definitive diagnosis from the pathologist are as high as after a surgical excisional biopsy, but this is often not realistic.

The primary goal of the pathologist should be to determine whether the needle biopsy sample contains lesional material that warrants further clinical intervention, usually a surgical biopsy. The diagnosis made on the needle core biopsy sample must be employed in the context of clinical and radiologic findings. Radiologists, surgeons, oncologists, and the patient must be prepared to accept an inconclusive report if the pathologist determines that the sample does not permit a specific diagnosis.

Differential diagnostic problems often encountered include:

- Reactive changes versus recurrent carcinoma after lumpectomy
- Benign sclerosing lesions ("radial scar") versus infiltrating carcinoma
- Papilloma versus papillary carcinoma
- Fibroadenoma versus cystosarcoma
- Atypical duct hyperplasia (ADH) versus intraductal carcinoma (DCIS)
- DCIS versus DCIS with (micro)invasion

Three principles provide guidance in the use of needle biopsy for the diagnosis and treatment of nonpalpable breast lesions. They are:

- Anything can turn up.
- What you see is what you have.
- What you have may be all there is; or it may not be all there is.

DIAGNOSIS OF CARCINOMA

Image-guided core biopsy has proven to be a reliable technique for assessing many characteristics of mammary carcinoma (Figure 10.2). However, it is not a substitute for

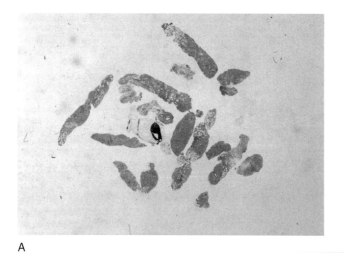
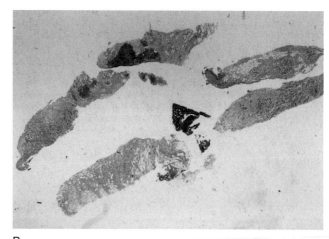

A

B

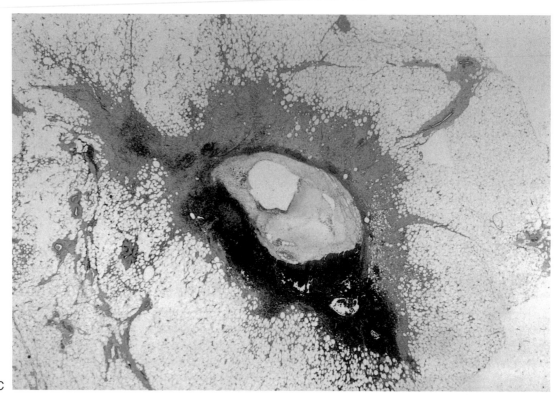

C

FIGURE 10.1. Image-guided needle core biopsy specimens. (**A**) Fibroadenoma. Multiple samples of varying size obtained with a 14-gauge needle. (**B**) Invasive duct carcinoma. Five samples and blood clot obtained with an 11-gauge needle. (**C**) Biopsy site. The central cavity from which needle core samples containing intraductal carcinoma were obtained is surrounded by reactive changes and hemorrhage in this excisional biopsy. No residual carcinoma was found.

the complete sampling of the excised tumor specimen. Concordance between needle core and surgical biopsies for the presence or absence of invasion was reported in 92% of 63 tumors after both procedures were performed.[7] Sharifi et al. reviewed 79 invasive carcinomas for which needle core biopsies and surgical excision specimens were available.[8] The classification of the tumor was the same in both specimens in 64 cases (81%). Eleven of 15 nonconcordant cases involved classification as infiltrating duct

carcinoma versus infiltrating duct and lobular carcinoma. The mixed pattern was reported in eight needle core biopsies with three having a final classification of infiltrating duct carcinoma in the excisional specimen. Among 65 tumors diagnosed as infiltrating duct carcinoma in the core biopsy, eight were classified as mixed duct and lobular tumors in the excised tissue, one was diagnosed as infiltrating lobular carcinoma, and two were classified as tubular carcinoma. Difficulty distinguishing between infiltrating

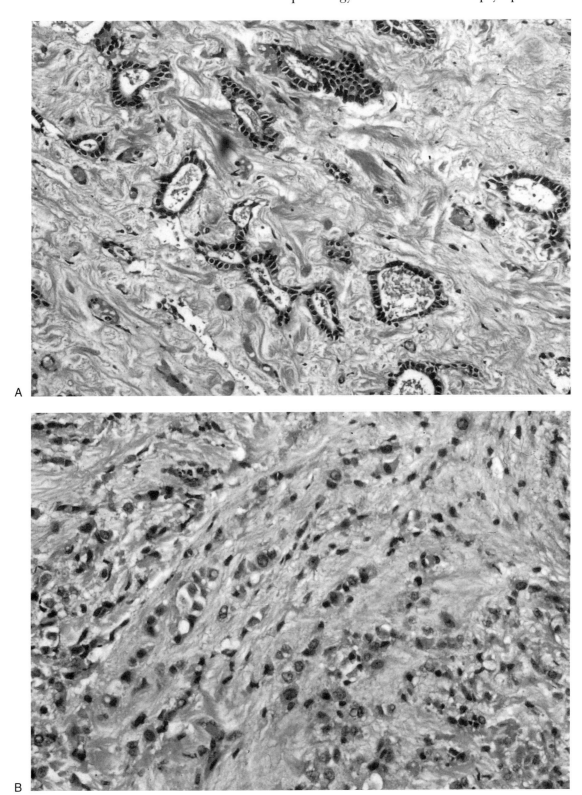

FIGURE 10.2. Invasive carcinoma. (**A**) Tubular carcinoma. Well-differentiated glands with round and angular shapes are shown in this low-grade form of ductal carcinoma. (**B**) Invasive lobular carcinoma. Small, discohesive cells in linear arrays are shown.

174   /   P.P. Rosen

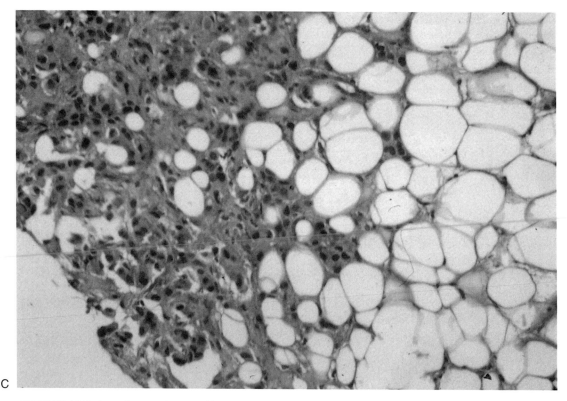

C

FIGURE 10.2. Invasive carcinoma. **(C)** Invasive duct carcinoma. Poorly differentiated carcinoma in fat.

duct and lobular carcinoma is most likely to arise when tubule formation is not seen in the core biopsy specimen.[9]

Comparison of the grading of carcinomas in needle core biopsy and surgical excisions revealed a tendency to assign a lower grade to the needle core biopsy in four studies.[8–11] Sharifi et al. found discrepant histologic grading in 75% of cases[8] and a 20% discordance rate was reported in a second review.[10] The mitotic index was more often underscored than overscored in needle core biopsies.[8,10]

Needle core biopsies have not been effective for reliably detecting the presence of lymphatic tumor emboli. In one report no lymphatic tumor emboli were seen in needle core biopsies from 17 infiltrating carcinomas that had lymphatic invasion.[8] In the same investigation needle core biopsy was relatively unsuccessful for predicting the presence of extensive intraductal carcinoma.

LOBULAR CARCINOMA IN SITU

Needle core biopsy yields lobular carcinoma in situ (LCIS) or atypical lobular hyperplasia (ALH) in about 1% of cases (Figure 10.3). Liberman et al. reported finding LCIS in 14 (1.2%) of 1315 biopsied consecutive lesions.[12] Surgical excision performed in 13 cases yielded intraductal carcinoma in 3 (23%) and infiltrating lobular

carcinoma in 1 (7.8%). The infiltrating carcinoma and one intraductal carcinoma in surgical excisions were preceded by needle core biopsies with florid LCIS that featured marked duct distension. These results suggested that about 25% of patients with LCIS in a needle core biopsy may harbor intraductal or invasive carcinoma.

Two subsequent studies also found intraductal or invasive carcinoma in a substantial number of excisions after a core biopsy revealed LCIS. Shin and Rosen reported that 23% of patients had either intraductal carcinoma or invasive carcinoma in an excision after a core biopsy with LCIS.[13] A larger series of patients with LCIS and ALH diagnosed in needle core biopsies performed for mammographic indications was reported by Lechner et al.[14] This multiinstitutional study of 32,424 biopsies revealed 89 (0.3%) examples of LCIS and 154 (0.5%) instances of ALH. Surgical biopsies were performed on 58 (65%) of the LCIS lesions, yielding the following: invasive lobular carcinoma in 8 (14%), invasive ductal carcinoma in 2 (3%), tubular carcinoma in 8 (14%), intraductal carcinoma in 2 (3%), LCIS in 23 (40%), ADH in 2 (3%), ALH in 4 (7%), and various benign findings in 8 (14%). Surgical biopsies performed in 84 cases after ALH was diagnosed in a needle core biopsy yielded invasive lobular carcinoma in 2 (2%), invasive duct carcinoma in 3 (4%), intraductal carcinoma in 4 (5%), LCIS in 18 (21%), ADH in 18 (21%), ALH in 13 (15%), and various benign findings in 32 (38%).

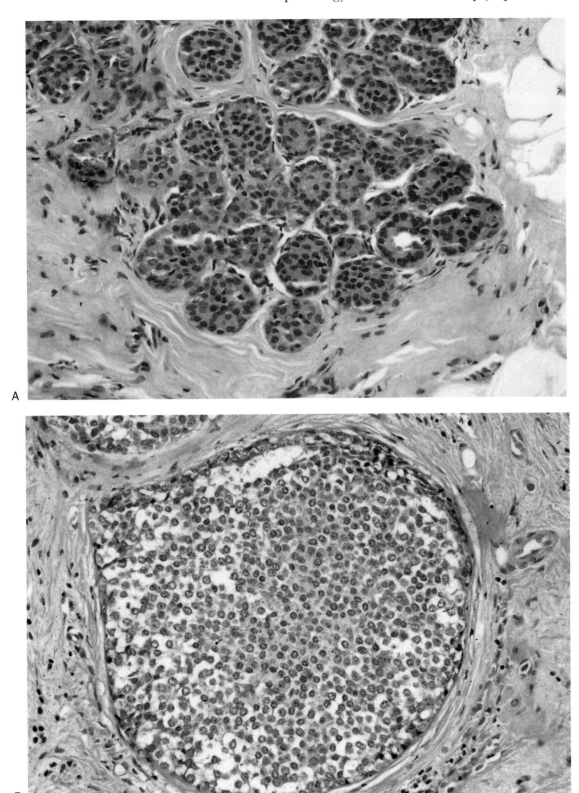

FIGURE 10.3. Lobular carcinoma in situ. (**A**) Intralobular component. The lobular glands are filled with and distended by carcinoma cells. (**B**) Florid ductal component. The distended duct is filled by small carcinoma cells that display loss of cohesion. This form of lobular carcinoma in situ may develop central necrosis with calcification, leading to detection by mammography.

On the basis of the data presently available, this author is of the opinion that excisional biopsy would be prudent to fully explore the site of a needle core biopsy that discloses LCIS. Excisional biopsy is essential if florid LCIS is found in a needle core biopsy. In the author's experience, this form of LCIS is more likely to have microinvasive foci than conventional LCIS. Cases studied by the author have shown loss of E-cadherin expression, a marker typically expressed in ductal carcinomas. The prognostic significance of florid LCIS with respect to the risk for subsequent invasive carcinoma has not been determined. In the typical case, the most florid areas tend to be located toward the center of the lesion, with more conventional LCIS at the periphery, where it may be found near or at the margin of resection.

Excisional biopsy is recommended for ALH if there are associated atypical proliferative lesions such as atypical columnar cell duct hyperplasia, if the mammographic indication for the needle core biopsy has not been entirely removed or if the patient is in a group at high risk for breast carcinoma. It is important to recognize that there is some variation among pathologists with respect to diagnostic criteria for ALH and LCIS. If the decision to perform an excisional biopsy hinges on this distinction, it may be advisable to obtain a second opinion review of the diagnosis.

PAPILLARY TUMORS

Papillary lesions present a challenging problem for diagnosis by needle core biopsy and subsequent clinical management (Figure 10.4). One series of 1077 consecutive lesions sampled by needle core biopsy included 34 papillary tumors (3%).[15] Seven lesions were classified as papillomas, and no carcinoma was detected in subsequent excisions or, when not excised, during 2 years of follow-up at the time of publication. Subsequently, one of the women who did not undergo excision developed invasive metaplastic carcinoma in and around the remnants of the papilloma. Immediate excision performed in two patients with a diagnosis of papillomatosis in the needle core biopsy revealed intraductal carcinoma that arose in spiculated radial sclerosing lesions. Among 10 cases with atypical papillary lesions in the core biopsy, 3 (30%) had intraductal carcinoma in the later excision. Papillary carcinoma was found in all subsequent excisions performed in seven patients who had papillary carcinoma in a needle core biopsy. Four were entirely in situ but three excised tumors (43%) had an invasive component. These results indicate that surgical excision should be performed when a core biopsy reveals an atypical papillary lesion or intraductal papillary carcinoma. Until more data become available with long-term follow-up, excisional biopsy would be prudent if the needle core biopsy reveals a papillary lesion or papilloma without atypia.

PROGNOSTIC MARKERS

Needle core biopsies provide tissue samples that are suitable for evaluating prognostic markers in nonpalpable lesions. Most marker studies are now performed by immunohistochemistry, and generally there has been good correlation between the results obtained in the needle core and subsequent surgical excision specimens. Jacobs et al. reported agreement between the two specimens in all of 56 cases examined by immunostaining for bcl-2, estrogen receptor, c-erbB-2, and p53.[16] A lower level of concordance for microvessel density was achieved using the factor VIII immunostain. In 61.2% of cases, the microvessel counts were higher in the core biopsy specimens and the counts differed by more than 10% in 85.7% of cases. In a similar analysis by Di Loreto et al. there was also a high degree of concordance for reporting of estrogen and progesterone receptors, p53, and c-erbB-2.[11] There was also a significant correlation for mitotic counts with a trend to report lower counts in the core biopsy sample.

FALSE-NEGATIVE DIAGNOSES

False-negative diagnoses by needle biopsy reflect problems in sampling and tissue preservation comparable to those encountered in FNA biopsy. In addition to failure to enter the lesion, the sample may be obtained from a carcinoma in which there is necrosis, desmoplastic fibrosis, or structural heterogeneity. Neoplastic cells in some tumors are particularly fragile and susceptible to distortion by the biopsy procedure ("crush artifact"). The resultant specimen can be uninterpretable in the worst instances. The yield is improved if more than one pass of the needle is made in the lesion with the best results obtained when five or more cores are obtained from a solid palpable tumor. Additional reasons for failure to obtain diagnostic samples are technical issues relating to targeting of lesions and failure to obtain calcifications.

When needle core biopsy is performed for a nonpalpable lesion that has calcifications, several steps can be taken to minimize the likelihood of a false negative report. Radiographs of the biopsy samples should be obtained at the time of the procedure and compared with the prebiopsy mammogram to determine whether the tissue specimens contain the lesional calcifications. An immediate postbiopsy mammogram is useful to detect calcifications that remain; and at this time the relationship of a localizing clip to the biopsy site can be determined, if such a clip has been inserted at the end of the biopsy procedure. It is helpful to the pathologist if the core biopsy samples demonstrated to contain calcifications in specimen radiographs are submitted separately from the samples without apparent calcifications. They should be designated samples with and without calcifications.

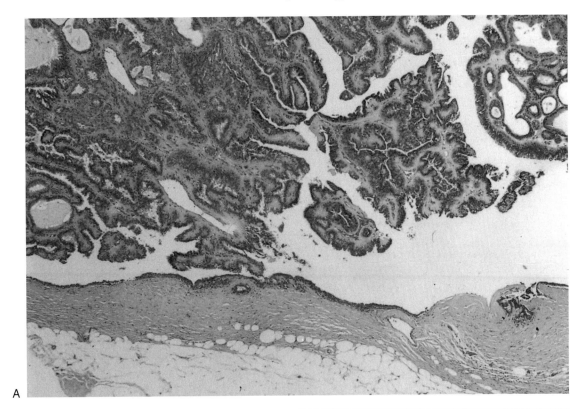

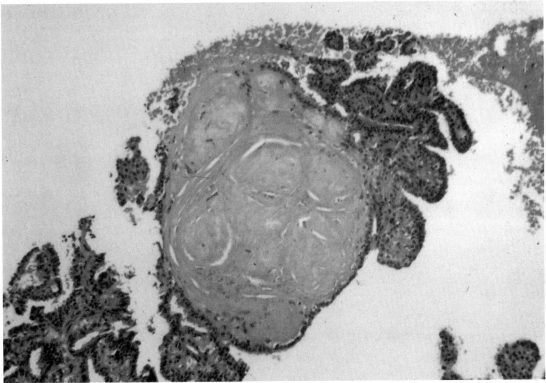

FIGURE 10.4. Papillary lesions. (**A**) Papilloma. Fibrovascular stroma is evenly distributed in the epithelial fronds of this cystic papilloma. (**B**) Papilloma. Collagenization of the stroma is shown in the central nodule around which there are papillary epithelial fronds.

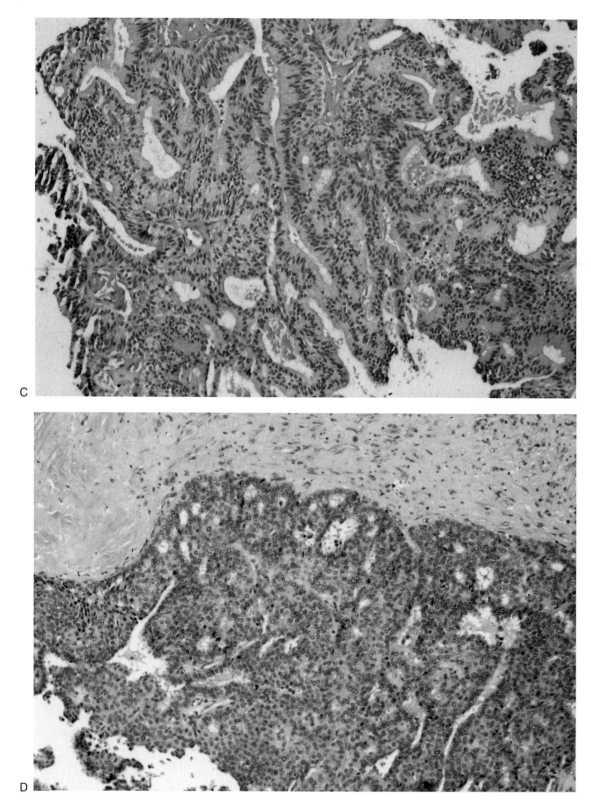

FIGURE 10.4. Papillary lesions. **(C)** Papilloma with atypia. Needle core biopsy specimen shows complex epithelial proliferation supported by fibrovascular stroma. **(D)** Solid papillary carcinoma. This needle core biopsy sample shows the circumscribed tumor border and solid growth pattern typical of this tumor (see Figure 10.8).

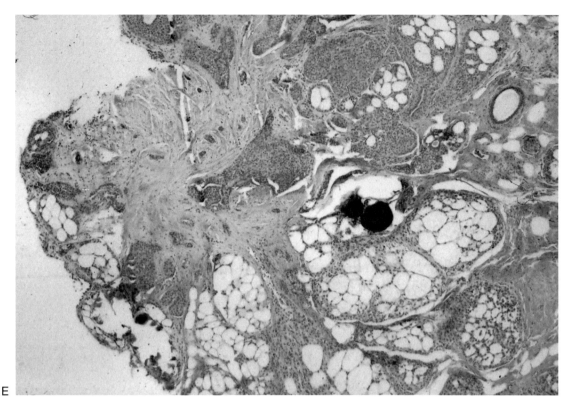

E

FIGURE 10.4. (E) Sclerosing papilloma with collagenous spherulosis. Degenerative change in the basement membrane material that accumulates in collagenous spherulosis predisposes to calcification that is detectable by mammography.

FALSE-POSITIVE DIAGNOSES

False-positive diagnoses are rarely documented in reported studies of needle core biopsy experience. They are probably less frequent than when surgical biopsies are examined by frozen section. Because the sample obtained by needle core biopsy is processed as paraffin embedded tissue, it is possible to prepare multiple sections and to perform special studies such as immunohistochemistry to assist in resolving diagnostic issues. A needle core biopsy of the breast should not be examined by frozen section unless there are exceptional clinical circumstances.

A false-positive diagnosis occurs when a needle core biopsy of a benign condition is misinterpreted as showing a malignant neoplasm. Since most malignant mammary tumors are carcinomas, this usually occurs when the sample in the needle core biopsy has been reported as in situ and/or invasive carcinoma but the excised lesion at the site of the core biopsy is benign, and on review both specimens are found to be histologically similar or there is no residual lesion at the biopsy site. A needle core biopsy that results in complete removal of carcinoma that is confirmed to be correct on review obviously does not constitute a false-positive diagnosis, although no carcinoma remains at the biopsy site. A nee-

dle core biopsy which reveals intraductal carcinoma when the excised tumor is invasive carcinoma is an instance of incomplete sampling but neither a false-positive nor a false-negative specimen.

The greatest risk for a false-positive diagnosis on a needle core biopsy lies in the interpretation of sclerosing proliferations such as sclerosing adenosis or radial sclerosing duct hyperplasia ("radial scar"). Mingling of proliferating epithelium and stroma in these tumors often simulates the appearance of invasive carcinoma. This process, sometimes described as "pseudoinvasion," can generally be appreciated in a tissue section of the entire lesion, but the small sample represented by a needle core biopsy could be misleading and interpreted as carcinoma. Examples of needle core biopsies of these lesions interpreted as tubular carcinoma or invasive lobular carcinoma have been encountered by the author (Figure 10.5). It is essential that the mammographic appearance and the radiologist's diagnostic impression be provided to the pathologist when such a lesion is the target of a needle core biopsy. In many instances, it is prudent practice to excise lesions with a spiculated mammographic configuration, even if the needle core biopsy is interpreted as benign; carcinoma may be focally present in these tumors.

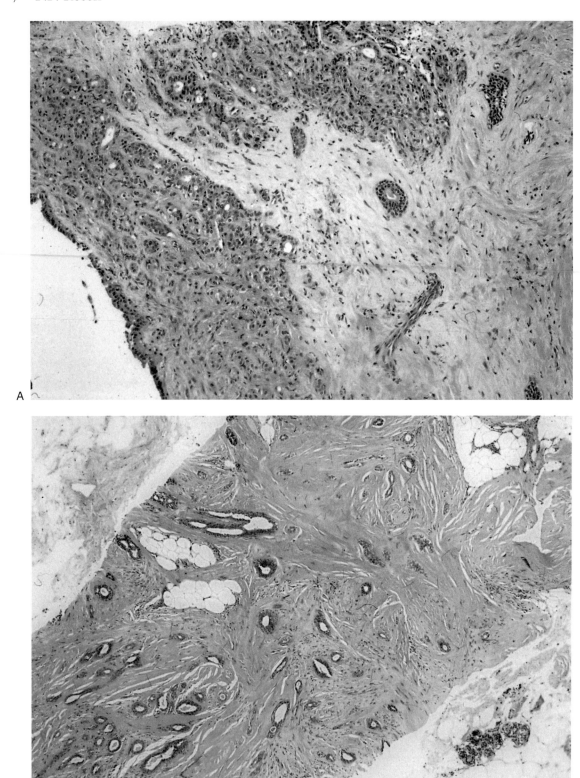

FIGURE 10.5. False-positive diagnoses. (**A**) Sclerosing adenosis mistaken for invasive carcinoma. The unusual location of sclerosing adenosis around a dilated duct (bottom left) contributed to misinterpretation of this needle core biopsy. (**B**) Radial sclerosing lesion mistaken for invasive carcinoma. Seen as an isolated fragment, this needle core biopsy sample was mistaken for tubular carcinoma.

ATYPICAL DUCT HYPERPLASIA

When ADH is reported in a specimen obtained by core biopsy, there is a substantial possibility that the lesion will ultimately prove to be carcinoma. In one series of 263 needle core biopsies, 26 lesions (10%) were reported to show atypical hyperplasia.[17] Twenty-two of the 26 patients had a surgical biopsy that revealed carcinoma in 12 (55%): 8 with intraductal and 4 with invasive carcinoma. Liberman et al. reported that the prior 14-gauge automated needle core biopsy diagnosis was ADH in 21 of 144 (15%) surgically diagnosed breast carcinomas.[18] Other studies have reported that 44%,[19] 48%,[20] 56%,[21] and 66%[22] of lesions with a 14-gauge automated needle core biopsy diagnosis of ADH proved to be carcinoma when excised surgically. These findings reflect the difficulty of distinguishing ADH from intraductal carcinoma in small biopsy samples. Improved sampling obtained with 14-gauge and 11-gauge vacuum-assisted biopsy devices results in carcinoma being diagnosed surgically after atypical 14-gauge and 11-gauge needle core biopsy samples in 18%[20] and 10–13%[20,23] of cases, respectively. The lower frequencies of carcinoma probably reflect more abundant sampling with the vacuum-assisted device.[24]

INTRADUCTAL CARCINOMA

When intraductal carcinoma was diagnosed with the 14-gauge automated needle biopsy device, 16% to 20% of patients proved to have invasive carcinoma at a subsequent surgical excision.[19,21,25] Vacuum-assisted core biopsy with 14-gauge or 11-gauge probes yielded a more specific diagnosis of intraductal carcinoma with invasion being found in 5% or fewer of subsequent surgical excisions.[19,23]

HANDLING OF THE SPECIMEN
BEFORE PATHOLOGY EXAMINATION

Paperwork submitted with the specimen container should specify the following: patient identification data; laterality; clinical indication(s) for the procedure, including relevant history; prior biopsies; clinical diagnosis; sites in the breast sampled; and specifics of the samples, such as the presence or absence of calcification. The needle biopsy cores should be placed in fixative promptly after the tissue has been obtained to preserve cytologic detail and minimize degradation of biologic markers, such as hormone receptors. For routine processing in a 24-hour period, 10% neutral buffered formaldehyde can be used.

Needle biopsy cores from a lesion with calcifications demonstrated by mammography should be assessed with a specimen radiograph. This procedure makes it possible to identify and segregate the core biopsy samples containing calcifications from those without demonstrable

calcifications. The cores with and without calcifications from each biopsy site can be placed in separate, properly labeled containers and immersed in fixative. Alternatively, the two sets of cores can be placed into separate tissue cassettes differentiated by color or labeling and submitted in a single container. The method chosen to separate specimens should be standardized within a given institution.

PATHOLOGIC PROCESSING
OF THE SPECIMEN

Each set of cores should be embedded in one or more paraffin blocks labeled to correspond to a specific specimen identity as described in the accompanying pathology requisition. A gross description should be recorded for each specimen documenting the number of cores, the range of length, and any other notable features. The entire specimen, including blood clot, must be embedded for histologic study. If the material corresponding to a specific sample is too abundant to examine in a single paraffin block, the cores should be separated into groups of approximately equal number and size.

Serial histologic sections are cut at 5- or 6-μm thickness from two or more levels in each tissue block, depending on the size of the sample. The sections are stained with hematoxylin and eosin for routine diagnostic purposes. It is preferable not to exhaust the tissue specimen in preparing initial histologic sections and to reserve material for additional studies, such as immunohistochemistry for hormone receptors or oncogene expression and other procedures that may assist in reaching a diagnosis.

PATHOLOGY REPORT

If calcifications were described in the needle core radiograph but none is initially evident histologically, the slides should be examined under polarized light for birefringent calcium oxalate crystals.[26] Radiographic study of the paraffin blocks may also be helpful to determine the location of calcifications.[27] Calcifications remain radiographically detectable in paraffin blocks for an indefinite period of time.

A detailed comparison of histological sections of needle core biopsy specimens and corresponding specimen radiographic studies revealed that calcifications smaller than 100 μm detected microscopically were not readily visible radiographically.[28] Consequently, histologically detected calcifications of this small dimension cannot be assumed to constitute the calcifications seen in a clinical mammogram. In the same study, calcifications described as linear and interpreted radiographically as having a "ductal" distribution had a ductal position histologically in 67% of the core biopsy specimens, whereas 24% were in the stroma and 9% were in other sites. Radiographically clustered calcifications also had a predominantly ductal location histologically.

The pathology report should describe the diagnostic features in a concise and clinically relevant form. It is not necessary to give a detailed microscopic description of the histological findings as long as the specific components are clearly identified. For example, it is sufficient to report a diagnosis of "fibroadenoma" without offering a microscopic description of the individual microscopic characteristics that define the lesion. Microscopic details may be added to the diagnosis to convey additional information, as, for example, in the diagnosis "fibroadenoma with cellular stroma: recommend excision to rule out phyllodes tumor."

Standardized forms listing the majority of potential diagnoses are a useful method for reporting breast pathology findings in many routine cases. Having such a checklist is an efficient method for recording the diagnosis in a comprehensive manner. A major drawback to the use of formatted diagnoses is the rigidity of the report, which usually gives equal weight to all components by presenting the findings in a predetermined sequence. In a particular case, certain diagnoses may require emphasis and should be given priority in the report. If the preformatted report does not have sufficient flexibility to permit rearranging the diagnostic components when necessary, the pathologist may choose to issue a nonstructured diagnosis. This is especially important if critical information cannot be conveyed by amplifying the formatted text with comments.

When carcinoma is diagnosed, the presence or absence of invasion must be noted. For in situ carcinoma, the diagnosis should state the type (ductal or lobular), nuclear grade, architecture if the carcinoma is ductal (e.g., cribriform, solid), and presence or absence of calcification. A high degree of concordance in the classification of intraductal carcinoma has been found between needle core and excisional biopsy specimens in the same patient. Major benign findings should also be cited.

If invasive carcinoma is diagnosed, the subtype of tumor (ductal, lobular, or special type, such as tubular or mucinous), associated in situ carcinoma, nuclear and histologic grade, and vascular invasion should be described, in addition to any significant benign proliferative lesions and the distribution of calcifications. Comparison of the grading of invasive ductal carcinomas in needle core and excisional biopsy specimens of the same tumor reveals a tendency to assign a lower grade on the basis of the needle core biopsy. Difficulty in distinguishing invasive ductal and lobular carcinomas may be encountered when tubule formation is not apparent in the core biopsy specimen.

If calcifications are the reason for biopsy, the etiology of the calcifications should be noted. If calcifications were biopsied and carcinoma is present, whether or not calcium is associated with the carcinoma should be noted in the report.

Needle core biopsy is highly accurate for the diagnosis of most breast lesions. However, it cannot be relied on to provide comprehensive data equal to what can be obtained from a surgically excision specimen. The pathology report for a breast needle core biopsy specimen must be integrated with other patient data including the clinical history, laboratory results, and physical and mammographic findings, to develop a treatment plan for the individual patient.[29]

PATHOLOGIC EFFECTS OF NEEDLING PROCEDURES SEEN IN SUBSEQUENT SURGICAL EXCISIONS

Virtually all excisional biopsy specimens obtained after needle core biopsy or needle localization contain foci of hemorrhage in the breast stroma. There is usually blood within the lumens of ducts and lobules not involved by the pathologic process as well as in epithelial structures in the lesional area.[30] Disruption of the epithelium in the lesion may result in displacement of epithelial cells into the needle track and into stroma of the surrounding tissue to produce a pattern that simulates invasive carcinoma (Figure 10.6).[30–32] This effect has been observed in benign as well as malignant lesions, and it can lead to the mistaken diagnosis of a benign lesion as invasive carcinoma (Figure 10.7). A granulation tissue reaction may be found around epithelium displaced from intraductal carcinoma if sufficient time elapses between the needling procedure and the excisional biopsy (Figures 10.7 and 10.8).[33] Displaced epithelium in vascular spaces is indistinguishable from intrinsic lymphatic or vascular invasion.[30,31]

Stromal epithelial displacement was found in three of five surgical biopsy specimens from patients with intraductal carcinoma and in three of seven papillary carcinomas studied by Boppana et al.[31] Tumor cell displacement has been observed after various needling procedures including wire/needle localization, FNA, core biopsy, suture placement, and local anesthetic injection and over a wide range of types and gauges of needles and wires. Seeding of carcinoma cells in the needle track has been described after needle core biopsy procedures with 14- and 19-gauge needles.[34,35]

Diaz et al. studied the frequency of epithelial displacement in needle core biopsy tracks after different types of procedures.[36] Epithelial displacement was detected more frequently at the site of image-guided 14-gauge automated gun biopsies (38%) than after 14-gauge vacuum-assisted biopsies (23%). Among cases of intraductal carcinoma where the biopsy site was available for examination, epithelial displacement was present in 6 of 18 (33%) after automated gun biopsy and 7 of 50 (14%) after vacuum-assisted biopsy. None of the post–vacuum-assisted specimens had "extensive" epithelial displace-

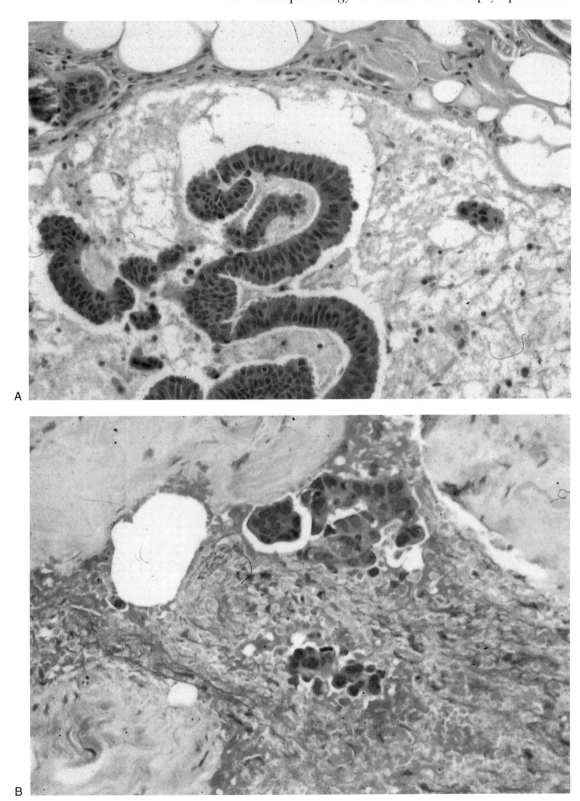

FIGURE 10.6. Displaced epithelium. **(A)** Displaced benign epithelium mistaken for mucinous carcinoma. These strips of epithelium dislodged from benign mucin-filled cysts were incorrectly interpreted as mucinous carcinoma in a lumpectomy obtained after a needle core biopsy. **(B)** Displaced intraductal carcinoma in a needle core biopsy track. This focus was interpreted as invasive carcinoma.

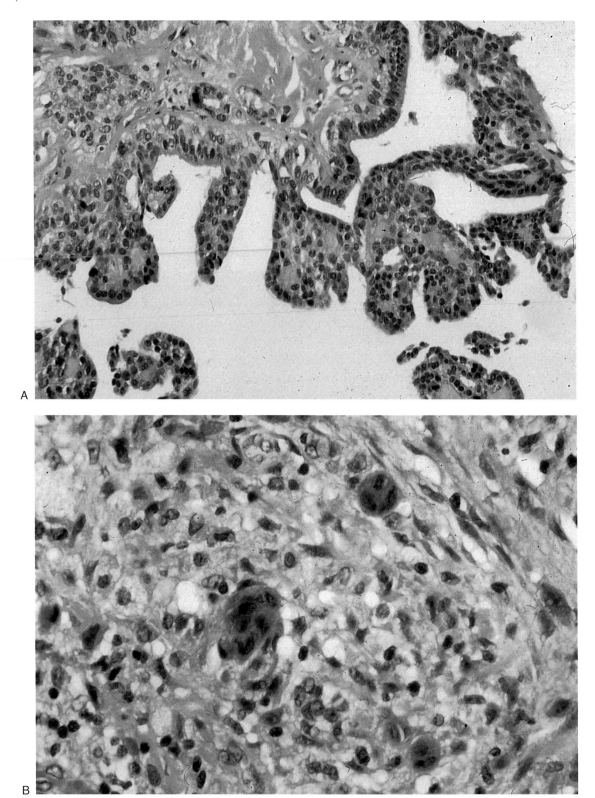

FIGURE 10.7. Displaced epithelium. **(A)** Papilloma. The needle core biopsy sample was a papilloma. **(B)** Displaced epithelium at the biopsy site. The excisional biopsy contained residual papilloma. This area of granulation tissue adjacent to the papilloma contains displaced clusters of papilloma epithelium that resemble invasive carcinoma.

ment whereas this description applied to 50% of cases with displacement after automated gun biopsy. The discrepancy between automated and vacuum-assisted biopsies was also present for invasive carcinomas, although it was less striking. Epithelial displacement was present in 38% and 37% of needle tracks after palpation-guided and stereotactic automated gun biopsies and in 30% after vacuum-assisted biopsies. Extensive displacement was less frequent after vacuum-assisted (7%) than after palpation-guided (18%) or stereotactic (13%) automated gun biopsies. Tumor displacement occurred significantly more often in ductal than in lobular or mixed ductal-lobular infiltrating carcinomas. Histologically low grade carcinomas tended to have extensive epithelial displacement less often (5%) than intermediate-grade (15%) or high grade (14%) lesions but the differences were not statistically significant.

Diaz et al. also assessed epithelial displacement in relation to the pathologic features of intraductal carcinomas.[36] When infiltrating carcinoma was present, the extent of intraductal carcinoma was not significantly related to the presence or absence of epithelial displacement. A trend to more extensive and more frequent epithelial displacement was noted for low grade forms than for intermediate- or high-grade forms of intraductal carcinoma, but the differences were not statistically significant.

Data collected by Liberman et al. also demonstrated a lower frequency of epithelial displacement associated with vacuum-assisted needle core biopsy.[37] The authors reviewed 28 consecutive patients diagnosed as having intraductal carcinoma in a vacuum-assisted image-guided needle core biopsy followed by surgical excision. The needle biopsy procedure employed a larger needle (11 gauge) than was used by Diaz et al. The median interval from needle biopsy to surgical excision was 27 days (range, 10–59 days) and the median number of core biopsy samples per case was 14 (range, 7–45). A needle track was present in each of the surgical excisions. The final diagnosis was intraductal carcinoma in 68%, intraductal and infiltrating carcinoma in 14%, and no residual carcinoma was present in 18%. No displaced carcinoma was detected, and two (7%) surgical excisions had displaced benign epithelium in granulation tissue.

The foregoing studies of Diaz et al. and Liberman et al. indicate that the frequency with which evidence of epithelial displacement can be detected in subsequent surgical excision specimens is related to the type of biopsy instrumentation used and possibly also to the gauge of the biopsy needle. The operational characteristics of vacuum-assisted stereotactic biopsy instruments concentrate sample acquisition in a localized region, employing negative (vacuum) pressure to draw tissue from around the probe into the biopsy chamber. It is likely that the majority of displaced epithelial fragments that occur in the biopsy site are drawn into the needle and removed with the core biopsy sample rather than remaining in the needle track. This effect is enhanced by the larger sample size acquired with an 11-gauge needle, as demonstrated by Liberman et al.[37]

The clinical significance of displaced epithelial cells in a FNA or core needle biopsy track remains to be determined. Since surgical excision is performed in most patients diagnosed by these procedures as having atypical lesions or carcinoma, displaced atypical or carcinomatous cells are removed in almost all cases. Thus far, no data have been presented suggesting that displaced benign epithelial cells constitute a precancerous hazard.

Cells cytologically compatible with coexisting in situ invasive carcinoma in lymphatic or vascular channels are indistinguishable from intrinsic lymphatic invasion associated with infiltrating carcinomas that have not been subjected to a needling procedure. Presently, no method exists for distinguishing cells that might have been displaced into vascular spaces by a needling procedure from cells in lymphatic spaces attributable to "intrinsic" invasion. The presence of carcinoma cells in lymphatic or vascular channels should be described in the pathology report.

Lack of information about the fate of displaced epithelial cells in the stroma or in vascular spaces, particularly carcinomatous cells, has contributed to uncertainty about the clinical significance of this finding. Diaz et al. reported a detailed analysis of the relationship of postneedle biopsy interval to the frequency of detectable epithelial displacement in a subsequent excisional biopsy.[36] As the interval between the procedures increased, the number of detectable needle tracks decreased, as did the amount of tumor displacement. The median interval in cases where no track was detectable (26 days, range 2–117) was larger than the intervals for specimens in which the tracks had, respectively, no displacement (17 days, range 0–128), minimal displacement (14 days, range 0–125) or extensive displacement (10 days, range 0–76). Extensive carcinomatous displacement was found in 17% of cases with an interval of 0–14 days, 8% when the interval was 15–28 days, and 1% of cases with an interval of more than 28 days. These data suggested that the majority of carcinoma cells displaced into the stroma did not survive and that the disappearance of the cells increased with increasing passage of time after the core biopsy procedure. Nonetheless these observations do not exclude the possibility that displaced epithelial cells could survive in a dormant state for a considerable period of time in some circumstances before becoming clinically active. Delayed clinical activity of intrinsic metastases is not unusual, and it is not beyond consideration that the same phenomenon could occur with cells displaced by a procedure such as needle core biopsy.

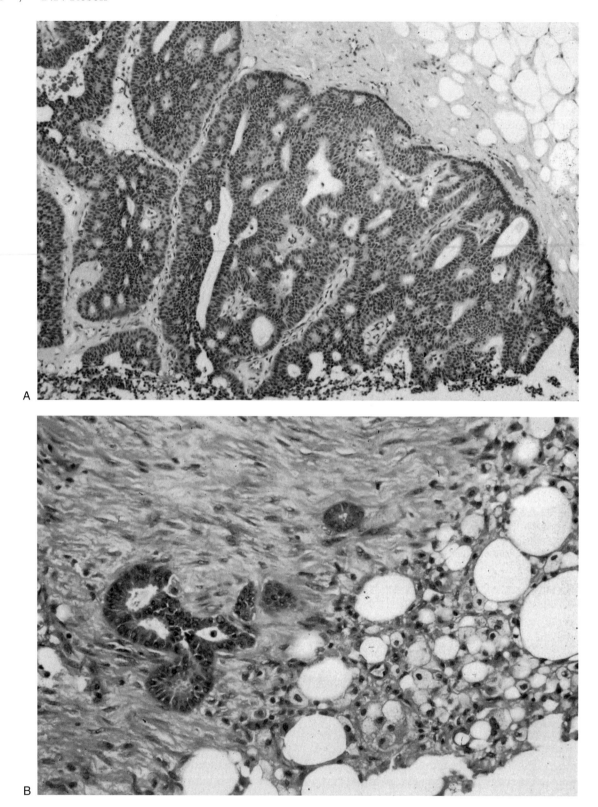

FIGURE 10.8. Displaced epithelium or microinvasion. (**A**) Solid papillary carcinoma. This is the excised solid papillary carcinoma from which a needle core biopsy sample was obtained (Figure 10.3B). (**B**) Possible microinvasion. Carcinomatous glands in an area of fibrosis and fat necrosis that could be microinvasion or displaced epithelium.

REFERENCES

1. Smeets HJ, Saltzstein SL, Meurer WT, Pilch YH. Needle biopsies in breast cancer diagnosis: techniques in search of an audience. J Surg Oncol 1986;32:11–15.

2. McMahon AJ, Lutfy AM, Matthew A, et al. Needle core biopsy of the breast with spring-loaded device. Br J Surg 1992;79:1042–1045.

3. Dowlatshahi K, Yaremko ML, Kluskens LF, Jokich PM. Nonpalpable breast lesions: findings of stereotaxic needle-core biopsy and fine-needle aspiration cytology. Radiology 1991;181:745–750.

4. Jackson VP, Reynolds HE. Stereotaxic needle-core biopsy and fine-needle aspiration cytologic evaluation of nonpalpable breast lesions. Radiology 1991;181:633–634.

5. Parker SH, Lovin JD, Jobe WE, et al. Nonpalpable breast lesions—stereotactic automated large core biopsies. Radiology 1991;180:403–407.

6. Janes RH, Bouton MS. Initial 300 consecutive stereotactic core-needle breast biopsies by a surgical group. Am J Surg 1994;168:533–537.

7. Liberman L, Dershaw DD, Rosen PP, et al. Stereotaxic core biopsy of breast carcinoma: accuracy at predicting invasion. Radiology 1995;194:379–381.

8. Sharifi S, Peterson MK, Baum JK, et al. Assessment of pathologic prognostic factors in breast core needle biopsies. Mod Pathol 1999;12:941–945.

9. Dahlstrom JE, Sutton S, Jain S. Histological precision of stereotactic core biopsy in diagnosis of malignant and premalignant breast lesions. Histopathology 1996;28:537–541.

10. Azam M, Raju U. Correlation of histologic grading of invasive ductal carcinoma in needle core biopsies and follow-up surgical excisions. Am J Clin Pathol 1998;110:517–518.

11. Di Loreto C, Puglisi F, Rimondi G, et al. Large core biopsy for diagnostic and prognostic evaluation of invasive breast carcinomas. Eur J Cancer 1996;32A:1693–1700.

12. Liberman L, Sama M, Susnik B, et al. Lobular carcinoma in situ at percutaneous breast biopsy: surgical biopsy findings. AJR 1999;173:291–299.

13. Shin, SJ, Rosen PP. Excisional biopsy should be performed if lobular carcinoma in situ is seen on needle core biopsy. Arch Path 2002;126:697–701.

14. Lechner MD, Park SL, Jackman RJ, et al. Lobular carcinoma in situ and atypical lobular hyperplasia at percutaneous biopsy with surgical correlation: a multi-institutional study. Radiology 1999;213:106.

15. Liberman L, Bracero N, Vuolo MA, et al. Percutaneous large-core biopsy of papillary breast lesions. AJR 1999;172:331–337.

16. Jacobs TW, Siziopikou KP, Prioleau JE, et al. Do prognostic marker studies on core needle biopsy specimens of breast carcinoma accurately reflect the marker status of the tumor? Mod Pathol 1998;11:259.

17. Liberman L, Cohen MA, Abramson AF, et al. Atypical ductal hyperplasia diagnosed at stereotaxic core biopsy of breast lesions: an indication for surgical biopsy. AJR 1995;164:1111–1113.

18. Liberman L, Dershaw DD, Glassman JR, et al. Analysis of cancers not diagnosed at stereotactic core breast biopsy. Radiology 1997;203:151–157.

19. Burbank F. Stereotactic breast biopsy of atypical ductal hyperplasia and ductal carcinoma in situ lesions: improved accuracy with directional, vacuum-assisted biopsy. Radiology 1997;202:843–847.

20. Jackman RJ, Burbank FH, Parker SH, et al. Atypical ductal hyperplasia diagnosed by 11-gauge, directional, vacuum-assisted breast biopsy: how often is carcinoma found at surgery? Radiology 1997;205:325.

21. Jackman RJ, Nowels KW, Shepard MJ, et al. Stereotaxic large-core needle biopsy of 450 nonpalpable breast lesions with surgical correlation in lesions with cancer or atypical hyperplasia. Radiology 1994;193:91–95.

22. Acheson MB, Patton RG, Howisey RL, et al. Histologic correlation of image-guided core biopsy with excisional biopsy of nonpalpable breast lesions. Arch Surg 1997;132:815–818.

23. Liberman L, Smolkin JH, Dershaw DD, et al. Calcification retrieval at stereotactic, 11-gauge, directional, vacuum-assisted breast biopsy. Radiology 1998;208:251–260.

24. Jackman RJ, Burbank F, Parker SH, et al. Atypical ductal hyperplasia diagnosed at stereotactic breast biopsy: improved reliability with 14-gauge, directional, vacuum-assisted biopsy. Radiology 1997;204:485–488.

25. Liberman L, Dershaw DD, Rosen PP, et al. Stereotaxic core biopsy of breast carcinoma: accuracy at predicting invasion. Radiology 1995;194:379–381.

26. Stein MA, Karlan MS. Calcifications in breast biopsy specimens: discrepancies in radiologic-pathologic identification. Radiology 1991;179:111–114.

27. Rebner M, Helvie MA, Pennes DR, et al. Paraffin tissue block radiography: adjunct to breast specimen radiography. Radiology 1989;173:695–696.

28. Dahlstrom JE, Sutton S, Jain S. Histologic-radiologic correlation of mammographically detected microcalcification in stereotactic core biopsies. Am J Surg Pathol 1998;22:256–259.

29. Morrow M. When can stereotactic core biopsy replace excisional biopsy? A clinical perspective. Breast Cancer Res Treat 1995;36:1–9.

30. Youngson BJ, Liberman L, Rosen PP. Displacement of carcinomatous epithelium in surgical breast specimens following stereotaxic core biopsy. Am J Clin Pathol 1995;103:598–602.

31. Boppana S, May M, Hoda S. Does prior fine-needle aspiration cause diagnostic difficulties in histologic evaluation of breast carcinomas? Lab Invest 1994;70:13A.

32. Lee KC, Chan JKC, Ho LC. Histologic changes in the breast after fine-needle aspiration. Am J Surg Pathol 1994;18:1039–1047.

33. Gobbi H, Tse G, Page DL, et al. Reactive spindle cell nodules of the breast after core biopsy or fine-needle aspiration. Am J Clin Pathol 2000;113:288–294.

34. Harter LP, Curtis JS, Ponto G, Craig PH. Malignant seeding of the needle track during stereotaxic core needle breast biopsy. Radiology 1992;185:713–714.

35. Grabau DA, Andersen JA, Graversen HP, Dyreborg U. Needle biopsy of breast cancer: appearance of tumour cells along the needle track. Eur J Surg Oncol 1993;19:192–194.

36. Diaz LK, Wiley EL, Venta LA. Are malignant cells displaced by large-gauge needle core biopsy of the breast? AJR 1999;173:1303–1313.

37. Liberman L, Vuolo M, Dershaw DD, et al. Epithelial displacement after stereotactic 11-gauge directional vacuum-assisted breast biopsy. AJR 1999;172:677–681.

CHAPTER 11

Medical Legal Aspects of Interventional Procedures of the Breast

R. James Brenner

With a developing consensus predicated on evidence-based clinical trials that mammographic screening for breast cancer favorably impacts mortality rates in a statistically significant manner, it is not surprising that compliance with this procedure continues to grow in countries offering either service-based or population-based screening mammography programs. Most states and the federal government in the United States mandate reimbursement for the procedure, and countries around the world are seeking to duplicate the success realized in many European trials conducting screening programs.

The multitude of lesions encountered in a screening mammography program require a deliberate approach toward analysis with regard to the likelihood of malignancy, so that downstream costs regarding management of screening-detected lesions will be sufficient to sustain appropriate action. For example, while stereotactic core breast biopsy procedures have been shown to be cost-effective when compared to surgery, the cost differential has been lessened by employment of newer technology in the marketplace.[1,2] Moreover, cost-effective analyses also show a negative impact when the same interventional procedures are used indiscriminantly as an alternative to imaging surveillance.[3] However, when intervention is indicated, the breast imager becomes an invaluable health care provider.

Interventional procedures of the breast for nonpalpable lesions necessarily require image guidance, usually provided by trained radiologists. Other medical specialists also perform such procedures. Under most circumstances, the level of care required for interventional breast

procedures is independent of the operator, and performance is evaluated, in a legal context, without regard to specialty.[4]

The field of breast imaging and intervention has attracted interested physicians from different backgrounds. Workshops at national meetings for both surgical and radiology specialties, for example, offer educational instruction regarding breast ultrasound and interventional procedures. Physician assistants and nurse practitioners play an increasing role in the clinical evaluation of women with breast problems. Consumer coalitions and manufacturers of medical equipment are involved with both the legislative and regulatory process regarding breast disease evaluation. Congressional and executive support for increased reimbursement for breast imaging is fundamental to implementation of new technologies and procedures. The U.S. Food and Drug Administration (FDA), pursuant to the enabling legislation of the Mammography Quality Standards Act, is carefully considering the overseeing of accreditation programs for stereotactic biopsy, having held hearings regarding current circumstances of practice.[5]

The optimism created by improved clinical outcomes for early detection and treatment of breast cancer combined with the large number of procedures that are generated consequent to demand for such services has created an environment where accountability for success is translated not only into medical environments, but also the legal environment. Delay in diagnosis of breast cancer, according to the Physician Insurance Association of America (PIAA), a consortium of physician-owned liability carriers, is the leading reason that physicians are sued for so called "medical malpractice."[6] Together with the overall increased legal exposure of those performing interventional procedures,[7,8] interventional breast procedures are likely to be subject to frequent legal scrutiny. Given the increasing employment and range of such procedures, as well as the various backgrounds of those engaged in their performance, it is worth reviewing basic legal concepts germane to this field. By understanding the legal context in which mishappenstances arise, it should be possible to plan accordingly to prevent many of the untoward legal consequences which apply to clinical practice. This is the essence of risk management, the most important facet of which emphasizes proper medical care.

BASIC LEGAL PRINCIPLES

American law represents a combination of different legal fields or specialties, each with different rules of evidence and procedure. Criminal law, for example, represents the interest of society, so that such cases are often denoted as "State v . . . " or "People v . . . " Because criminal conviction may mean loss of civil liberties, the highest standards of proof are required. Physicians are rarely subject to such charges in standard medical malpractice cases, except in two circumstances. The first involves such heinous behavior that criminal sanctions may be sought. A number of states have employed criminal procedures, for example, in dubious cases of life support withdrawal.[9] The second is more relevant to this discussion and involves issues of criminal fraud and abuse. An increasing number of actions have been sought by the federal Inspector General's office or similar state agencies for the filing of false claims or improper business relationships. For example, referral practices which violate "anti-kickback" statutes and do not fall under a "safe harbor" exception may be guilty of criminal conduct.[10] While this form of prosecution is beyond the primary scope of the current discussion, the overuse of interventional procedures such as stereotactic biopsy may invite future scrutiny regarding the relationships among providers.

Most medical malpractice cases come under the category of civil law and, more specifically, tort law. Tort law defines the relationships between or among individuals (or parties) where restitution is the primary compensatory remedy, assessed as payment of money.

Civil law is derived from two sources: statutory law and common law. Statutory law is that body of law passed by lawmakers at the local, state, and national level, presumably representing a consensus of opinion by society of approved methods of conduct. Radiation safety provisions may be prescribed by local ordinances. Licensure laws and laws regarding different kinds of informed consent are usually governed by state law or jurisdiction. The Mammography Quality Standards Act (MQSA) was passed by Congress in 1992,[5] and implemented in October 1994 as a national statutory law; with its reauthorization in 1998, new rules propagated by the FDA prescribed new forms of conduct that are expressly stated standards of care. Statutory law is interpreted and implemented by regulatory agencies. As mentioned, the FDA regulates the practice of mammography and may extend regulatory standards to the performance of stereotactic biopsies. The effect, for example, might be to establish an obligate number of cases which must be performed each year—similar to accrediting procedures such as the one for mammography administered by the American College of Radiology.

Most law regarding medical malpractice is not covered by statutes and is referred to as common law. Derived during the eighteenth century from English common law, American common law embodies a series of decisions by judges and juries that are meant to establish parameters for conduct by individuals. Common law is based on a legal principle of *stare decisis* whereby decisions rendered by appellate courts establish legal precedent to be followed in that jurisdiction or locale when similar facts or situations arise. Appellate decisions and statutes are published for purposes of reference and, although binding only in the specific jurisdiction, may be relevant to other locales. By contrast, decisions made by trial courts in a particular case are predicated upon specific fact situations, and, as such, do not serve as precedents.

The torts which are of importance to the breast interventional radiologist include battery and negligence, the latter associated with sometimes subtle implications. These legal aspects of practice will be considered from both an educational as well as a risk-management perspective.

INTENTIONAL TORTS: BATTERY

An intentional tort is a prohibited act that one party intends to commit on another party and that in fact occurs. Neither motive nor actual harm need be shown to prevail in this kind of legal action.

Battery is the unlawful, nonconsensual, and deliberate touching of another person and thus is an intentional tort. Incidental or normal touchings, such as in a crowded room, lack sufficient intent to provide legal remedies. In fact, battery may be subject to both civil and criminal remedies, as in the case of a shooting. Thus, when certain medical cases are subject to legal action, the issue of criminal battery may arise, though such cases are rare.

Unpermitted touchings do not necessarily require expert opinion to establish their legal sufficiency, so that lay judges or juries may make such determinations. Moreover, intentional torts such as battery are often awarded punitive damages—a multiple of the damages shown to result from the legal harm—to serve as a deterrent to such behavior.

Most medical liability insurance policies do not cover either the defense expenses or indemnification of actions brought against physicians for battery. Under most circumstances, however, battery is part of a number of "causes of action" sought by a plaintiff, which generally include negligence. The latter tort is the basis for primary coverage provided by liability carriers.

INTENTIONAL TORTS: CONSENT

A published survey of interventional breast procedures performed by radiologists—largely consisting of preoperative needle localizations, cysts aspirations, and ductography—found that majority of radiologists did not obtain consent before performing these procedures.[11] While such procedures may be considered minimally invasive, they constitute, as defined above, battery. The consent obtained for a surgical procedure, even if needle localization is included in that consent, is unlikely to be legally sufficient in defense of an untoward event when the radiologist performing the procedure is not involved in the process of obtaining the consent. That radiologists are rarely sued for battery under these circumstances probably reflects the favorable outcome and relatively small potential damage award which would result from such a legal action. Plaintiff attorneys, whose remuneration is usually derived as a percentage of the compensated monetary award, have little incentive to appropriate their own resources for such cases. Nonetheless, legal exposure remains and may come into play in a derivative manner.

Suppose, for example, that a preoperative needle localization is performed without consent. Predictably, a finite percentage of cases—often averaging 2% to 3%—will result in failed surgical recovery of the lesion.[12] In pursuing an action for negligence—bona fide or not—against the surgeon and radiologist, the plaintiff attorney may discover an additional legal "cause of action" for battery if no consent was obtained.

Liability in this context is eliminated by the obtaining of consent to perform the procedure. This is based on the legal doctrine of *volenti non fit injuria* or "to he/she who consents there is no injury." This doctrine remains the fundamental defense to a charge of battery. Any invasive procedure may be considered legal battery and, as mentioned, does not require a poor outcome for legal redress. Obtaining consent defeats such a charge.

Sometimes it is difficult to identify where "lawful touchings" in medicine end and battery begins. No matter how trivial the procedure, intervention is not generally covered under "implied consent" doctrines, which apply only to the obtaining of X ray or other images.[13] Many procedures such as physical examination or simple phlebotomy may seem so inherent a part of clinical

practice that courts may recognized implied consent.[14] For example, an ultrasound examination where a transducer is placed on the patient is unlikely to be subject to battery, although exceptions may occur, especially during transvaginal ultrasound procedures. Consider the issue of contrast enhanced imaging, where the need for consent is unlikely to be sought for the venipuncture, but more likely to be sought for the injection of iodinated contrast. Some facilities seek consent for mammography, which is unlikely to be necessary. Those facilities may ask the patient to acknowledge the risk of bruising, implant rupture, or other untoward effects. The sufficiency of this request is dubious if the examination is not performed properly. If performed properly, the consent is not likely to be of value, even if an untoward consequence occurs.

A discussion of the law of consent and the various special types of consent applicable to a variety of situations (e.g., minors, emergency) is beyond the scope of this discussion and has been reviewed elsewhere.[13] Those performing interventional breast procedures should be familiar, however, with the ramifications of different forms of consent.

It is also necessary to recognize that exceeding the consent obtained—absent exigent circumstances—may also constitute battery. Thus, where a sonographically defined mass demonstrates internal echos, and the radiologist cannot determine if the appearance represents a complicated cyst or solid mass, the decision for intervention may arise. A consent for simple cyst aspiration may be inadequate if fluid is not obtained and the procedure is simply converted to a large-bore core needle biopsy. Anticipating such circumstances and obtaining alternative or contingency consent may obviate the need to reinstitute a process of obtaining another consent for the second procedure. Excessive contingencies, however, may not be valid, and will likely be subject to the test of reasonableness. In this context it should be noted that obtaining a second consent for the latter procedure while the patient is draped and residing on the interventional table may be subject to invalidation of the consent by the doctrine of duress.

In general, issues such as the above are subordinated to a more frequent issue, which requires the obtaining not only of consent but of informed consent. This issue falls under a different tort, that of negligence.

LAW OF NEGLIGENCE: GENERAL PRINCIPLES

The law of negligence governs most medical malpractice cases and is concerned with the conduct of physicians, rather than the outcome of their actions. Nonetheless, by deed and doctrine, it is the outcome—moreover an adverse outcome—which brings the issue of conduct to the attention of the court. Unlike battery, intent is not a component of analysis for a case of negligence. Although negligence has a pejorative connotation, it is a term of art in law, requiring definable elements to be shown in order to prevail.

Common law notions of negligence emerged historically from decisions of judges that were directed toward those professions deemed to be providing a public calling, decisions which were meant to provide for the safety and welfare of the citizens. Proof of medical negligence usually requires expert opinions to establish standards of care and the likelihood of a departure from such standards. The standard of care represents that conduct which a reasonable and prudent physician would have shown under similar circumstances.[14] It is independent of background, so that the care which should be rendered during interventional procedures is the same, whether performed by a specially trained breast imager, a general radiologist, or a physician of another specialty, such as surgery.

Experts testifying to standard of care issues are called upon to help the court (e.g., trial judge or jury) determine issues of fact, not law. In other words, the issue before the court relates to whether or not conduct was in conformance with an objective standard of care. Practice guidelines or published standards are not tantamount to standard of care for two reasons. First, such documents or treatises are frequently consensus statements, often without sufficient evidence-based data. As such, those involved in the development of such guidelines cannot be individually cross-examined or interviewed by attorneys in the case. Thus, these positions are not admitted per se into evidence. Nonetheless, experts may declare them as a basis—in part or in whole—for their position. Therefore, such guidelines will be judged in this light and may carry considerable influence. Second, most courts recognize the "alternative school of thought" doctrine. Where conduct departs from a given prescribed method (e.g., a guideline or standard) and has a rationale basis, then such conduct may be reasonable. Indeed, the test of negligent conduct focuses not on strict adherence to a given approach or successful outcome but, rather, on reasonableness. Recall, however, that statutory standards require no expert opinion and, as discussed before, represent an unequivocally prescribed manner of conduct.

The tort of negligence is defined by four elements: duty, breach of duty, causation, and damages. In other words, if the defendant breaches a recognized duty and if it bears a substantial relationship to injury, then negligence will be found. The court is not generally concerned with matters which require no compensation, so that actual damages usually need to be shown to proceed. The concept of negligence has been defined in the legal literature as follows: "One who undertakes gratuitously or for consideration to render services to another which he should recognize as necessary for the protection of the other person or things, is subject to liability to the other for physical harm resulting from his failure to exercise such care or perform an undertaking if such failure to exercise such care increased the risk of such harm."[15]

The first element of negligence is duty. One need not accept a referral for an interventional procedure, especially if clinical circumstances are sufficiently compelling that a greater likelihood of harm will occur. Declining to perform such a procedure needs to be deliberated, not only because of the possibility that an adverse outcome will occur without such a procedure, but also because of the potential adverse interaction between the referring physician and radiologist. As will be shown later, each case needs to be evaluated on its merits. However, once the referral is accepted, the interventionalist has engaged a duty which must be attended in a reasonable manner. If that duty is breached and if it is a "cause in fact" and "proximate cause" of injury, then negligence has occurred. Because there is often no manner by which to undo such harm (e.g., the delayed diagnosis of breast cancer), the law approaches compensation from a perspective of restitution. Money damages are awarded when the elements of negligence have been established as a "best" feasible attempt to "make the plaintiff whole" to the extent possible.

There are three primary areas of negligence that concern the breast interventional radiologist: the acceptance and performance of the procedure itself; the obtaining of consent for the procedure; and the responsibility for follow-up communication and recommendations for management that involve the patient, the radiologist, and the referring physician.

Accepting and Performing the Procedure

Accepting a referral would appear to be a natural extension of the role of a radiologist. Interventional procedures depart from this approach in that requests for intervention may be generated based on the performance of an image-detected abnormality by a different imaging center. The evaluation from another center (and even the same center) may be incomplete.

Two studies illustrate this issue. In a group of patients referred for preoperative needle localization, 8.8% (53/603) of cases were canceled based on either clearly benign findings on re-review or, more importantly in the context of this discussion, the absence of a true lesion.[16] A similar study identified 16% (89/572) of cases referred for stereotactic biopsy that were canceled for similar reasons.[17]

Consider the notion that stereotactic biopsies must be performed while imaging a given target in one view only. However, a lesion that has been identified in only one view during a diagnostic examination has a real possibility of representing a summation artifact and not a real lesion.[18] Accepting a case—absent extenuating circumstances—and performing a stereotactic biopsy with insufficient rationale raises two potential problems. First, there may be a concern for a fraud and abuse issue or false claim.[10] Second, if there is a complication from the procedure and if the case is reviewed such that it can be established that there was no bona fide indication for a biopsy, negligence may be found. Although uncommon, lawsuits have been instigated for unnecessary surgery or surgery not justified by the clinical circumstances.[19,20]

In like manner, sonographically guided biopsies accepted by the radiologist must usually be reconciled with either a definable mammographic abnormality or a palpable finding. On the other hand, ultrasound performed for one area may inescapably identify another noncystic area. Because feasibility studies are presently lacking in the published literature for sonographic surveillance of ultrasound-only-detected lesions, sonographic biopsy may be necessary under these conditions. This is one of the adverse consequences which may be realized with a large area or even whole breast ultrasound, a subject beyond the scope of this discussion.

It may initially appear unreasonable that the interventionalist is responsible for reevaluating an imaging study performed elsewhere and referred for image guided biopsy. However, when one undertakes an interventional procedure, the conduct is predicated upon targeting a real lesion, and the inability to substantiate the presence of a lesion may undermine the rationale of the intervention. Sometimes interventionalists will need to reevaluate the lesion in a diagnostic sense prior to intervention. At other times the procedure might need to be canceled until the case is properly evaluated at either the index institution or another. This invites patient dissatisfaction and may be avoided by requiring films be submitted prior to scheduling the procedure for full evaluation. On the other hand, such strict requirements often interfere with cordial clinical–radiology relationships. However, because the image-guided interventional procedure may only involves the radiologist in most circumstances, this requirement may be more easily implemented.

A more difficult set of circumstances arises for preoperative localizations. Often films are not previewed, and a number of other services are affected, such as surgery and anesthesiology, when cases are either delayed or canceled. In addition, patient preparation has occurred so that the radiologist is faced with more complicated circumstances. Nonetheless, adherence to basic radiology principles cannot be circumvented. When lesions have not been sufficiently identified on two orthogonal projections and both the existence and location of the presumed lesion are in question, then preoperative localization should not be performed, except under extraordinary circumstances which are governed by mutual understanding among the surgeon, radiologist, and patient, and included in informed consent. Figure 11.1 demonstrates a needle placed into a lesion and presumed to be in the upper outer quadrant without having been convincingly demonstrated; it resulted in failed surgery. Reevaluation of the lesion identified the exact location—at considerable distance from the presumed location—and reexcision was performed with recovery of a small cancer.

Competency in the performance of a procedure is difficult to measure. Clinical studies often attempt to help establish an anticipated time course for developing sufficient skill of a "reasonable interventionalist under similar circumstances." For example, only one published study has adduced the number of stereotactic biopsies that must be completed to demonstrate reasonable proficiency.[21] Consensus guidelines recommend a certain number of procedures to be performed on an annual basis to profile continued competence. Presumably skills obtained during supervised residency lend themselves to different circumstances, so that the acquisition of new skills or modification of old ones may be facilitated by additional tutorials, continuing education courses, and even short fellowships. Many approved continuing education courses offer "hands-on" workshops for developing or improving skills in interventional breast procedures.

Establishing competence in a new procedure to the satisfaction of anyone challenging such skill, as may occur after an adverse event, is an important component of risk management. When the conduct is suspect, documentation of prior experience, education, and familiarity with the parameters of widespread clinical trials form the basis of such a position. In addition, early experience may be accompanied by informed consent, which includes disclosure to the patient of the new incorporation of such procedures into regular clinical practice.

Success is not guaranteed in any procedure, nor does the law of negligence require a favorable outcome. Conduct, not outcome, is at issue in such cases, as discussed earlier. The occurrence of complications is a risk of any invasive procedure and is discussed when informed consent is obtained. As part of this process, a deliberate plan should be in place to resolve a complication, if it occurs. This planning needs to identify the person responsible for treating the complication and often the procedures to be followed if a complication occurs.

Many interventionalists are trained and suited to treat complications secondary to radiology procedures. When this is not the case, it is important to establish an approach regarding appropriate transfer of care to resolve complications. For example, the diagnosis and monitoring of a pneumothorax after a needle that has been inserted into the breast and violated the pleural space can be assessed and remedied if necessary in a straightforward manner but may result in unnecessary problems if left without monitoring. Protocols and informed consent form the basis for such approaches, and alerting the patient to the availability of urgent care centers or emergency departments may add an additional measure of safety if untoward consequences arise.

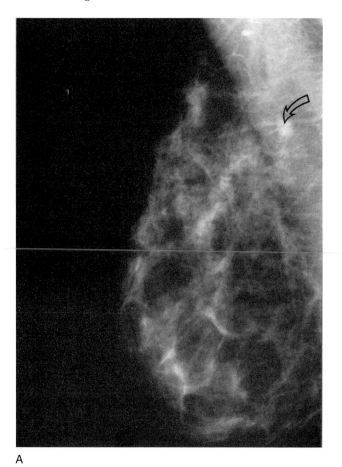

A

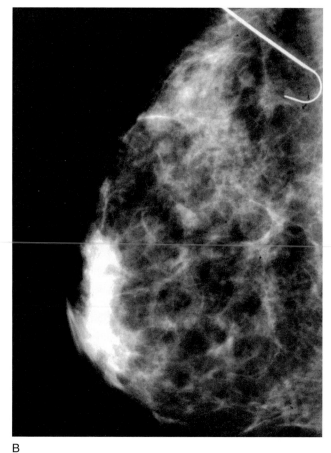

B

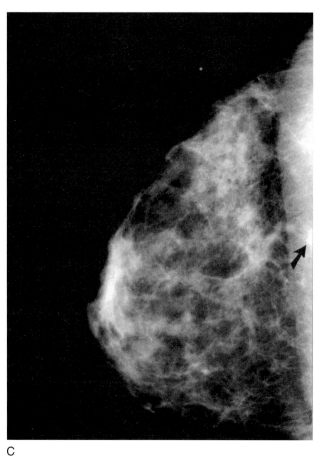

C

FIGURE 11.1. Preoperative needle localization of nonpalpable cancer. New spiculated 7 mm lesion is seen easily on the right mediolateral oblique view (curved arrow) (**A**) and is thought to be located among several nodular densities in the upper outer quadrant where the localization wire was placed (**B**). Failed surgery prompted reevaluation, which demonstrated that the lesion in fact is located at the 12 o'clock position of the breast, near the chest wall (arrow) (**C**). Localization of this focus was successful in recovering the lesion 4 months later. (*From* Frankel SD, Steven D, Brenner RJ. Interventional radiology and the law: breast procedures. Semin Intervent Radiol 2001;18:415–424, with permission).

Informed Consent

As discussed earlier, simple consent, appropriately obtained, is a complete defense to the charge of battery. Most lawsuits involving consent are instigated not under the theory of battery but, rather, of negligence. It is the duty of the radiologist to obtain reasonable consent from the patient. Because most interventional procedures are elective, this usually means informed consent.

Issues regarding informed consent, unlike simple consent, may require expert testimony and are more difficult concepts to understand. Informed consent has been defined classically by a federal appellate court as the disclosure of material risks and complications and the alternatives available.[22] This definition is a derivative of the formula expressed by a jurisprudential commentator, Judge Learned Hand, where the standard of care regarding disclosure may be seen as a determination of the product of the severity of the complications and their incidence. Thus, any serious complication or any mild complication with a high frequency must be disclosed.

Disclosure is assessed differently, depending on a given state jurisdiction. Several states maintain a "reasonable patient" standard such that compliance with proper consent is judged by what a reasonable patient would expect to know to make an informed decision. Other states use a "reasonable physician" standard, evaluating proper consent by measuring the parameters of what a reasonable physician in similar circumstances would disclose. These nuances may have a determining influence on the outcome of a case, and radiologists should familiarize themselves with their own state requirements.[13] Most medical malpractice cases are tried under state jurisdiction and laws which govern the practice of medicine in that locale. The patient standard emphasizes disclosure, an approach that may be preferred if, for any given set of circumstances, the physician is in doubt regarding the disclosure of a risk in that jurisdiction.

The manner of disclosure is important to avoid unnecessary anxiety and potentially adverse effects of a patient refusing an important procedure. The approach requires a Blanca, and sometimes finesse, in disclosing risks clearly, without undue fear. The difficulty of this approach is evidence by one published study indicating that 121 of 1513 (8%) of radiologists surveyed had been involved with informed consent litigation.[23]

Much attention has been paid to the production of proper informed consent form. Certainly, procedure-specific forms are preferred but are often not necessary and do not lend themselves easily to the multitude of types of procedures performed in an imaging department. Obtaining informed consent is a process, and emphasis needs to be placed on a meaningful discussion between the physician performing the procedure and the patient. The written consent form is important—but as evidence of the discussion between physician and patient, not as proof. The signed consent form is therefore not synonymous

with or tantamount to informed consent and is, in fact, subordinate to the discussion with the patient. A regular, repetitive recitation of known risks, best validated by a protocol and witnessed by other persons, is the essence of the process. Together with a signed form, a factual basis for reasonable conduct is established by this kind of approach. Informed consent often requires disclosure of alternatives and occasionally the consequences of not undergoing the procedure. Although exceptions occur to the obtaining of informed consent, they are generally not applicable to elective procedures performed in interventional breast work.

The person performing the procedure should obtain the consent. Residents, colleagues, or other persons may not substitute for the person performing the procedure. Often, details of the procedure may be related by other providers so that the discussion time is shortened between the interventionalist and the patient. This approach is permissible, so long as the essence of the consent is obtained by the physician involved. Tissue sampling and preoperative localizations by image guidance require additional consideration in this context. As has been documented in clinical studies and discussed in this text, tissue sampling procedures are associated with a finite percentage of nondiagnostic yields, and reasonable preoperative localizations are associated with a finite percentage of failed surgical recovery.[12,21] Disclosure of these possibilities is an important component of the consent process.

Reasonable Management

Radiologists have for some time been involved with image-guided biopsies. Fine-needle aspiration biopsy of pancreatic or hepatic lesions in hospitalized patients has become part of routine clinical practice. These situations lend themselves to a "closed loop" analysis because the patient is in the hospital and the order for such a biopsy has been placed. Thus, obtaining results is usually an inherent part of the hospital management plan. Accountability for proper quality assessment and communication is often part of a normal quality assurance program required by the Joint Commission on the Accreditation of Healthcare Organizations.

Tissue sampling biopsies and deliberate planning may require special attention for breast interventionalists because most procedures are performed on an outpatient basis and lack many of the internal controls mentioned for inpatient services that preempt untoward consequences. A reconsideration of fundamental aspects of such procedures is therefore useful.

Historically, the role of the radiologist has been seen as subordinate to that of the clinician. In California, for example, a radiologist's role is defined as a consultant, with the state's appellate court indicating that interference with the clinician–patient relationship may invite unnecessary problems.[24] Other courts have taken a different view. The evolving role of the interventionalist may redefine some aspects of these relationships, regardless of jurisdiction.

Unfortunately, some "experts" may contend that one approach is not only favorable, but required to meet a standard of care issue, a misleading position in this and other contexts. It has been criticized. Indeed, the general legal principle of "alternative schools of thought" support the reasonableness of more than one approach which can be sufficiently validated.

Usually a treating physician refers a patient to a radiologist for an interventional procedure. In these circumstances the report needs to be directed to the referring clinician. Although current regulations of the MQSA now require that reports of mammography results in lay terms also be sent to the patient, this requirement does not currently apply to the interventional procedure. Different circumstances dictate reasonable conduct.[25] When radiologists accept self-referred patients with no other treating physician, pathology results will be sent directly to the radiologist who is responsible for communicating the result to the patient and for future management referrals.[26] When the radiologist serves in a consultative role, he or she should also review results—in addition to the results being sent to the referring primary physician—for two reasons. First, the results need to be reconciled with the imaging findings in order to ensure the reasonable success of the procedure. Second, because the radiologist is the primary performer of the procedure and inherently involved with its outcome, positive results or results requiring further surgery should prompt a communication to the referring physician, who may not know when the procedure was done and thus be unaware of forwarded results.[27] When the results are benign, there is little significant downside if the response to results is delayed. However, if further surgery is required—as is the case with cancer or florid atypical ductal hyperplasia—then ensuring that results are communicated to the treating physician becomes a more important task. When results have not or cannot be communicated by the referring physician to the patient or by the radiologist to the referring physician—extraordinary circumstances which should be documented—then the interventionalist should communicate the results to the patient or to another physician who has agreed to care for the patient following appropriate transfer of care. This approach incorporates a major legal principle of foreseeability which will help govern the interventional radiologist's analysis of the situation; that is, if it is reasonably foreseeable that further treatment is necessary, the conduct of the radiologist as consultant should be modified accordingly.[25] Contingency planning, either by protocol or by individual case review, will prevent untoward consequences in this regard.

A physician who recognizes that a clinical circumstance is beyond his or her competence to provide adequate care has a duty to refer the patient for further care. The role of the radiologist, either in the subordinate role as a consultant or a primary role if accepting self-referred patients, follows from this legal duty.

There are several derivative torts or civil actions which follow from these circumstances, torts with which the interventional radiologist should be familiar.[28]

1. *Abandonment.* When the care of the patient either suffering a complication of a procedure or subject to results which require further care (e.g., surgery) is not attended to, the tort of abandonment arises. Patients are free to leave the care of a physician at any time, but when additional care is required—especially exigent care—the physician cannot simply delegate such duties. Depending on the severity of the situation, the radiologist must assist in providing a plan or direct referral for the patient's care. This is particularly important for self-referred patients. Under most circumstances, care for patients under the treatment of other physicians may and even should be coordinated through their offices.

2. *Negligent referral.* When a physician refers a patient to another treating physician or facility which the referring physician knows or has reason to know is not suitably competent to resolve a medical situation and an untoward event occurs, then the facility or physician may be liable for negligence, and the physician who referred the patient may be liable for "negligent referral." Again, this situation most commonly is applicable to treating clinicians or radiologists accepting self-referred patients. Patients, however, may seek the radiologist's opinion, and thus all referrals should be made with an awareness of the need for reasonableness, whether offered formally or informally, as even the latter may be subject to legal redress.

CONCLUSIONS

Data regarding the legal exposure of the radiologist performing interventional procedures is difficult to obtain as published studies usually reflect the exposure of interventionalists in general or the liability incurred by radiologists performing breast-imaging procedures. Given the high incidence of lawsuits involved in both of these endeavors, potentially high legal exposure exists in this field. As mentioned earlier, the two efforts of diagnostic evaluation and intervention are often inseparable for a given case. Recognition of the legal principles which govern the practice of both radiology and intervention should therefore both alert practitioners to potential hazards and should prompt approaches and systems that avoid untoward events. The evolutionary role of the radiologist involved in breast interventional procedures may serve as a paradigm for the developing profile of the entire professional specialty.

REEFERENCES

1. Liberman L, Fahs MC, Dershaw DD, et al. Impact of stereotaxic core breast biopsy on cost of diagnosis. Radiology 1995;195:633–637.
2. Liberman L, Sama MP. Cost-effectiveness of stereotactic 11-gauge directional vacuum-assisted breast biopsy. AJR 2000; 175:53–58.
3. Brenner RJ, Sickles EA. Surveillance mammography versus stereotaxic core biopsy for probably benign breast lesions: a cost comparison analysis. Acad Radiol 1997;4:419–425.
4. Skeffington v Bradley, 366 Mich 552, 115 N.W.2d 303 (Mich 1962).
5. Mammography Quality Standards Act of 1992, PL 102–539.
6. Physicians Insurers Association of America. Breast Cancer Study of 1995. Washington DC: Physicians Insurers Association of America, 1995.
7. Texas Medical Association. Medical professional liability: an examination of claims frequency and severity in Texas. Houston, TX: Texas MedicalAssocation, Tonn & Associates, 1994.
8. Bowyer EA. High radiology losses to invasive procedures. Risk Management Foundation Forum 1985;6:1–8.
9. McCormick B. Don't criminalize medical judgement. Am Med News 1993;36:6.
10. Morrison AW. An analysis of anti-kickback and self-referral law in modern health care. J Legal Med 2000;21:351–394.
11. Reynolds HE, Jackson VP, Musick MS. A survery of interventional mammography practices. Radiology 1993;187: 71–73.
12. Jackman RJ, Marzoni FA. Needle localized breast biopsy: why do we fail? Radiology 1997;204:667–684.
13. Reuter SR. An overview of informed consent for radiologists. AJR 1987;148:219–227.
14. Brenner RJ, Eth S, Trygstad CW. Defining the risks of venipuncture (letter). N Engl J Med 1976;295:53–54.
15. Restatement (second) of Torts, Section 323 (a).
16. Meyer JE, Sonnenfeld MR, Greenes RA, et al. Cancellation of preoperative breast localization procedures: analysis of 53 cases. Radiology 1988;169:629–630.
17. Philpotts LE, Lee CH, Horvath LJ, et al. Canceled stereotactic core-needle biopsy of the breast: analysis of 89 cases. Radiology 1997;205:423–428.
18. Brenner RJ. Asymmetries of the breast: strategies in evaluation. Semin Roentgenol 2001;33:201.
19. Kinikin v Heupel, 305 NW2d 589 (1981).
20. Hume v Bayer, 178 NJ Super 370, 428 A2d 961 (NJ, 1981).
21. Brenner RJ, Fajardo L, Fisher PR, et al. Percutaneous core biopsy of the breast: effect of operator experience and number of samples on diagnostic accuracy. AJR 1996;166:341–346.
22. Cantebury v Spence, 464 F2d 772 (DC Cir, 1972).
23. Hamer MM, Morlock F, Foley HT, et al. Medical malpractice in diagnostic radiology: claims, compensation, and patient injury. Radiology 1987;164:262–266.
24. Townsend v Turk, 266 Cal App 3d 278, 1266 Cal Rptr 821 (1990).
25. Brenner RJ. Medicolegal aspects of breast imaging: variable standards of care relating to different types of practice. AJR 1991;156:719–723.
26. Monsees B, Destouet JM, Evens RG. The self-referred mammography patient: a new responsibility for radiologists. Radiology 1988;166:69–71.
27. Brenner RJ. Interventional procedures of the breast: medicolegal considerations. Radiology 1995;195:611–615.
28. Brenner RJ. Breast cancer evaluation: medical-legal and risk management considerations for the clinician. Cancer 1994; 74(suppl):486–491.

CHAPTER 12

Quality Control, Quality Assurance, and Accreditation

D. David Dershaw

The use of objective criteria to assess the level of quality in a practice is valuable in establishing and maintaining a high level of patient care. The utilization of a quality control program designed by an accrediting organization and the documentation that such a program is being followed makes it possible for a facility to receive certification that it adheres to the standards established by that organization. This accreditation by recognized bodies is helpful in assuring patients that the quality of care delivered by a practice meets the requirements of these organizations and may also be helpful in reimbursement and medicolegal situations.

GENERAL CONCEPTS IN QUALITY CONTROL AND QUALITY ASSURANCE

Quality control (QC) and quality assurance (QA) should be ongoing programs involving a variety of measures of monitoring the level of care given by a facility and each of its members. Documentation makes it possible for independent auditors to determine what level of monitoring has been performed, and it also is helpful in ensuring that scheduled tasks are performed at designated intervals.

Quality assurance is the total program at a facility, encompassing equipment maintenance, quality of patient care, and patient outcome. This program is the responsibility of a designated physician. It is designed to maximize the likelihood that every biopsy performed is appropriate to patient care, that the necessary images and tissue samples have been obtained during the procedure to optimize the possibility of correctly managing the clinical issue, that the procedure is done as safely and cost effectively as possible, and that information obtained from the biopsy is correctly interpreted and made available for

rapid patient care. A comprehensive QA program includes continuing medical education, outcome data, preventive maintenance measures, and routine equipment testing.

Quality control is part of an effective QA program. It is designed to ascertain if equipment is functioning correctly. A QC program involves acceptance testing, establishing the baseline performance of equipment, identifying changes in the level of equipment performance before they become clinically obvious, and documenting that equipment problems have been corrected.

The personnel requirements, QC tests, and record keeping requirements for the American College of Radiology (ACR) stereotactic accreditation program are outlined in the QC manual for that program[1] and are reviewed in this chapter. The QA concepts and many of the tests are based on those outlined in the QC manual for the ACR mammography accreditation program.[2]

PERSONNEL

Specific personnel should be designated to be responsible for specified areas of the QA program. Any program must include a physician, a technologist, and a medical physicist. Adequate time should be made available to each of these professionals to accomplish the goals specified for them in establishing and maintaining the QA program. In addition to these individuals, a QA committee may be organized to oversee the QA program. This committee may include any persons involved in the care of the patients undergoing these interventional procedures. Therefore, surgeons, nurses, support staff, and others can be included in this committee, helping to optimize quality of care and patient satisfaction.

The ultimate responsibility for the QA program rests with a designated *physician*. The tasks of each member of the QA team should be overseen by this physician, and the end result of the QA program is this physician's responsibility. It is up to this physician to be certain that medical personnel participating in these biopsy programs are adequately trained and have appropriate continuing medical education credits for the procedures in which they are involved. The physician is responsible for ensuring that a QA program is in place, that those involved in this program are instructed in their responsibilities, that a technologist and medical physicist are selected as the designated persons for performing their QC tests, and that they have sufficient time to fulfill these duties. This physician should make certain that the materials needed to perform these tests are available, that the results are checked, and that feedback is given to the technologist and physicist about their results. Finally, the physician is also responsible for making sure that appropriate records are kept concerning personnel qualifications, radiation safety and protection, QC and QA, and other appropriate data.

Within the QA program of stereotactic and sonographically guided breast biopsy, the physician should accumulate data for the entire program and for each physician performing these procedures, including the number and type of biopsies done, number of complications, types of complication, and the instrumentation involved. Additionally, the outcome of each biopsy should be recorded, as well as the number of biopsies that need to be repeated and the reason for each. These reasons include nonconcordance of the biopsy results with imaging findings (presumed miss), inability of the pathologist to make a definitive diagnosis due to the small amount of tissue retrieved (e.g., phyllodes versus fibroadenoma, papillary lesion, radial scar, ductal atypia), and other reasons for repeat biopsy. Also, records should be kept of the results of repeat biopsies, as well as results of histopathologic analysis at the time of definitive treatment of carcinomas. Analysis of these data should make it apparent if a physician within the group has an unacceptable rate of complications or misses at biopsy. If this is the case, then additional training might be indicated or it might be deemed appropriate to have these procedures performed by other physicians.

In the ACR stereotactic breast biopsy accreditation program, these procedures can be performed by individual physicians or by a physician team. If performed by an individual physician, the physician must meet the requirements for mammography interpretation as outline by the U.S. Food and Drug Administration under the Mammography Quality Standards Act (MQSA) or have evaluated at least 480 mammograms every 2 years with an MQSA qualified physician and have 15 CME credit hours in stereotactic biopsy (or 3 years of experience performing at least 36 stereotactic biopsies), as well as 4 CME credit hours in medical radiation physics. Additionally, this physician should have performed at least 12 stereotactic biopsy procedures on his own or at least 3 hands-on biopsies under a physician who is qualified to interpret mammograms under MQSA and has performed at least 24 stereotactic biopsies. The physician must perform at least 12 biopsies annually, have 3 hours of category I CME credits in stereotactic breast biopsies, and obtain 3 additional CME hours every 3 years. Individual physicians who are working together (e.g., surgeon and radiologist) have requirements as a group that are equivalent to the requirements for individual physicians performing these biopsies. The accreditation program of the ACR should be contacted for details by those interested.

Radiologic technologists who participate in stereotactic biopsies at accredited facilities need to be certified by the American Registry of Radiological Technologists or licensed by their state. They must perform mammography regularly, doing at least 200 mammograms every 2 years. Additionally, they are required to have 3 hours of category A CEU in stereotactic biopsy before accreditation and obtain an additional 3 hours every 3 years. They must also perform at least 12 stereotactic biopsies each year.

Medical physicists who are utilized by accredited facilities must meet the qualifications outlined in the final rules by the U.S. Food and Drug Administration under MQSA. They must be licensed or approved by a state or certified in diagnostic radiological or imaging physics by the American Board of Radiology or the American Board of Medical Physics (or by another certifying body with equivalent standards). They must also have at least a master's degree in physical science, 20 semester hours of physics, 20 contact hours of training in conducting surveys of mammography facilities, and experience in conducting mammography surveys of at least 10 units and one facility. The physicist must have at least 15 hours of CME in mammography physics every 3 years and 3 hours of credits in stereotactic breast biopsy unit physics. Additionally, the physicist is required to have performed at least one hands-on stereotactic breast biopsy physics survey under the guidance of a qualified medical physicist and continue to perform at least one survey independently each year.

The ACR has also established an accreditation program for sonographically guided breast biopsies. Facilities seeking accreditation through this program must meet the requirements for accreditation for breast sonography. Additionally, requirements for training, initial and continuing experience for physicians performing these biopsies are similar to those outlined for stereotactic breast biopsy.

TECHNOLOGIST'S QUALITY CONTROL TESTS FOR STEREOTACTIC BIOPSY

The performance of these tests requires a technologist who is interested in their results, is trained to perform them accurately, and who has been given sufficient time in her schedule to perform these tests and record their results. A detailed description of each test is contained in the *Stereotactic Breast Biopsy Quality Control Manual* of the ACR.[1]

Before each patient is placed in the stereotactic biopsy unit, zero alignment testing should be performed, if this is required by the manufacturer.

Daily quality control testing includes:

• localization accuracy test (in air)

Additionally, for facilities using using film-screen imaging rather than digital imaging:

• darkroom cleanliness
• processor quality control

Weekly testing for all facilities should be done with:

• phantom images

Facilities using film-screen imaging are also required to perform weekly tests for:

• screen cleanliness
• viewbox and viewing conditions

Monthly tests include:

• visual checklist

Facilities using digital imaging should perform monthly assessment of:

• hardcopy output quality

Quarterly testing of facilities using a film-screen imaging is required for:

• analysis of fixer retention in film

Semiannual testing at all facilities is required for:

• compression
• repeat analysis

For those facilities using film-screen imaging, semiannual analysis should be performed to test:

• darkroom fog
• screen-film contact

Daily tests need only be performed on days when stereotactic biopsies are being done. Tests should also be done before a program is initiated. Additionally, they should be repeated more frequently if a problem is encountered and corrective action needs to be taken. In that setting, they should be used to document that the intervention has been effective in correcting the problem.

The localization accuracy test in air is designed to ensure that the system accurately places the tip of the biopsy probe at the correct point in space. A calibration needle is required to perform the test. This needle is placed in the biopsy gun in the prefire position (Figure 12.1). If necessary, the technologist should zero the needle *z*-position. The needle tip should be placed at a known position, and a stereotactic pair of images is obtained. The position of the needle tip is then calculated by the stereotactic unit and compared with the known position

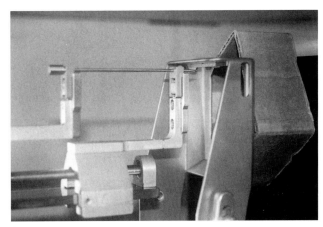

A

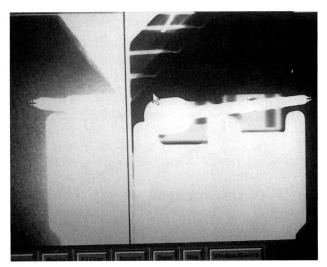

B

FIGURE 12.1. Localization accuracy test. **(A)** The test needle is placed in the gun holder at a designated position. **(B)** A stereotactic pair is obtained, and the location of the needle tip (marked with a + on each image) is calculated by the computer. This should correspond to the known position of the tip. If it does not, localization is not accurate, and appropriate corrective steps need to be taken. This test is performed daily before any biopsies are done.

of the needle tip. The needle tip should be within 1 mm of the known location of the tip in each axis, unless greater accuracy is recommended by the unit manufacturer. The results of the test should be recorded each day.

Phantom image quality testing is done to be certain that the system is at least equal to the image quality of diagnostic mammography equipment. The test requires a commercially available phantom, which is designed to simulate a 4.2 cm compressed breast composed of 50% glandular and 50% fatty tissue. The phantom is placed in the breast support system of the unit, the system is set up for imaging a 4.2 cm compressed breast (using either phototiming or manual timing), and the phantom is exposed (Figure 12.2). The image is then processed. For film, the central background optical density is measured and recorded. The number of test objects seen is then calculated and recorded. For digital image receptors, if the ACR MAP phantom is used and the field of view of the receptor is too small to accommodate the size of the phantom, it should be divided into quarters and imaged in four separate sections. The digital images should be viewed in a darkened room on the monitor of the unit. They should be assessed for artifacts, as well as scoring the phantom for the ability to identify specks, fibers, and masses. The image can be windowed and leveled, and magnification can be used to optimize visualization. Results should meet recommended minimum requirements and should be recorded.

For digital imaging units, hardcopy output quality is tested to be certain that it is consistent over time and that it matches the grayscales on the CRT monitor. A densitometer is required, as is a test pattern or phantom image having a wide range of grayscales (Figure 12.3). The test pattern is exposed, and the image should be displayed each time at the same window and level. The image is then printed on film, which is processed and then viewed under optimal viewing conditions. The optical density of the film should be measured at four sites, using the same location each time the test is conducted. The grayscale on the film and the monitor should then be compared. Results are recorded. Optical densities at the four sites on the film should be within 0.20 of control levels. The contrast and brightness of the film image and that on the monitor should also be comparable.

The visual checklist for proper equipment functioning (Table 12.1) is designed to ascertain that the mechanics of the equipment are working properly and safely. All items that are appropriate for a unit should be checked at least monthly, and the results recorded.

Testing of compression is performed to determine if the pressure is adequate to hold the breast in stable posi-

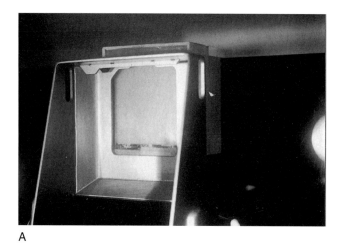

A

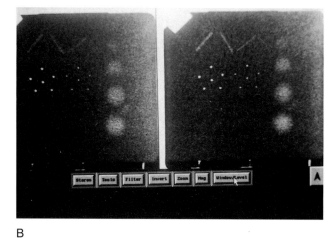

B

FIGURE 12.2. Phantom image quality testing. (**A**) A phantom is placed between the compression paddle and the image receptor, and a stereotactic pair is obtained. (**B**) On a digital image receptor, the image is windowed and leveled to optimal parameters. Visualization of specks, fibers, and masses is graded. Image quality should be similar to that of diagnostic mammography. If it is not, it might not be possible to see some target lesions during the biopsy procedure.

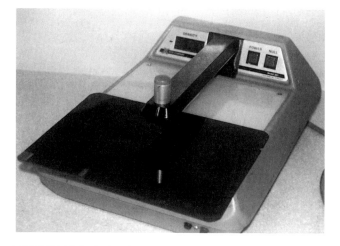

FIGURE 12.3. A densitometer is used to calculate film density in several quality control tests.

TABLE 12.1. *Visual checklist for stereotactic breast biopsy units*

Are X-ray tube locks and detents properly functioning?
When the table is locked, is it nonmovable relative to the compression paddle?
Do image receptor locks function properly?
Does the light field work correctly?
Is the collimation or diaphragm the correct size?
Do all moving parts move properly and smoothly?
Are foot switches functioning correctly?
Is adequate compression obtainable?
Is compression force consistent throughout the procedure?
Are coordinates correctly zeroed?
Is immobilization of the biopsy device adequate to prevent recoil?
Are needle guides secure and free of movement?
Are paddles in good condition (e.g., no cracks, sharp edges)?
Is the operator properly shielded from radiation?
Can the patient be observed during an X-ray exposure?
Are technique charts posted and readily available?
Are cleaning supplies on hand and used regularly?
Is the equipment blood-free?
Is the monitor clean (if a digital system is used)?
Are other tests routinely recommended by the manufacturer carried out?

tion during the biopsy and to be sure that the compression pressure is not excessive. The test requires a flat, analogue type bathroom scale or a digital scale designed specifically for this test. Padding, such as towels, should also be used to protect the compression paddles from the surfaces of the scale. The bathroom scale and padding are positioned (or taped into place on prone tables), and the compression device is applied to the scale using automatic or power compression until it stops (Figure 12.4). The compression force is measured. Additional, manual compression is then applied until it stops, and this is also measured. The compression force should be sustainable for at least 5 minutes. Compression force should be adjusted to a maximum of 25–40 pounds in the power drive mode. It may exceed this level under manual compression. Results should be recorded.

An analysis of the number and reason for repeat images, repeat analysis, is designed to determine the number of repeated images obtained for each technologist. This identifies the causes of repeat imaging with the goal of decreasing this number, thereby decreasing the patient radiation dose and the cost of the biopsy procedure. In order to perform this study, the number of images usually obtained during a stereotactic biopsy must be known. The number of rejected films or images for each technologist and the reason for each is tabulated. For film-screen imaging these include patient motion, poor positioning, films that are too light or too dark, and artifacts.

If film is used, the rejected films for stereotactic biopsy should be saved separately from other repeat films stored, and the reason for each repeat should be recorded. The percentage of repeats as a percentage of the total number of stereotactic films should be calculated, and the percentage of repeats for each reason should be determined. For digital imaging a worksheet should be used to record the number of repeated images and the reason for each. For digital imaging repeat exposures may be due to patient positioning, patient motion, noisy images (underexposed), improper detector exposure, incorrect patient identification, equipment failure (X-ray equipment or software), and blank image. The ACR recommends that the repeat rate should be less than 20%, and that this percentage should be based on at least 150 patient examinations or 1000 exposures.

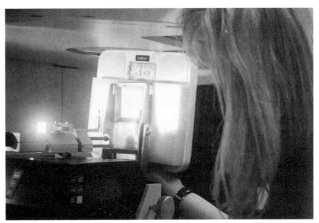

A

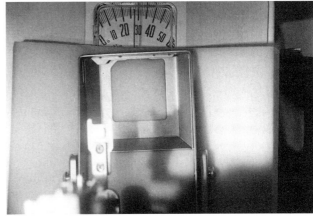

B

FIGURE 12.4. Compression testing. (**A**) An analogue bathroom scale has been placed between the image receptor and the compression paddle. Foam rubber is positioned between the compression paddle and the scale as padding to protect the paddle. (**B**) Compression force should be no more than 25–40 pounds in the power drive mode. It should be sustainable for 5 minutes.

MEDICAL PHYSICIST'S QUALITY CONTROL TESTS FOR STEREOTACTIC BIOPSY

The goal of testing stereotactic biopsy units by a qualified medical physicist is to be certain that the equipment will function at a level comparable to that of mammography equipment. Depending upon the imaging receptor used, the equipment will need to be tested for digital and/or screen-film imaging. The results of these tests should be communicated in a written report to the physician responsible for the facility. If corrective actions are required, they should be documented. The medical physicist should also routinely review the results of quality control testing done by the radiologic technologist. If necessary, recommendations for actions based on the results of these tests should be made.

The medical physicist is responsible for acceptance testing at the time the stereotactic unit is initially installed and for annual retesting of the unit. The tests to be conducted by the medical physicist include:

- Unit assembly evaluation
- Collimation assessment
- Focal spot performance and system limiting spatial resolution
- kVp accuracy and reproducibility
- Beam quality assessment (half-value layer measurement)
- Exposure control performance assessment
- Patient dose and exposure reproducibility
- Image quality assessment
- Artifact evaluation
- Localization accuracy
- Image uniformity:
    for screen-film: uniformity of screen speed
    for digital imaging: digital receptor uniformity

The goal of unit assembly evaluation is to determine that the stereotactic biopsy unit is properly functioning so the patient is safe from mechanical hazards. The medical physicist should be certain that the unit is mechanically stable under normal conditions. All moving parts should move smoothly and only when intended to move. The image receptor should be securely in place. If screen-imaging is done, the cassette should be easily put in place and removed. Breast compression should be measured by the unit within an accuracy of ±5 mm and should be reproducible within ±2 mm. Personnel and patients should not be exposed to sharp or cracked edges. Technique charts should be posted. Appropriate radiation shielding for the equipment operator should be in place. The biopsy probe holder should hold the probe accurately.

Evaluation of collimation should determine that radiation does not extend beyond the edges of the image re-

ceptor and that the biopsy window and X-ray field are aligned. Testing requires tape, four coins, cassettes and film, and a millimeter ruler. Coins are taped inside the compression plate window so that their outer edges touch the edge of the biopsy window (Figure 12.5). The part of the image next to the chest wall should be identifiable. The X-ray tube is positioned at 0°. If screen-film or digital imaging is used, a cassette with film is put in place so that the center of the cassette is behind the biopsy window and extends beyond the window in all directions. If screen-film imaging is done, a cassette with film should also be in position in the cassette holder. An exposure is then taken with technique adequate to expose the film behind the biopsy window and either the digital receptor or the film in normal position in the image receptor. ACR suggests a technique of Mo/Mo, 25 kVp, 20 mAs. Both images should be processed, and an optical density above 1.0 should be present on all film images. The entire coins should be seen on the film that was positioned just behind the biopsy window. The outer edges of the coins indicate the size of this window. The coins should be fully visualized on the film placed behind the biopsy window. If the edges of all four coins are not seen, then the collimation needs to be adjusted. The radiation field should be fully contained within this cassette field. For screen-film imaging the radiation field should also be fully contained within the image receptor, except at the chest wall side where it can extend up to 2% of the source-to-image distance beyond the chest wall. For digital imaging, the radiation field can extend beyond the image receptor on all sides but not by more than 5 mm. This calculation is made by comparing the size of the radiation field on the digital image versus the film image. If these measurements are not met, appropriate adjustments should be made.

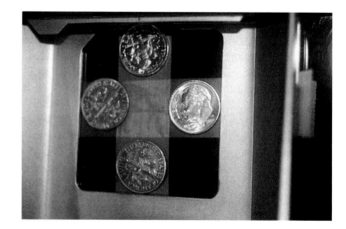

FIGURE 12.5. Collimation testing. Testing is done with four coins taped inside the compression plate biopsy opening. The edges of the coins should abut the edges of the opening on all four sides. When an image of these coins is obtained without angulation of the tube, the four coins should all be completely visualized. If not all seen completely, collimation is too tight and should be adjusted.

Focal spot performance is tested by measuring limiting spatial resolution with a high-contrast resolution pattern positioned perpendicular and parallel to the anode-cathode axis. The test requires a line-pair test pattern that can measure at least 20 lp/mm for film and 10 lp/mm for digital imaging, film in a ready-pack or cassette, a lead marker to mark the cathode-anode axis, a magnifier with 10× to 30× magnification capability, and a ruler. The test object is placed 4.5 cm above the image receptor, appropriately oriented and positioned within the field-of-view to test parallel or perpendicular to the cathode-anode axis. A lead marker is placed in the field-of-view to indicate the axis orientation. The X-ray settings should be at the most common kVp used and with an mAs to obtain a background optical density of 1.0–1.5. The bar pattern is viewed using magnification, either with a magnifying lens or with the electronic magnification available on the digital unit. It is considered to be resolved if any portion of the pattern shows clearly the correct number of bars. For imaging done parallel to the cathode-anode axis, resolution of at least 13 lp/mm should be obtained. For imaging done perpendicular to this axis, resolution should be at least 11 lp/mm. Spatial resolution should be consistent on repeated testing. If there is degradation, it should be corrected.

Testing for kVp accuracy and reproducibility requires a device that can measure kVp with an accuracy within ±1.5 kVp and a precision of 0.5 kVp within the mammographic range. The test should determine that the kVp is accurate within ±5% of the indicated kVp and that it is reproducible with a coefficient of variation ≤ 0.02. Using the manual exposure mode, the most frequently used kVp should be selected. Four exposures should be made, and the measured kVp is recorded. If other clinically important kVps are used, a single exposure at each of these settings is made. Average the four kVp readings and compare with the nominal setting. Standard deviation and the coefficient of variation are calculated. Measurements should be within the range noted above. If they exceed it, service personnel should check the equipment.

Beam quality is tested to ascertain that the half-value layer of the X-ray beam is appropriate to keep the patient dose low while maintaining adequate image contrast. The test requires an ionization chamber and an electrometer calibrated at mammographic X-ray beam energies and five sheets of 0.1 mm thick 99.9% pure aluminum of type 1145 alloy or 99% pure type 1100 alloy of a size adequate to cover the ionization chamber. Results recorded with type 1100 alloy can be 7.5% lower than those obtained with 1145 alloy and should be corrected to those that would be obtained with 1145 alloy. The test is conducted centering the ionization chamber in the X-ray field 4.5 cm above the breast support surface. The most commonly used target filtration and kVp should be selected; mAs should be selected to give an exposure of approximately 500 mR. An exposure should be made without any aluminum filtration. Exposures are repeated initially with 0.2 mm of aluminum filtration and then with additional 0.1 mm of filtration for each additional exposure. This is continued until the ionization chamber reading reaches less than one-half of the unfiltered, initial exposure reading. This should be repeated for all target-filter and kVp settings used clinically. The half value layer is calculated according to an established formula. Measurements at a given kVp should be within recommended parameters or service personnel should be called to correct the equipment.

Testing of the ability of the equipment to maintain appropriate film density or detector signal levels over a variety of breast thicknesses is also performed. This can test either automatic exposure control (AEC) or manual exposure performance. Testing requires a phantom composed of either acrylic or BR-12 that consists of at least four 2 cm thick elements that can simulate breast thicknesses of 2 cm, 4 cm, 6 cm, and 8 cm. Lead numbers and a densitometer are also needed. Images are acquired using either manual or phototimed technique for phantoms of four thicknesses, and the optical density at the center of the films is recorded. For digital (ROI) systems, the signal at the center of the image is measured using a region-of-interest (ROI). There should be a constant film optical density or mean signal throughout various thicknesses, and these should be obtained with exposure times of less than 2 seconds.

Patient radiation dose is measured as entrance exposure and average glandular dose. This should be measured for a typical exposure for a 4.2 cm compressed breast composed equally of fat and glandular tissue. Testing equipment needed includes an appropriate phantom and an ionization chamber and electrometer accurate at mammographic X-ray beam energies. With the phantom and ionization chamber in place, four exposures should be made using clinical exposure techniques. Entrance exposure (and mAs for AEC exposures) should be recorded for each. Using these data, the average glandular dose can be calculated. Also, the variation in exposure and mAs reproducibility can be calculated. The coefficient of variation for these should not exceed 0.05. If the variation is beyond this, the unit should be serviced. The average glandular dose to the breast at the techniques used for this testing should not exceed 3.0 mGy. If the dose is excessive, techniques should be modified to bring the dose into an acceptable range. If techniques are changed, the phantom image quality needs to be retested.

Image quality is assessed to be certain that it is at least comparable to that obtained in mammography and that the quality does not deteriorate over time. The same phantom used in radiation dose testing is utilized. If the phantom cannot be fully imaged in one exposure, four exposures (one for each quadrant of the phantom) should be made. Optical density of the image is measured. The ability to see fibers, specks, and masses on the image should be

206 / D.D. Dershaw

scored in a darkened room if read off of a monitor or with the image masked on a viewbox if film is used. A magnifying lens of the same type as that used clinically can be used to score the images. Electronic magnification can be used in scoring images on a monitor. The image should meet acceptable published scores. The image of the phantom should also be assessed for artifacts. Because the medical physicist may be more adept than the radiologic technologist at phantom image scoring, images obtained by the technologist should also be reviewed at the time of this testing. Scoring should also be reviewed with the technologist. If images do not meet established criteria, the reason for this should be ascertained and corrected.

Images also need to be assessed to identify artifacts and localize their source. For screen-film systems, two images are obtained with the cassette turned 90° to itself before the second exposure. Films are run through the processor in the same orientation in which they were taken (at 90° to each other). When the films are positioned identically for viewing, processor artifacts will be at right angles; cassette, film, and X-ray equipment artifacts will be oriented in the same direction. The source of these should be identified and corrected. Testing for artifacts with digital receptors requires only a single exposure. The image should be displayed with high contrast so that minimal changes in the grayscale are evident at the edges of the image. Areas of information dropout (white spots), nonuniformity, and other artifacts should be searched for. If they compromise image interpretation, they should be corrected. Artifacts that occur intermittently can be more difficult to isolate and correct. However, if they occur, efforts should also be made to eliminate the source of these artifacts.

Testing is also done to ascertain if the biopsy probe tip is accurately positioned for tissue acquisition. The localization accuracy test requires a gelatin phantom with targets that are <5 mm in diameter. A stereotactic pair is obtained of the target, and lesion location in the x, y, and z axes is calculated. The biopsy probe is positioned at the calculated site, and on a stereotactic pair it should be located within the lesion. A postfire stereotactic pair is also obtained, and this should demonstrate the probe tip positioned beyond the target. Examination of the specimen obtained during testing should demonstrate that the target has been harvested from the phantom. For fine needle aspiration sampling, a test image with postfire postioning is not obtained, and examination of the specimen may not be appropriate. If the specimen is not sampled during this test or if inspection of the images shows probe positioning to be unsatisfactory, the unit should be serviced.

Medical physicist testing should also be done to determine if the quality of the image is uniform throughout the area of the exposure. For screen-film systems, the uniformity of the screen speed is tested. This testing requires the film and cassettes used during stereotatic biopsy imaging, a phantom, and a densitometer. Cassettes should

be labeled with lead markers so the films obtained from each cassette can be identified. Images should be obtained with each cassette using the most commonly used radiographic technique for stereotactic biopsy so that the center of the image of the phantom reaches an optical density of at least 1.40. The first cassette that is used in this test should be exposed three times, at the beginning, middle, and end of testing the cassettes. All three films (control films) used during this repeated testing should be developed, along with all the other films obtained during the test. The standard deviation of the optical density of the control films should be calculated and should be no more than 0.05. If the value exceeds this number, the test is invalid. If it is within this range, then the maximum and minimum optical densities from all the cassettes should be determined. The difference in the maximum and minimum should not exceed 0.30. Any cassette that does not fall within this range should be corrected or discarded.

Uniformity of digital image receptors should be tested to be certain there is no image distortion, disruption in fiberoptics, lens malalignment, or CCD element dropout. Testing requires a screen-film contact mesh (or ROI measurements) and a 4 cm thick piece of acrylic or BR-12 to cover the image receptor. A digital image is obtained using the usual technique for a 4 cm compressed breast. If possible, signal means and standard deviations should be calculated using ROIs in the center and corners of the image. From this, the signal-to-noise ratio is computed in each ROI by dividing the mean signal by the standard deviation. The signal-to-noise ratios in each corner should be within ±15% of the measurement obtained in the center of the image. If measurements are beyond this range, receptor inhomogeneity needs to be corrected. Images are

StereoGuide Technique Chart

Mode	Thickness (cm)	kVp set	mAs set	Exposure Time (sec)	ESE (R)	AGD Glandular Dose (mrad)
512	2.0	28	16	0.2	0.15	52
	3.0	28	40	0.5	0.40	91
	4.0	28	72	0.9	0.74	131
	4.5	28	96	1.2	1.00	160
	5.0	28	152	1.9	1.62	228
	6.0	31	140	2.0	2.03	262
	7.0	34	140	2.0	2.78	335
	8.0	34	210	3.0	4.32	451

The above table is approximate and the mAs and kVp should be adjusted according to positioning and breast texture to have acceptable image quality.

AGD-Average Glandular Dose, 50% fatty/50% glandular breast

This technique chart follows the 1998 ACR preliminary guidelines, which require that the average signal levels remain within ±20% of the 4cm thickness signal level (3088) from a patient thickness of 2 cm through 8 cm and that ideally the exposure duration be less than 2 seconds.

FIGURE 12.6. A chart of recommended radiographic techniques is supplied by manufacturers and should be posted near the control panel of the stereotactic unit so that it is available for quick reference.

then obtained with the mesh as close to the image receptor as possible, covering the entire image receptor. A 4 cm layer of acrylic is placed between the compression paddle and the mesh, and compression is applied. A digital image is obtained using manual technique for a 4 cm compressed breast. The edges are inspected for geometric pincushioning. The image should then be adjusted until it consists of black dots on a white field. The image is examined for areas of non-uniformity. Servicing the unit is recommended if excessive geometric pincushioning extends more than 1 cm beyond the edge of the field of view, if areas without black dots occupy more than 10% of the image, or if a line without black dots extends more than one-fourth of the length of the image.

Stereotactic biopsy facilities are recommended to have posted a technique chart for kVp and mAs for varying thicknesses of compressed breast (Figure 12.6). These are available from manufacturers. Accredited facilities should have their accreditation certificate posted so that it is readily seen by patients.

QUALITY CONTROL FOR SONOGRAPHICALLY GUIDED BIOPSY

As with other biopsy procedures, results of sonographically guided biopsies should be maintained to assess the successful performance of the facility and individual physicians performing these procedures. Data identical to those kept for stereotactic biopsies should be maintained. The data include the number of procedures performed, number of carcinomas found, numbers of inconclusive studies and the reasons for each, as well as the numbers and types of complications.

Equipment quality control is designed to maximize the safety and performance level of equipment used in these procedures. A quality control program should be outlined in the facility's policy and procedures manual, and adherence to this program should be documented.

A suggested quality control program for sonographically guided breast biopsy includes testing by the medical physicist and technologist. Medical physicist's tests include (Figure 12.7):

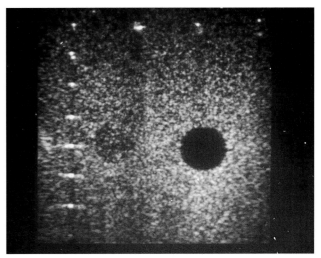

A

B

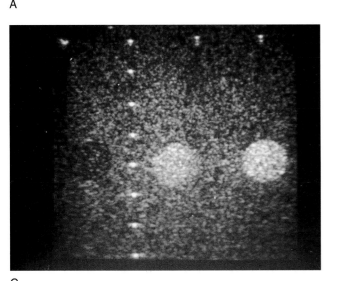

C

FIGURE 12.7. Phantom testing for sonography. **(A)** A standardized phantom is scanned with optimized time gain curve to assess spatial resolution and system noise. **(B, C)** Imaging of the phantom requires moving the transducer to obtain images of the entire phantom. Horizontal and vertical rows of specks make it possible to determine system resolution, depth of visualization, and system accuracy. Masses of varying echogenicity can be used to assess field uniformity and the ability to resolve masses of minimal difference in echotexture. An anechoic mass can be used to determine system noise.

- maximum depth of visualization assessment
- verification of horizontal and vertical distance accuracy
- field uniformity
- assessment of ring down
- lateral resolution
- evaluation of electrical-mechanical cleanliness

These tests should be performed annually.
   Radiologic technologist's tests include:

- universal infection control procedures for each biopsy
- quarterly assessment of distance calibration
- quarterly assessment of grayscale photography

It is recommended that all physicians involved in these procedures meet certain minimum standards of training.[3] For the ACR accreditation program, these are defined as initial training in an accredited diagnostic radiology residency program including 3 or more months of diagnostic ultrasound or postgraduate training in ultrasound that includes the performance of at least 500 ultrasound examinations, including breast ultrasound, under the guidance of a qualified physician; or 2 years or more experience performing ultrasound during which time at least 500 general or 100 breast ultrasound examinations were done. Maintenance of competence requires performance of at least 12 sonographically guided breast biopsies annually, regular performance of breast ultrasound, and 3 hours of category I CME credits in sonographically guided breast biopsy every 3 years. Because imaging and performance of the biopsy are deemed to be the direct responsibility of the physician, training requirements are not stipulated for medical physicists or technologists.

It should be noted that accreditation of a facility for the performance of sonographically guided breast biopsy by the ACR requires that the facility also be accredited in the performance of breast sonography.[4]

INFECTION CONTROL

Incorporated into each facility's program for performing breast biopsies should be an infection control program. The policies of this program should be included in the facility's procedure and policy manual. They should include procedures to control the spread of infection, adherence to universal precautions, and the use of clean or sterile techniques appropriate to the procedure being performed.

Technologists should be taught the concepts involved in infection control (Figure 12.8). The techniques of infection control should also be reviewed with physicians involved in these procedures. They include hand-washing and sterile technique. Also, facilities should be available and be used for the safe and appropriate disposal of contaminated waste and sharp objects.

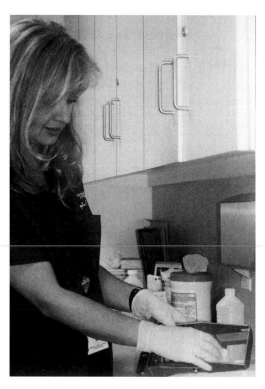

FIGURE 12.8. Infection control. Technologists should be trained in sterile technique and in infection control. Appropriate cleaning and sterilization of equipment should be performed each time the system is used. These procedures are needed for the safety of staff, as well as patients.

CONCLUSIONS

The incorporation of a quality assurance program into a breast interventional practice makes it possible to objectively assess the quality of care being administered to patients. These programs involve meeting objective criteria for both equipment and personnel. Outcome data assessment makes it possible to evaluate the quality of patient management. Documentation of these procedures ensures that they are adhered to. Facility accreditation gives independent verification of the quality and safety of care provided by a facility.

REFERENCES

1. Hendrick RE, Dershaw DD, Kimme-Smith C, et al. Stereotactic Breast Biopsy Quality Control Manual. Reston, VA: American College of Radiology, 1999.
2. Hendrick RE, Bassett L, Botsco MA, et al. Mammography Quality Control Manual. Reston, VA: American College of Radiology, 1999.
3. ACR Standard for the Performance of Ultrasound Guided Percutaneous Breast Interventional Procedures: Standards 2000–2001. Reston, VA: American College of Radiology, 2000;171–175.
4. ACR Standard for the Performance of Breast Ultrasound Examination: Standards 2000–2001. Reston, VA: American College of Radiology, 2000;389–392.

Index

Note: Page numbers followed by *f* or *t* denote figures or tables, respectively.